CONSULTATION-LIAISON PSYCHIATRY

SEMINARS IN PSYCHIATRY

Series Editor

Milton Greenblatt, M.D.
Chief, Psychiatry Service
Veterans Administration Hospital
Sepulveda, California
and Professor of Psychiatry
University of California, Los Angeles

Other Books in Series:

CONSULTATION-LIAISON PSYCHIATRY

Edited by

Robert O. Pasnau, M.D.
*Associate Professor of Psychiatry
and Chief, Psychiatric Consultation-Liaison Service
University of California School of Medicine
Los Angeles, California*

GRUNE & STRATTON
A Subsidiary of Harcourt Brace Jovanovich, Publishers
New York   San Francisco   London

Library of Congress Cataloging in Publication Data
Main entry under title:

Consultation-liaison psychiatry.

    (Seminars in psychiatry)
    Includes bibliographical references and index.
       1. Psychiatric consultation.   2. Medicine, Psy-
chosomatic.   3. Medicine and psychology.   4. Psychiatry—Study and teaching.   I. Pasnau, Robert O.
[DNLM: 1. Psychiatry.   2. Psychosomatic medicine.
3. Referral and consultation.   WM90 C758]
RC455.2.C65C66   616.08   75-30562
ISBN 0-8089-0901-0

Grune & Stratton, Inc.
111 Fifth Avenue
New York, New York 10003

Library of Congress Catalog Card Number 75-30562
International Standard Book Number 0-8089-0901-0
Printed in the United States of America

This volume is dedicated to the memory of
I. Arthur Mirsky, M.D.,
teacher, mentor, and friend.

Contents

Preface

*"Health is that pattern of disease
which is accepted by a culture or society
in a particular historical time."*
          Eugene Pumpian-Mindlin, M.D.

The major reason for editing this book was my growing concern for the health of people and my fear that in spite of years of experience and knowledge, most physicians remain largely in the dark about the interaction of mental and physical health. As we enter the fourth quarter of the twentieth century, health care once again has become the watchword of medicine. And in psychiatry, liaison psychiatry has emerged as a recognized area of special interest in the delivery of health-care services within the broader framework of psychiatry as a branch of medicine. This book is an attempt to assess the relationship of liaison psychiatry to general psychiatry and at the same time to clarify what liaison psychiatry is all about, what its premises are, and what it is striving for and how.

Nowhere is Mindlin's definition of health more useful than in the culture called the hospital. In medicine, concepts of what is healthy are continually being revised in response to the development of new knowledge as well as the demands from the consumers, i.e., the patients. As these ideas and attitudes change, so must the awareness of the psychiatrists who work in these environments. Often it is the psychiatrist himself who is responsible for changing the idea of what is health by bringing, from his background in behavioral science, knowledge which can be applied in the larger medical setting.

This volume deals with four major aspects of consultation-liaison psychiatry. After a broad overview of the development and scope of psychiatric liaison by its major contemporary spokesman, Dr. Z. J. Lipowski, its first section reaffirms the conceptual and investigative links between liaison psychiatry and the broader field of psychosomatic medicine. As Lipowski points out, consultation-liaison psychiatry is the clinical practice based conceptually upon psychosomatic medicine and the belief that there is multicasualty of all illnesses. This requires that biological, social, economic, and psychological factors be considered in providing all health care. Research in this area has been pronounced over the past twenty years. This research has encompassed human and animal psychophysiological studies as well as clinical and epidemiological investigations. The chapters in this section explore some of the parameters of the current research and serve as a general reference for the reader who may wish to delve further into any special area of interest.

The second set of chapters deals with what has come to be known as liaison psychiatry. This field of clinical practice has been greatly expanded in the past decade to include much more than the older "consultation" activities of psychiatrists in general hospitals. Borrowing from social psychology, community psychiatry, and even systems theory, liaison psychiatry has focused on education, prevention, and systems approaches in detection as treating the elements in the environment which promote health or produce the reverse. Anyone working in this field is aware that it is hazardous duty. I have used the term "troubled marriage" to describe both the sense of frustration and disharmony which is often attendant and the sense of hopefulness that with adequate "counseling" and problem-solving the marriage can and must survive. Because of the great pressures for such a union, both within and outside of medicine, it would indeed be unfortunate if the psychiatrists, divided in their opinions on their professional role as they are, failed to meet the challenge. This section describes some of the successes and opportunities and problems and their solutions of liaison psychiatrists who have each spent many years working in their areas of special interest and expertise.

In the third set of chapters I have included some of the older areas of concern to consultation psychiatry. Even though contemporary liaison psychiatry has moved beyond the traditional concept of psychiatric consultation, per se, the perennial problems remain. Much new data has been accumulated since the publication of volumes a decade ago in this area, and I believe that it is important to refine our consultation skills even as we broaden our liaison efforts. Nonetheless, this section contains a sample of such problems, but the sample sufficiently demonstrates the requirement of skill and knowledge which must be brought to the clinical situation by the liaison psychiatrist.

The fourth section reflects my personal interest in medical education and represents the second major reason for putting together this book. As far as I know, the role of liaison psychiatry in the education of medical students, family practitioners, psychiatric residents, and practicing physicians has received only the passing interest and attention of medical educators. The problems for educators as well as students are very great. The authors in this section, all of whom have had many years experience in medical education, address themselves with considerable thoughtfulness to this subject. It is my firm belief that the place to teach psychiatry in the medical school is on the wards and clinics of the general hospital and that it is the liaison psychiatrist who makes the best medical educator. It is apparent that without educating liaison psychiatrists, either during their residency or beyond, medical education in psychiatry must be inadequate to prepare the future physician in the practice of medicine. There is a clear need to refine the techniques, spell out the goals, and evaluate the results in the years to come.

Finally, this book is written for students, residents, and any practicing physicians who, in the course of their work, discover that they wish to have a practical guide to contemporary liaison psychiatry. It is my hope that by reading this volume they will be better prepared to stand in the doorway between psychiatry and the rest of medicine, as Dr. Peter Knapp has said, interpreting what is happening in behaviorial science to the nonpsychiatric physician and what is happening in the rest of medicine to the psychiatrist.

Robert O. Pasnau, M.D.

Contributors

Daniel B. Auerbach, M.D.
Assistant Professor of Psychiatry
University of California at Los Angeles
School of Medicine
Los Angeles, California
and Chief, Consultation-Liaison Psychiatry
Veteran's Administration Hospital
Sepulveda, California

Norman Q. Brill, M.D.
Professor of Psychiatry
University of California at Los Angeles
School of Medicine
Los Angeles, California

Joshua S. Golden, M.D.
Associate Professor of Psychiatry in Residence
and Assistant Dean for Student Affairs
University of California at Los Angeles
School of Medicine
Los Angeles, California

Klaus D. Hoppe, M.D.
Associate Professor of Clinical Psychiatry
University of California at Los Angeles
School of Medicine
and Member and Faculty Instructor
Southern California Psychoanalytic Institute
Los Angeles, California

Kay Jamison, Ph.D.
Assistant Professor of Medical Psychology
University of California at Los Angeles
School of Medicine
and Consultant UCLA Multidisciplinary Pain Clinic
Los Angeles, California

Robert O. Jones, M.D., FRCP(C), FAPA, FACP
Professor of Psychiatry
and Head, Department of Psychiatry
Dalhousie University
Halifax, Nova Scotia

Harold I. Kaplan, M.D.
Professor of Psychiatry
and Director, Psychiatric Education and Training
New York Medical College
and Attending Psychiatrist
Flower and Fifth Avenue Hospitals
New York, New York

Chase Patterson Kimball, M.D.
Associate Professor of Psychiatry
Departments of Psychiatry, Medicine, and Behavioral Science
University of Chicago
Chicago, Illinois

Z. J. Lipowski, M.D.
Professor of Psychiatry
Dartmouth Medical School
Hanover, New Hampshire

Robert E. Litman, M.D.
Adjunct Professor of Psychiatry
University of California at Los Angeles
School of Medicine
Los Angeles, California

L. Robert Martin, M.D.
Professor of Medicine
and Chief, Division of Family Practice
University of California at Los Angeles
School of Medicine
Los Angeles, California

Charles McCreary, Ph.D.
Assistant Professor of Medical Psychology
University of California at Los Angeles
School of Medicine,
and Consultant, Multidisciplinary Pain Clinic
and Consultant, Orthopedic Clinic
University of California at Los Angeles Hosptial
Los Angeles, California

Daniel H. Naftulin, M.D.
Associate Professor of Psychiatry
and Chief, Consultation-Liaison Service
Department of Psychiatry
Cedars-Sinai Medical Center
Los Angeles, California

Robert O. Pasnau, M.D.
Associate Professor of Psychiatry
and Chief, Psychiatric Consultation-Liaison Service
University of California at Los Angeles
School of Medicine
Los Angeles, California

Commander Richard H. Rahe, M.D., MC, USNR
Head, Stress Medicine Divisions
Naval Health Research Center
San Diego, California

Burton Roger, M.D.
Assistant Clinical Professor of Psychiatry
University of California at Los Angeles
School of Medicine
and Liaison Psychiatrist, Renal Dialysis Unit
University of California at Los Angeles Hospital
Los Angeles, California

Robert T. Rubin, M.D.
Adjunct Professor of Psychiatry
University of California at Los Angeles
School of Medicine
Harbor General Hospital Campus
Torrance, California

John J. Schwab, M.D.
Professor of Psychiatry
and Chairman, Department of Psychiatry and Behavioral Sciences
University of Louisville
School of Medicine
Louisville, Kentucky

David Shapiro, Ph.D.
Professor of Psychiatry
University of California at Los Angeles
Los Angeles, California

Edwin S. Shneidman, Ph.D.
Professor of Thanatology
and Director, Laboratory for the Study of Life-Threatening Behavior
Department of Psychiatry
University of California at Los Angeles
Los Angeles, California

Manuel Straker, M.D.
Professor of Psychiatry
University of California at Los Angeles
School of Medicine
and Chief of Psychiatry
Veteran's Administration Hospital
Los Angeles, California

Charles William Wahl, M.D.
Clinical Professor of Psychiatry
University of California at Los Angeles
School of Medicine
and Member and Instructor
Southern California Psychoanalytic Institute and Society
and Consultant, Veteran's Administration Hospital
Sepulveda, California
and Consultant, Olive View Hospital
Los Angeles, California

Avery D. Weisman, M.D.
Associate Professor of Psychiatry
Massachusetts General Hosptial
Harvard Medical School
and Principal Investigator
Project Omega
Massachusetts General Hospital
Boston, Massachusetts

Louis Jolyon West, M.D.
Professor and Chairman
Department of Psychiatry
University of California at Los Angeles
School of Medicine
and Director, The Neuropsychiatric Institute
University of California at Los Angeles
Center for the Health Sciences
Los Angeles, California

Joel Yager, M.D.
Assistant Professor of Psychiatry
and Director of Residency Education
Department of Psychiatry
University of California at Los Angeles
School of Medicine
Los Angeles, California

CONSULTATION-LIAISON PSYCHIATRY

Z. J. Lipowski

1

Consultation-Liaison Psychiatry: Past, Present, and Future

Consultation-liaison psychiatry has emerged as a recognized area of special interest within clinical psychiatry. One of its major roles is to maintain a link between psychiatry and medicine in the provision of comprehensive health care and in research on and teaching of psychosocial aspects of medicine. These issues of health care and psychosocial medicine are rapidly growing in importance and recognition as the whole matter of health care delivery undergoes a sweeping scrutiny in all of its key aspects: philosophical, ethical, organizational, social, and economic. Concurrently, the role of psychiatry and its practitioners is being reappraised, and there is a heated debate whether the practitioners should operate as health professionals within the orbit of medicine or go their own way as social reformers, community counselors and organizers, or wandering apostles of a mental health movement.

In this climate of change and questioning of our basic assumptions as professionals, medical and psychiatric, the practitioners of consultation-liaison psychiatry must also revise their professional roles, premises, and goals. They need to define their relationship to the various practitioners of the so-called community mental health consultation and delimit the boundaries of their field of professional activity. This chapter is an attempt at reassessment and clarification of what consultation-psychiatry is about, what its premises are, and what it is striving for, how, and for whom.

Expanded version of the article ''Consultation-Liaison Psychiatry: An Overview'' published in *American Journal of Psychiatry* 131:623–630, 1974. Copyrighted by the American Psychiatric Association 1974. Used with permission.

DEFINITIONS OF BASIC CONCEPTS

According to a 1970 nationwide survey of the activities of American psychiatrists[1] 68.4 percent of the respondents engage in consultation, which is estimated to account for 9.1 percent of their average work week. Less than 1 percent of the respondents spend 80 to 100 percent of their time in it. The term "consultation" is not explicitly defined in the survey, but it is implicitly distinguished from direct patient contact, teaching, research, and administration. Furthermore, psychiatrists are stated to engage in "consultation" in 18 different settings or locations defined for the purpose of the survey. These range from private offices through mental and general hospitals to schools, correctional institutions, colleges, community mental health centers, drug addiction and alcoholism centers, and so forth. The general hospital ranks second as the most common location where psychiatrists practice either fulltime or parttime; 22.4 percent of them work there, and 14.4 percent of their time is devoted to consultation.

These statistics indicate that the majority of psychiatrists in this country regard some part of their professional activity as "consultation." It is quite clear, however, that this term has more than one connotation. Regardless of how psychiatrists define it, they profess to practice consultation in every setting in which they work. Thus, ambiguity surrounds the concept of psychiatric consultation, hampering communication and fostering misunderstandings. A clarification is called for so that this integral aspect of psychiatry can increase its usefulness, be better taught, and lend itself to adequate evaluation.

Mental Health Consultation

Caplan defines consultation as "a process of interaction between two professional persons—the consultant, who is a specialist, and the consultee, who invokes the consultant's help in regard to a current work problem with which he is having some difficulty and which he has decided is within the other's area of specialized competence."[2] This definition contains three basic elements: an interactional *process;* two *participants*, one of whom is an expert; and a *purpose*, that is, help with a difficult work problem. A mental health consultation designates, according to Caplan, a special category of the general class of activity called consultation, namely, that which is a "part of a community program for the promotion of mental health and for the prevention, treatment, and rehabilitation of mental disorders."[2] The mental health consultants must possess relevant specialized knowledge and may include not only psychiatrists but also psychologists, psychiatric social workers and nurses, and so forth. The consultees, according to Caplan, include the whole range of "care-giving professionals" who lack specialized knowledge of psychiatry and yet play a significant part in preventing or treating mental disorders. Physicians, nurses, teachers, clergymen, lawyers, welfare workers, probation officers, and policemen are considered by Caplan as potential consultees. One might, by implication, extend this list to include practically every type of professional who deals with people in the conduct of his specialized activity and who might be baffled by their behavior and/or wish to promote their mental health.

There are problems with Caplan's definition, however. The promotion of mental health and the actual treatment of mental disorders are two different things. It is one purpose to promote mental health and another to deal with mental disorders, that is, those personal attributes, inner states, and overt behaviors that are currently regarded as abnormal or deviant. Emphasis on one or the other of these two proposed goals needs to be made explicit since they involve different concepts, skills, settings, and priorities for specific actions. Furthermore, it is necessary to distinguish between two classes of consultees, those trained for and directly involved with patient care and those who are not health professionals. This clarification is needed to demarcate the scope of mental health consultation and thus the role of the consultants.

Caplan's concept of mental health consultation may be criticized further. First, there is no concept of mental health that is either self-evident or generally agreed upon. Jahoda has reviewed six major approaches to mental health and underscored the paucity of relevant knowledge as well as the complexity of the criteria for the field.[3] She suggested that positive mental health is only one among many social goals and observed that mental health workers tend to display almost religious fervor and "see in it a panacea for all evil and all social problems or for the whole improvement of mankind." There is an obvious need for more empirical data and a realistic delimitation of goals in this field. Second, the designation "care-giving professionals" is so broad in Caplan's definition as to represent a *reductio ad absurdum*. It involves a skewed conception of the primary roles of the various professionals whose involvement with mental health is more or less incidental to the main roles assigned to them and for which they are trained—be they policemen, lawyers, or teachers. The consequence of this extended definition of the "clients" is that the role of the mental health consultants becomes blurred, diffuse and of unclear purpose. Third, the causes of what are currently viewed as deviations from mental health are multifactorial and poorly understood. They require more research rather than dissemination of vague and contradictory guidelines about their prevention. Fourth, a sizable proportion of mental disorders appear to be causally related to organic diseases, especially of the chronic type, for which no primary prevention is yet in sight and which provide a vast population in need of mental health care. Fifth, the number of available mental health experts and consultants is very limited, and their deployment must be a matter of carefully weighed priorities.

The foregoing arguments pertain to the issues of definition, scope, settings, participants, and purposes of mental health consultation. These matters have to be approached in the light of current social needs and not from the viewpoint of an utopian quest for a mental health millenium.

Psychiatric Consultation

For the purpose of this discussion psychiatric consultation rather than mental health consultation will be the terminology used. This is not quibbling with words. The designation "psychiatric" implies a primary concern with actual or suspected deviations from mental health as these are currently defined and classified rather than a primary concern with the promotion of vague and controversial notions of mental health as such. Thus, a psychiatric consultation is defined as *provision of expert advice on the diagnosis, management, and prevention of mental disorders by specially trained mental health professionals at the request of other health professionals and within the constraints of available knowledge and techniques.*

PARTICIPANTS

It follows from our definition that a psychiatric consultation involves, first, at least one *consultant* who is a trained expert in the area of mental disorders; second, one or more *consultees* who are health professionals concerned with patient care; and, third, the *primary beneficiary,* that is, the patient. The term "patient" in this context designates any individual who considers himself as, or has been found by a health professional to be, ill and thus aspires, rightly or wrongly, to the sick role. One of the commonest reasons for a psychiatric consultation in a medical setting is to help a nonpsychiatric physician decide if a particular person's insistence that he has a physical disorder is justified fully, partly, or not at all. In other cases it is the person's behavior that the consultee perceives as in some way deviant or abnormal, regardless if a physical illness has been diasnosed, that leads to a request for an expert opinion.

The consultant may be a psychiatrist or a psychiatrically trained nonmedical expert in disorders of mental functioning and behavior, such as a clinical psychologist, psychiatric social worker or nurse, a social scientist, or a psychiatric paraprofessional. The degree and specific area of the given consultant's expertise will vary according to the nature of his training and professional experience.

A consultee is, by the above definition, a trained provider of some aspects of patient care, be he or she a nonpsychiatric physician, nurse, social worker, and so forth.

SETTING

As already stated, the author advocates the use of the term "psychiatric consultation" in the context of the health care delivery system. Thus, the setting may be a hospital, a nursing home, a community clinic, a physician's office, or any health care facility in which a consultant meets a consultee, or a group of consultees, for the purpose of providing expert psychiatric advice on the care of patients.

It is misleading to set off sharply the hospital, or any other health care facility, from *the* community. Any health care facility is an integral part of the surrounding community, and its population flows continually between the two. Every hospital, or even hospital ward, is a community in its own right, as is every school, prison, or other collective of people who spend some time in a "formal" institution. Health care facilities and personnel are spread out outside of the hospital walls and so are the mental health professionals and consultants. The contrast of hospital versus community psychiatric consultation is spurious and a source of pointless controversies. What really matters is the purpose of the consultant's activities, that is, whether the focus is on the care of the sick or on the promotion of mental health.

PURPOSE

A psychiatric consultation has a twofold purpose: the achievement and maintenance of the best patient care and the avoidance, whenever possible, of the needless maintenance of the patient or the assumption of the sick role. This purpose is achieved directly through contact with the patient as well as indirectly by means of the advice and teaching given to the consultee. In any case, the patient is regarded as the key target and beneficiary of psychiatric consultation. A consultation may fail to benefit a particular patient, but this does not alter its basic purpose. Furthermore, a psychiatric consultation often involves members of the patient's family, his employer, and other individuals concerned with his functioning and well-being. Thus, the purpose of the consultation may be extended to enable the patient to return to his original community setting, to reduce potentially pathogenic social and occupational pressures on him, as well as to prevent psychiatric morbidity, which could result from the overall impact of his illness or disability on his family environment. These preventive goals of psychiatric consultation are increasingly strived for in all health care facilities. They make meaningless a sharp distinction between a patient-oriented, consultee-oriented, health-team-oriented, and community-oriented consultation. Diagnosis, management, rehabilitation, and prevention of emotional and behavioral disorders are the chief goals of a psychiatric consultant; and they are varied flexibly according to the demands of a given situation.

PROCESS

The process and techniques of a psychiatriatric consultation are dependent on the variables of setting, participants, and purpose. They may involve a diagnostic interview with the patient, discussions with a consultee or a health team to promote understanding and facilitate management of an individual patient or a particular category of patients, or a family interview. The consultant may simultaneously or sequentially perform the role of diagnostician, therapist, interpreter, or mediator. These techniques are identified and categorized separately only for the purpose of clarification; in the actual conduct of psychiatric consultation they are frequently interwoven. As a general rule, a consultant does not function as a therapist to the consultees in the performance of his consulting role. Here again, however, an extended consultation with a particular consultee, or group of consultees, may result in enhancement of not only their professional skills but also of their self-understanding and hence may achieve one of the goals of psychotherapy. To deny that this may and does happen would be intellectually dishonest. Yet, by definition, a consultant is primarily an invited expert adviser on mental health problems and not a therapist for the consultee.

The process of consultation is influenced by its goal. This may be to relieve an upset patient facing major surgery, for example, or to prepare another one to face terminal illness, or to motivate him to collaborate with a rehabilitation plan, or to help resolve an illness-related family crisis, or to reduce a conflict between a patient and his doctor or his medical care team, or to enhance an individual consultee's care-giving skills. Furthermore, the process is modified by the setting in which the consultation is taking place, be it a medical ward, an outpatient clinic or emergency department, a physician's office, or a place selected for a regular discussion with a group of consultees of their health-care-related problems. The consultant will adapt his method of approach to each situation. He may act as an interviewer, discussion leader, counselor, or teacher. These distinctions are relative and may be used in combinations. A consultant who confines himself to only one mode of consultation process restricts his role unduly and limits his effectiveness and scope of influence. This may be a deliberate strategy but not one to be stridently promoted and exclusively taught to future consultants.

Caplan rightly stresses that consultation is an interactional process.[2] This implies interaction between the participants. It follows that the attributes and aims of the consultant and consultee will influence the process of consultation. For example, the attitude, rank, experience, and interest of the consultee are all important variables that affect both his interactions with the psychiatric consultant and the outcome of the consultation. A consultee, say a physician, may disparage the consultant and what he represents but will request a consultation to try to be rid of a troublesome patient. Another consultee has a genuine interest in the patient and expects the consultant to help him understand and manage the patient better. Clearly, the interaction will be different in these cases. To talk about the consultation process in "global" terms without specifying its participants and goals is misleading and does not allow proper evaluation of the effectiveness of the consultation.

The discussion reflects the author's explicit bias and personal convictions. A psychiatric consultation is a multifaceted activity provided by psychiatrists and nonmedical psychiatrically trained mental health professionals in the framework of a comprehensive health care delivery system. Each consultant's expertise is limited and should be defined and applied only within the scope of the consultant's knowledge, skills, and competence. No individual can claim today to be an expert in all facets of human behavior and thus a potential consultant to just any individual, or group, wishing to improve his own professional functioning, solve his particular psychosocial problems, or influence others in the name of the promotion of mental health. This obvious stricture has to be emphasized in view of the current tendency to extend and dilute the concept of psychiatric consultation and the role of the consultant to that of peripatetic human engineer or an all-round fixer of faulty human functioning (be it an individual, group, or organization) of any kind and in every setting. This approach distorts the concept of psychiatric consultation as the rendering of expert advice that is inevitably limited by the constraints of our current knowledge in general and by the ubiquitous limitations of every consultant's expertise in particular.

Conclusion

The viewpoint is advocated here that the primary basis of operation for psychiatric, or mental health, consultants should be the health care system alongside other health professionals. There are at least two cogent arguments in support of this opinion. First, epidemiological studies have shown that 20 to 50 percent of both the physically and the psychiatrically ill suffer from concurrent organic and behavioral disorder.[4] This finding justifies the contention that comprehensive management, medical and psychiatric, is needed by vast numbers of the people seeking health care. Second, there is a widespread tendency today for people to define their distress and discontent, of whatever origin or kind, in terms of disturbed health, to communicate such distress in the language of the body, and to seek help from health care providers. This ubiquitous trend has immense medical, social, and economic implications. It leads people to expect relief and counsel from physicians for the whole range of what are basically psychosocial concerns. The doctors cannot cope with the magnitude of these problems, which transcend their competence and their conception of their professional role. As a result, the physicians attempt to approach and treat psychosocial problems as bona fide medical problems, and then there is the consequent rising costs of medical care, due to needless diagnostic tests and/or hospitalizations. This approach not only helps to create chronic pseudopatients, but it also fails to meet the seekers' expectations of relief from their existential difficulties and stresses. Employing mental health consultants in all health care facilities could help identify nonmedical problems early and lead quickly to managing them appropriately. Thus a better service would be provided, and overutilization of health professionals and health care facilities would be reduced with consequent savings of time and cost.

The preceding definitions delimit the scope of consultation-liaison psychiatry. They do not prevent anyone from defining "mental health consultation" in any way he wishes or from promoting any concept of mental health in nonmedical settings. It is proposed, however, that these different concepts should be clearly distinguished to avoid confusion between consultation-liaison psychiatry and other modes of consulting activities in which some mental health workers may engage outside of the health care delivery system.

AN HISTORICAL PERSPECTIVE OF CONSULTATION-LIAISON PSYCHIATRY

Since the 1930s consultation-liaison psychiatry has developed as an outgrowth of general hospital psychiatric units.[5] The development of these units represents a landmark in the history of psychiatry and has led to fundamental changes in the management of psychiatric patients. The continued growth of general hospital psychiatry has done much to overcome their isolation from the community and from general health care and to open psychiatry to the advances in the medical and behavioral sciences. As a result, there has been a diversification of therapies, research, and theories. In turn, the entry of psychiatry into the mainstream of medicine has fostered changes in medical education and in the management of the physically ill in the direction of comprehensive medicine.[6]

The first viable general hospital psychiatric unit in the United States was opened in the Albany Hospital (New York) in 1902.[7] In 1974 there were about 800 such units and 22.4 percent of all psychiatrists worked there.[8] The provision of psychiatric consultations to the medical and surgical wards and clinics has been a major concern from the beginning.

Consultation-liaison psychiatry was given additional impetus by the emergence in the twenties of psychosomatic medicine. In 1929 appeared Henry's classical paper on "Some modern aspects of psychiatry in general hospital practice."[9] It marks the beginning of consultation-liaison psychiatry as it is practiced today. This article has not lost its relevance. The emphasis on careful observation rather than inspired guessing, on jargon-free communication, and on flexibility on the choice of therapy is still valid. Henry's observation that physicians tend to dismiss as irrelevant patients' complaints that are not directly pertinent to physical illness is still largely true.

In 1934 the Rockefeller Foundation funded the establishment of five psychiatric liaison departments in university hospitals. One of them was organized at the Colorado General Hospital.[10] Another, at the Columbia University Medical Center, was led by Flanders Dunbar, one of the pioneers of psychosomatic medicine. She and her collaborators helped expand the theoretical basis on which consultation-liaison work rests.[11] Dunbar forecast optimistically that "the time should not be too long delayed when psychiatrists are required on all our medical and surgical wards, and in all our general and special clinics." That prediction, made in 1936, is still unfulfilled and its realization is nowhere in sight. Yet progress has been made, particularly since the end of World War II. Kaufman and his collaborators deserve much credit for this. They organized model psychiatric services, with particular stress on close liaison with the medical and surgical wards and clinics, at the Mount Sinai in New York in 1945.[12, 13, 14] Liaison psychiatrists were to play a key role in building a bridge between psychiatry and medicine by virtue of their clinical and teaching activities. Kaufman and Margolin spelled out the goals of this teaching in 1948.[14] They emphasized indoctrination of physicians in psychoanalytic psychology and psychosomatic medicine. These teaching objectives which have been modified and expanded since then, will be discussed later in the chapter.

The years since 1945 have brought a gradual growth of consultation-liaison psychiatry in all its aspects. A 1966 survey showed that 76 percent of all psychiatric training centers in the United States offered instruction in consultation work.[15] Although more recent figures are unavailable, informal inquiries indicated that most postgraduate training programs in psychiatry demand that the residents spend some time consulting on the medical and surgical floors.

An extensive literature in the field of consultation-liaison psychiatry has developed. Of particular general interest are a general review,[16] a handbook,[17] a reference guide,[18] and a critical review of consultation research.[19] Some of this literature deals with mental health consultation in settings other than the medical ones, which are the focus of the present chapter. Despite certain shared assumptions and techniques, medical-psychiatric consultation work differs from that in nonmedical settings, such as schools, social and correctional agencies, industry, and so forth. The chief differences are (1) operation in the context of health care delivery both administratively and conceptually, (2) adherence to the psychosomatic approach, one which proposes that human health and disease result from an *interaction* of biological, psychological and social factors, and (3) focus on people whose psychiatric problems are related to physical illness and disability and/or those who communicate their distress in terms of somatic symptoms.

Much of the literature on consultation-liaison psychiatry is descriptive, but several notable works stand out as attempts to conceptualize the consultant's mode of operation, assumptions and aims.[20, 21, 22, 23, 24] These articles should become recommended reading for psychiatric trainees.

The current role of consultation-liaison psychiatry has been succinctly, if incompletely, summed up by the American Hospital Association:

The development of liaison psychiatric services is based on the acknowledged fact that psychiatry applied in general or specialty medicine contributes to the quality of care provided, affects hospital utilization, and results in a savings of the physician's time. . . . The liaison psychiatrist often serves the unserved, by helping to ensure the identification and appropriate management of mental and emotional aspects of illness throughout the hospital.[25]

The statement acknowledges the contribution of consultation-liaison psychiatry to improved patient care and to preventive medicine and psychiatry. This recognition comes after 40 years of an uphill struggle to establish and maintain psychiatric consultation services in the general hospitals. There is reason to believe that despite obstacles these services are here to stay and will develop further.

THE SCOPE OF CONSULTATION-LIAISON PSYCHIATRY

Consultation-liaison psychiatry has been defined as that area of clinical psychiatry that encompasses clinical, teaching, and research activities of psychiatrists and allied mental health professionals in the nonpsychiatric divisions of a general hospital.[16] This definition is already too narrow. While it is true that the medical and surgical wards, outpatient clinics, and emergency departments of general hospitals provide the main operational base for the liaison psychiatrists, their activities are gradually spreading beyond the hospital walls. Consultation-liaison psychiatry's scope has expanded to include collaboration with all categories of health professionals in all types of health care facilities, be they community health clinics, rehabilitation centers, convalescent hospitals, nursing homes, or doctors' private offices.

The designation "consultation-liaison" psychiatry reflects a twofold role for this area of psychiatry. The consultation aspect refers to the provision of expert advice on all aspects of mental health to the other health professionals — physicians, nurses, social workers, and so on. The liaison role is more complex. At a more abstract level it connotes mediation between psychiatry and the rest of medicine. The liaison psychiatrist acts as an interpreter and bridge builder between two conceptual domains and professional groups. He attempts to integrate in his clinical and teaching activities the conceptions and knowledge belonging to the behavioral and biological sciences and approaches to patients, respectively. He also maintains a link and promotes collaboration between the mental health and the other health care professionals. This activity is based on the belief that health care delivery and the management and prevention of all forms of illness are best served by a comprehensive approach to patients, one that integrates in practice the psychosocial, biological, and ecologic aspects of health and disease.

In a more concrete sense, liaison implies mediation between patients and those taking care of them. This involves explanation, interpretation, and maintaining communication. The consultant brings to bear his knowledge of individual and group psychodynamics as well as his skills in interviewing and communicating to perform this mediating function. The commonest occasion for consultation liaison is the breakdown of communication with resulting conflicts between a patient and one or more members of the clinical team. Poor communication and conflicts interfere with optimal patient care and may at times disrupt the function of a ward as a therapeutic community.[21, 26] Conflicts may arise in the context of a doctor-patient relationship, between patients and nurses, and within the medical team itself. It is one of the functions of the liaison psychiatrist to identify the sources of disruptive interpersonal conflicts that interfere with efficient management of patients and to help attenuate them. Particularly useful for both liaison and teaching is a regular conference attended by the consultant assigned to a given medical service or unit and the therapeutic team. This provides a forum for discussion of patients as well as the strains within the team. Staff's problems related to uncooperative and hostile patients, their reactions to the severely ill and dying, idiosyncratic countertransference reactions, and many other issues related to patient care may be discussed with the consultant. To perform this role, the consultant must maintain close contact with the ward or clinic to which he is assigned. This cannot be accomplished if the number of consultants available is just sufficient to provide formal consultations only.

Consultation and liaison are mutually complementary activities. In some hospitals these two functional components are separated. The liaison service is involved in teaching and research but does not provide psychiatric consultations, which are left to other members of the department of psychiatry. Such an arrangement has serious flaws since the liaison work is most effective if the same personnel provides consultations on request. A consultation should encompass three interlocked focuses: the patient, the consultee, and the therapeutic group.[16] This implies that consultation is most effective if the consultant has personal contact with both the patient and those taking care of him. Further, no consultation is complete unless the patient's relationships with his social environment, apart from the health professionals involved, is taken into account.[27] A patient's management is truly comprehensive if it includes communication with and knowledge about the patient's family and, to a lesser extent, other significant people in his social milieu. This is crucial in all cases of prolonged convalescence and chronic or fatal illness.

The aim of the extended social view in patient management generally, and in psychiatric consultation-liaison work particularly, is the prevention of psychiatric morbidity related to the impact on the patient of the social and economic consequences of his illness as well as to the influence of his disability and illness behavior on his family. Numerous studies have established that people tend to become ill and seek medical help and hospitalization at times of social stress and that such stress may contribute to various forms of deviant illness behavior, such as psychogenic invalidism, noncompliance with physician's advice, and overutilization of health and social welfare facilities.[28] The attitudes and behaviors of the patient's family members play a key role in bringing about these undesirable behavior patterns. A patient's illness and illness-related behavior may be a source of psychological stress and psychiatric morbidity for his spouse and other family members.[29]

Demonstration of the importance of identifying and managing the psychological, social, and economic consequences of all types of severe and prolonged physical illness and disability is one of the major contributions of consultation-liaison psychiatry to the practice and teaching of medicine. Since the most prevalent forms of serious illness today are chronic, such as cardiovascular diseases, the importance of the psychosocial factors in medicine is being increasingly recognized. At the same time medical training, with its heavy emphasis on narrow specialization and the biological aspects of disease, does not prepare physicians adequately to recognize and deal with the influence of these factors on their patients. By default this role is often relegated to the liaison psychiatrists and allied mental health professionals. It is in this area that psychiatrists can discharge their responsibilty to medicine, which Engel so eloquently advocates.[30]

ASSUMPTIONS AND AIMS

No organized form of human activity can survive in an ideological vacuum. Here "ideology" implies a set of beliefs, assumptions, and formulated aims that furnish an organized activity with a raison d'etre that justifies its continuation in the eyes of its practitioners and outside observers. If an ideology, as defined, becomes diffuse, vague, and full of contradictions and is increasingly challenged by vocal critics, the purpose and legitimacy of the activity based on it are questioned. As a result, the practitioners' sense of meaningful commitment is undermined. As expressed in "fashionable" jargon, the practitioners are in a state of "identity crisis." This condition is experienced by some psychiatrists today, as highlighted by the formation of a task force in 1973 to define the terms "psychiatrist" and "mental illness."[31] The liaison psychiatrist is also potentially vulnerable to confusion about his professional identity. Working as he does at the boundary between two professions and two distinct conceptual approaches to man and his ills, he is often treated with reserve by colleagues on either side of the territorial fence. They are liable to consider him as neither fish nor fowl and as a troublemaker whose border-crossing activity disturbs complacent cultivation of prosperous professional gardens. Thus, the liaison psychiatrist epitomizes the current ambiguity of the role of psychiatry in general. An attempt to spell out the ideological base of consultation-liaison psychiatry may have validity for the specialty as a whole.

Consultation-liaison psychiatry is firmly embedded in psychosomatic medicine. Since the latter designation has become ambiguous, its contemporary connotation needs to be restated.[16, 32, 33] Psychosomatic medicine is often erroneously identified with a search for psychogenesis of chronic somatic disorders of unknown etiology vaguely called ''psychosomatic.'' The main investigative techniques as well as the resulting explanatory hypotheses about the putative causal psychological factors of these disorders were derived from psychoanalysis. Between 1930 and 1950 the most conspicuous and vocal psychosomaticists were engaged in research and theorizing along thses lines. Their thinking was clearly formulated in Alexander's book *Psychosomatic Medicine*[34] but their influence faded away soon afterward having bogged down in methodological problems. Today their conception of psychosomatic medicine is obsolete. Yet Alexander has made an enduring contribution by formulating the theoretical and practical postulates for comprehensive medicine and psychiatry. His prediction, made in 1958, about the direction psychiatry would follow has been partly fulfilled and remains germane: ''A growing integration of the biologic, psychodynamic, and sociologic approaches, and the emergence of comprehensive psychiatry which no longer attempts to solve the great mystery of human behavior from one single restricted point of view.''[35]

Consultation-liaison psychiatry has developed as a clinical activity and teaching applying to the psychosomatic approach. The liaison psychiatrist attempts in his daily work to collect and integrate complex information relevant to the diagnostic process and to the planning of comprehensive management of patients. The general systems approach has provided him with a workable conceptual framework for organizing data derived from several levels of abstraction: psychological, physiological, sociological, and ecological.[22, 23]

The ultimate aim of consultation-liaison psychiatry is promotion of optimal care of the sick. To achieve this goal an organizational structure is needed to coordinate the diverse roles, functions, and activities of the mental health professionals working in medical settings.

ORGANIZATION OF A CONSULTATION-LIAISON SERVICE

To be effective and provide continuity of service the consultants should work as a team. Lack of organizational structure is liable to make the provision of service haphazard and subject to the vagaries of availability of consultants.

Further, an established consultation-liaison service is indispensable for maintaining morale among the consultants and for the negotiation and coordination of service, teaching, and research. One critic has observed that circumscribed consultation services have stultified the development of "full liaison" between medicine and psychiatry and that in the future all full-time members of a psychiatric faculty should be required to spend some time teaching on the medical and surgical floors.[36] This suggestion is a well-meaning invitation to bedlam. To suggest that all psychiatrists would be able and willing to perform such work without proper training and interest in it betrays ignorance of the realities of liaison psychiatry. Many competent psychiatrists prefer to stay away from the often uncomfortable and trying conditions of work in the medical wards and clinics. Some are unable to establish a working relationship with other physicians and are not able to communicate adequately with them. Others shy away from the exigencies of work with the physically ill, disabled, or dying. While psychiatric consultation services need not monopolize psychiatric clinical work and teaching on the medical wards, they should provide a core of psychiatrists and other mental health professionals who are committed to liaison work, are trained for it, are acceptable to their medical and surgical colleagues, can coordinate clinical and teaching activities, and are willing to keep abreast with the advances in medicine. To expect all psychiatrists to fulfill these criteria is as unrealistic as to claim that all physicians are capable and willing to deal with psychosocial problems of their patients.

An ideal consultation-liaison service should be an administrative unit based in the psychiatric department of a general hospital or psychiatric division of a community health clinic. It should be staffed by full-time as well as part-time psychiatrists and include at least one psychiatric liaison nurse,[37] social worker, and psychologist. The person in charge should be a psychiatrist experienced in consultation-liaison psychiatry. Each of the professionals on the staff brings to the team his or her particular expertise. A consultation-liaison service is not an experiment in community living in which all roles are interchangeable. Each member does what he is trained to do and makes a useful contribution within his competence. Some functions will overlap, as in carrying out psychotherapy, in teaching or research. The head of the unit has to coordinate all of these activities. In addition, he must be able to communicate and negotiate with other physicians in their language and on an equal footing; that is why it is recommended that the chief of staff be a consultation-liaison psychiatrist. This "elitist" arrangement reflects a pragmatic approach to the distribution of responsibilities according to acquired knowledge and skills.

The size and composition of a consultation-liaison service will vary, depending on the size of the hospital or clinic, availability of consultants, funding, and other factors. Many consultants have developed close liaison with a wide range of specialties and therapeutic settings, including medicine,[38] surgery,[39] pediatrics,[40] neurology and neurosurgery[41] intensive care units,[42] oncology,[43] hemodialysis units,[44] emergency departments,[45] outpatient clinics,[46] and rehabilitation.[47] such special liaison facilitates continuity of service, development of a close working relationship with staff, acquisition of expert knowledge about a given specialty, treatment, or therapeutic environment, and opportunity for collaborative clinical research.

A common problem bedeviling consultation work is the vulnerability of the service to the attitudes toward it of the chiefs of the medical and psychiatric departments. A change in one of these key administrative positions may spell generous support or, on the contrary, isolation and neglect of the service. Only a firmly established and respected consultation service may ride out changing fortunes. The role of the psychiatric department head is crucial in this regard; it would help if each chief of psychiatry considered liaison with other departments as one of the integral functions and commitments of psychiatry.

To advocate the team approach as the optimal organizational principle for a psychiatric consultation-liaison service has obvious economic implications. At present, most such services rely on government grants and/or fee-for-service payments to psychiatric consultants by the insurance companies. Nonpsychiatric members of the team receive a salary whose source is usually grant money. Since such monies are increasingly difficult to obtain, the whole question of funding a consultation-liaison team must be solved.

Under the prevailing system of practice no psychiatrist could earn an average income by doing consultation-liaison work only. Much of the work, if done properly, is time consuming. It involves not only interviews with patients for which a charge is made, but also discussions with consultees and teaching. Although these activities are an inherent part of liaison, they usually are not remunerated. The best solution is a salary for a block of time—regardless of how that time is spent. It would seem reasonable that the nonpsychiatric department to which the consultant is assigned should contribute at least part of such a salary, but this seldom occurs.

SOURCES OF FRUSTRATION FOR THE TEAM

Conditions of work and economic factors may account for the fact that relatively few consultation-liaison psychiatrists remain in this area of clinical psychiatry for more than several years. One who has worked as a liaison psychiatrist for more than 10 years is considered a ''grizzled veteran.'' There are several sources of frustration and discomfort in this type of work. Mendelson and Meyer have written about countertransference problems of the consultants.[48] Relationships with the consultees is another problem. A consultant has to put up with much indifference and varying degrees of suspicion and hostility on the part of his colleagues. Their negative attitudes are often expressed in a subtle and jovial manner. Sometimes it is the effusively cordial medical colleague who hampers and deprecates the consultant's work most effectively. Senior physicians' disparaging remarks about psychiatry or assertions that every physician can deal effectively with emotional disorders tend to influence medical residents and students. As a result these young physicians may regard the liaison psychiatrist as an intruder. Too often consultation may be requested, but the consultant's conclusions and recommendations are ignored. Problems of communication are common, and some consultees are indifferent to psychological and social information about their patients.

It requires patient and tact on the consultant's part to persevere in his work despite such frustrating attitudes. It may require some years of close liaison with a particular department for a consultant to become accepted as someone who has something useful to offer and whose assistance is actively sought and has advice followed. Much depends on the consultant's own attitude and ability to demonstrate his usefulness to the consultees. The consultant must constantly consider the sensitivity of many of his medical colleagues to statements that may sound critical of them.[49] Psychiatrists are often unaware of the extent to which their words are scanned by others for signs of opprobrium, for some surreptitiously gleaned ulterior motive, or for evidence of incompetence. Use of psychodynamic terms is particularly liable to give rise to such misinterpretations. The less the consultant talks like a stereotype psychiatrist ridiculed in cartoons and jokes, the more practical and helpful he is, the more he is likely to be respected and listened to. A consultant whose manner and way of talking puzzle or offend the consultees—one who fails to offer practical advice intelligibly—will remain ineffective and be called only to see the most disturbing patients in order to effect their transfer to a psychiatric facility.

Another source of frustration for the consultant stems from the fact that many patients referred for psychiatric consultation from medical wards and clinics do not ask for the service and often resent it. This attitude is usually the result of the inadequate preparations of the patient by the consultee.[50] To make matters worse, the conditions in which the patient has to be interviewed on a medical ward are often uncomfortable and lacking in privacy.

To persist in his work the consultant needs support and professional satisfaction. The former should be provided by his department of psychiatry. The position of a consultant is strengthened if he has some clinical and teaching responsibilities in the department—for example, if he acts as a consultant to a psychiatric inpatient ward or clinic, carries out intensive psychotherapy, and tutors psychiatric residents. In this way he can maintain his professional ties with psychiatry and bring his special experience and psychosomatic viewpoint to bear on the teaching in and the functioning of the psychiatric unit. The professional satisfaction comes from viewing liaison work as an opportunity for effective therapeutic and teaching activity, and as an intellectual challenge to apply one's knowledge to ever new and highly complex clinical problems. The broader the consultant's theoretical interests are the more satisfaction can he derive from his work.

FUNCTIONS OF CONSULTANTS

All consultants are engaged in clinical activities; most of them teach; some engage in research; and many pursue all three forms of activity. Taken together, these three functions—clinical work, teaching, and research—define a consultant's professional role.

Clinical Work

In addition to liaison discussed earlier, diagnostic and therapeutic activities comprise a consultant's clinical function. Requests for psychiatric consultation are divided about equally between help with diagnosis and management of patients. In most cases a consultee's request for aid in diagnosis leads to advice on management or disposition of the patient. For the purpose of this discussion, however, these two aspects of consultation will be considered separately.

Diagnostic problems that most commonly face the consultant can be separated into several categories. First, the patient has somatic complaints for which no adequate organic explanation can be found regardless if he is known to suffer from a physical illness or not. The symptoms may indicate the presence of a psychiatric disorder. On such a diagnosis depends in part the advice on treatment. Depression is the psychiatric disorder most often accompanied by somatic complaints and encountered among medical patients. Hysterical anxiety and hypochondriacal neuroses as well as schizophrenia may all present with somatic complaints, but they are less common. In addition, one encounters somatic complaints to which no clear-cut diagnostic label can be assigned, unless one resorts to that nosological wastebasket called "psychophysiologic disorders."[51] Second, a patient may display for him uncharacteristic behavior, that is, either accentuation or alteration of his usual personality traits, and the consultee wants to know if this change is a manifestation of cerebral disease, functional psychiatric disorder, or an unclassifiable behavioral response to physical illness, interpersonal stress, or both.[4, 27] This diagnostic area requires familiarity with subtle psychological manifestations of an early cerebral disorder and of many systemic diseases, such as cancer, that may give rise to psychological symptoms.[52] Third, a patient may present an obvious psychiatric disorder that the consultee may or may not correctly diagnose but of whose presence he is aware. Fourth, the patient displays deviant illness behavior, such as self-destructive non-compliance with medical advice, excessive dependence on, or, on the contrary, boisterous disregard or gross denial of illness, a given-up attitude, factitial illness, overt suicidal tendencies.[4]

Such a broad range of diagnostic problems is not encountered to an equal extent in other areas of psychiatric practice. Much of the clinical material that a consultant to medicine encounters is not discussed in textbooks. Many of the symptoms, somatic and behavioral, have no known neurophysiological substrate, and their significance is unclear. Some of the somatic symptoms represent metaphors couched in body language. Others suggest increased or decreased awareness of the somatosensory information input that may be endowed with idiosyncratic symbolic meanings, labels, and interpretations by the patient. This is a largely unexplored area at the boundary of the physical and the mental. It is of more than theoretical interest since more than one-half of patients presenting in medical outpatient clinics and at least one-third of inpatients complain of somatic symptoms of unknown etiology.[16, 28] Such complaints are labeled "psychosomatic" or "functional," both ambiguous terms covering our ignorance. Lack of reliable diagnostic guidelines to identify these symptoms results in a vast number of costly laboratory tests being carried out to exclude organic pathology.[53] Early psychosocial evaluation of every patient who does not present an acute medical problem should result in reducing the cost of investigations and of hospital admissions and thus contribute to containment of the rising cost of health care delivery.

A consultant's diagnostic work is complex and time-consuming. The only diagnostic tools available are the interview and clinical observation. The consultant often has to take a comprehensive history, including a detailed functional inquiry, and supplement it by additional information from family members, primary physicians, employers, and others who have had contact with the patient. A liaison social worker is of great help in securing this type of information and mediating between physicians, patients, and the patients' relatives, employers, and other concerned persons. The consultant has to collate a great deal of data in arriving at a comprehensive diagnostic assessment, which is the basis of management planning. He must avoid fitting a patient's somatic symptoms too readily into a plausible cause-and-effect sequence of intrapsychic conflicts, defense mechanisms, and recent life changes. Psychiatric training has often fostered inspired guesswork rather than careful data gathering, observation, and diagnostic reasoning. A consultant should not practice the deceptive art of psychodynamic speculation based on sparse factual material. His is an area of psychiatry with a fair degree of public accountability. What he learns about the patient, how he interprets this information, and what practical action he recommends are recorded and open to scrutiny. Inferences and recommendations of the consultant are promptly tested and highly visible. His competence, knowledge (and gaps of knowledge), capacity for expeditious information gathering and logical reasoning, ability to make decisions and communicate them clearly, and therapeutic efficacy are all open to scrutiny when he is called to consult.

Diagnosis is inseparably linked to guidelines for action. A consultation is useless if it does not result in practical recommendations. Diagnostic labeling and imaginative psychodynamic interpretations are by themselves of no value to the consultee. The consultant has to suggest further investigations, if any, advise in concrete terms on the psychological approach to the patient, and recommend specific therapies, such as psychotherapy, psychotropic drugs, and so forth. At times he may undertake treatment himself. Medical wards and clinics are a suitable setting for brief psychotherapy.[54] Psychiatrists used to long-term psychotherapy tend to belittle the therapeutic potential of such an intervention. The author has been impressed over the years with the effectiveness of clearly focused brief psychotherapy in medical settings. Many a patient faced with the threat, uncertainty, novelty and ambiguity occasioned by physical illness, obscure somatic symptoms, and hospitalization is more open to an incisive scrutiny of his values, goals, relationships, and coping strategies in such settings. Many, if rightly approached, welcome an opportunity to talk with someone who conveys empathy with their predicament and willingness to spend time listening and talking.

The interview is best started by an inquiry into the history, antecedents, and circumstances surrounding the onset of the patient's presenting symptoms. This helps dispel his suspicion that the psychiatrist is only interested in psychological data—searches for evidence that the patient is mentally deranged and that his distress is all "in his head." The consultant can obtain not only diagnostically valuable history, both medical and psychiatric, but he can also unobtrusively extend the scope of his inquiry into psychological and social areas. By shifting freely between directive and associative interviewing techniques he not only gathers information but also provokes reflection and self-examination in the patient. The patient may become aware of personal problems and continue to reflect on them with resulting choice and decision-making long after one or several interviews with the consultant. In some cases an overriding current problem will be the focus of therapy. This may be preoperative anxiety, shock at learning the diagnosis of a chronic or fatal illness, grief over loss of a body part or function, conflict with staff, a crisis in family relationships, an acute psychosis, or suicidal impulses or attempt.

Thus, the consultant's therapeutic intervention is focused on the currently most pressing problem, usually coupled with attempts at bringing about attitude changes transcending the immediate crisis. There is neither a sharp dividing line nor incompatibility between so-called crisis intervention and long-range preventive and change-evoking aims. This therapeutic approach reflects a current trend in psychiatric practice. Its hallmarks are (1) choice of therapy best suited for a given patient's both immediate and long-term needs, (2) clear definition of therapeutic goals based on thorough psychiatric assessment, (3) flexibility in the conduct of therapy, and (4) incisive intervention by the therapist to achieve his goals expeditiously. Present trends in health care delivery will increasingly favor this type of therapeutic approach. The experiences since the introduction of medicare that includes psychiatric care in Canada make it clear.[55]

Some consultants use treatment modalities other than individual psychotherapy. Group psychotherapy has been successful for special categories of patients, such as survivors of myocardial infarction,[56] victims of severe burns, or patients with orthopedic problems requiring prolonged hospitalization. Marital couple therapy, family therapy, behavior modification techniques, biofeedback, and hypnosis have been employed for specific medical problems and their psychosocial complications.[32] Psychiatric therapies have been used for a whole range of illnesses: acute and life-threatening ones, such as myocardial infarction; chronic ones, such as multiple sclerosis, hypertension, or ulcerative colitis; and terminal diseases. Every patient presents a different therapeutic challenge influenced by his illness and its potential for reversibility and compensability and by his coping capacity. The consultant must evaluate the patient's response to his illness and his available resources for coping with it as a precondition for an individually tailored therapeutic intervention aimed at bringing out the most adaptive coping strategies of which the patient is capable. Every management plan involves assessment of the patient's personality, his particular conflicts, his coping style and strategies, liabilities and assets. Basic to the plan, of course, are the nature of the organic pathology and related deficits, the symptoms, and the prognosis. Further, the medical and surgical therapies involved, the characteristics of the environment in which the patient is treated, and the impact of his illness on his family relationships, his social roles, and his sources of gratification must all be evaluated. There is no room in this approach for preconceived notions that sufferers from a given somatic disorder, or those having a particular personality structure, demand standard therapeutic strategy and goals.

A thorough familiarity with psychotropic drugs and especially with their potentially deleterious effects on various somatic disorders (such as coronary heart disease, hypertension, hepatic and renal diseases) is indispensable. So is the knowledge of the interactions of the psychotropic drugs with those prescribed for various physical illnesses. Drug treatment of psychiatric emergencies, such as psychotic excitement, delirium, panic, or rage, falls within a consultant's competence.[32]

Teaching

Practically every liaison psychiatrist acts as a teacher. His teaching may not be formal; one can teach by providing a model role and example. Psychiatric consultants to medicine have become increasingly more involved in planning and carrying out teaching programs of psychiatry and the psychosocial aspects of medicine to medical students and residents, physicians, nurses, social workers, and physicians' assistants.[57] Particularly important is the teaching of medical students.[32] The liaison psychiatrist is in a favorable position to teach psychiatry as it applies to the daily practice of medicine. He can demonstrate at the bedside, in clinical conferences, in seminars, and during informal discussion groups the techniques of interviewing, the making of a comprehensive diagnosis, and management planning as well as the application of psychiatric treatment modalities. Some medical students elect a rotation on a liaison service so that they can observe and carry out, under supervision, psychiatric consultations on medical and surgical patients. At the Dartmouth-Hitchcock Medical Center every senior medical student rotating through medicine is expected to act as a consultee, that is, initiate a referral for psychiatric consultation, be present during the interview, and discuss the results of the consultation and the recommendations with the consultant. The student observes the consultation process and learns to appreciate the potential and limitations of psychiatric consultation. Hopefully, he will learn how to use such consultations in his future practice. With the increasing emphasis on team work and integrated community health clinics, current trends in health care delivery will make such collaboration necessary, and our teaching should prepare the students for it.

At the postgraduate level, experience on a well-functioning and adequately staffed consultation-liaison service has much to offer to the senior psychiatric resident.[58, 59] He learns to view patients comprehensively rather than segmentally. The psychosomatic approach is no less relevant to psychiatric practice than it is to medicine. The need to take into account every patient's somatic functioning as well as his psychodynamic, social, and economic aspects serves as a useful antidote against a narrow professional bias to which psychiatrists are as prone as their medical colleagues. Regardless of what particular facet of psychiatry the resident will choose to pursue, he should have the experience of dealing with the physically ill and those who present their psychosocial problems in the form of somatic complaints.

On a liaison service he learns to apply his psychiatric knowledge expeditiously, express his findings and recommendations in plain English, and collaborate with nonpsychiatric health professionals. The type of psychiatry practiced by consultants discourages vagueness, use of jargon to cover ignorance, free-floating speculation, and fanatical adherence to a single theory or therapeutic technique. It encourages open-mindedness, respect for observation and clear thinking, flexibility, and a truly eclectic approach to psychiatric practice. Ignorance, muddleheadedness, and wooly jargon are more visible on a liaison service than on other psychiatric services.

Current trends are likely to result in the psychiatrist's being increasingly used as a consultant to and a team member of integrated health care facilities. Training should prepare our residents for these roles. Experience on a liaison service is well suited to promote diagnostic, therapeutic, and communicative skills that will be useful in the years to come.

Clinical Research

The spread of general hospital psychiatric units and the resulting closer links with general medicine have been a powerful stimulant to psychiatric research. Psychiatrists have gained access to first-rate laboratory facilities and to rich clinical material. The spirit of scientific inquiry pervading teaching general hospitals presented the psychiatrists working in them with an irresistible challenge. Recent advances in psychopharmacology and the neurobiology of psychiatric disorders are largely the result of psychiatry's closeness to the medical sciences. At the same time the traditional focus on individual psychodynamics and psychopathology as well as psychiatry's links with the behavioral sciences have added a missing dimension to medical research, education, and practice: they have added a humanistic perspective.

Consultation-liaison psychiatrists have made a major contribution to this mutually enriching rapprochement. Their research endeavors have been many and varied. The work of Engel and his colleagues of the Rochester group provides an impressive illustration of the scope and far reaching theoretical and clinical implications of this research. Starting with the classical studies of delirium in the midforties, the Rochester group has investigated the psychophysiology of fainting and hyperventilation, psychological characteristics of the pain-prone patients, conversion reactions, psychological aspects of ulcerative colitis, psychological antecedents, in the form of the giving-up—given-up syndrome, of all types of illness (physical and psychiatric), psychosocial factors influencing the onset of myocardial infarction and the patient's behavior following the onset of its symptoms, and many other subjects. The impact of the work by only one group of liaison psychiatrists over the last 30 years on both medicine and psychiatry remains to be evaluated.[60, 61, 62, 63, 64]

Other consultants have pioneered research on the attitudes toward death and the experience of dying; on the psychiatric aspects of the new medical technology, such as chronic hemodialysis, organ transplantation, open-heart surgery, ileal bypass surgery, chronic cardiac pacemakers, and so on; on psychological reactions to and psychiatric complications of the whole gamut of physical illnesses, their treatment, and therapeutic environments; on the neurophysiological, neuroendocrine, and immune mechanisms intervening between social situations and events and their psychophysiological and pathological consequences; on the hospital ward as a social milieu; on the process of consultation and crisis intervention.[19, 32, 33]

This incomplete list allows the claim that closer liaison between psychiatry and medicine has opened up a vast and still largely untapped area of scientific inquiry. It is on the borderlands between the various scientific disciplines concerned with man, especially on the interface of the medical and behavioral sciences, that some of the most exciting research possibilities lie today. This is particularly true of the most prevalent chronic diseases, such as coronary heart disease, hypertension, cancer, and schizophrenia. It would mean the loss of a great opportunity if psychiatrists failed to grasp this challenge and instead withdrew into a new isolationism. Future growth of our field will depend on psychiatric educators and the training that they provide. Such training must encompass human biology and behavioral sciences, psychopathology, psychophysiology and human ecology, psychological development and psychodynamics of individuals, and the functioning of the body in health and disease.

PROBLEMS OF EVALUATION

An important albeit neglected area of research calling for separate discussion is that of the evaluation of the outcome and effectiveness of medical-psychiatric consultation. A review of consultation research by Mannino and Shore highlights the paucity of evaluation studies.[19] A consultant's impression, or even fervent conviction, that his work is useful offers no acceptable substitute for systematic inquiry into its effectiveness. Relative scarcity of studies in this area stems from lack of adequate methodology and from shortage of manpower and funds necessary to carry out follow-up surveys.

To evaluate consultation work properly calls for clear definitions of its aims and criteria by which to judge the degree of their attainment. Two major aims of psychiatric consultation may be distinguished for this purpose: consultee satisfaction and patient satisfaction. The main difficulty concerns criteria for the evaluation of these outcomes. The most direct and simple strategy is to ask a sample of consultees or patients if they were satisfied with the consultation and found it useful. This method may involve either an interview or a questionnaire.[50, 65, 66, 67, 68] A review of the few studies using this approach indicates that 30 to 60 percent of the patients referred for psychiatric consultation found it helpful. Several variables appeared to influence patients' attitudes: (1) the manner in which the patient had been prepared for consultation by the referring doctor, (2) the patient's distinctive emotional reaction toward consultation, and (3) presence of dysphoric emotions (anxiety, depression) in the patient prior to consultation.

Satisfaction of referring physicians has been assesed indirectly by comparing the numbers of patients referred for consultation before and after the introduction of liaison with a particular medical service, or of a regular clinical conference. In both instances the volume of referrals increased.[69, 70]

Other evaluative approaches have focused on the overall adjustment of patients referred for consultation six months after hospitalization;[71] the outcome of psychiatric disorder for which the patient had been referred one year prior to a follow-up assessment;[72] and the discrepancy between the expectations of consultees and the services provided by the psychiatric consultants.[73]

In summary, adequate evaluative research of the outcome and efficacy of psychiatric consultation is wanting, and more studies are needed. An important issue that remains to be investigated concerns economic aspects of these consultations. Specifically, we need to establish whether consultations result in reduced costs of health care. Such saving could be expected to be brought about by fewer laboratory investigations, shorter hospitalization, and earlier return to work of those patients referred for psychiatric consultation as soon as their psychosocial problems are identified. We tend to believe that such outcome does prevail, but objective evidence is still lacking.

THE FUTURE

Consultation-liaison psychiatry embodies a set of assumptions, attitudes, skills, and activities that represent one of the dominant trends in psychiatry today. Its importance may be expected to grow as a result of the direction of scientific, social, and economic forces that presently influence the form of health care delivery. Recent writers discussing the future of psychiatry affirm this view. Arthur states, "In the future, perhaps psychiatrists and other specialists will function more in the role of consultants . . . . But to be a consultant one must indeed be better educated, know more, and be more competent than workers at the initial level."[59] This is echoed by West: "The neuropsychiatrist of the future will, in keeping with the liaison concept, work closely with colleagues in the other traditional clinical disciplines and also with those in such new specialties as family medicine, community health, and emergency medicine, to mention only three."[74]

To the current debate on the psychiatrist's professional role and on the future of our discipline the liaison psychiatrist can contribute a role model that has endured for 40 years in an often unreceptive climate. It is a model based on a broadly conceived psychosomatic and social-ecologic view of health and disease, of medical and psychiatric theory and practice. This model affirms the complexity and ambiguity of our knowledge of man and eschews the reductionist approaches that offer security to fervent believers in a single theory and practitioners of a single therapeutic technique. Liaison psychiatrists see themselves as neither social reformers, nor politicians, nor magic healers offering solutions to all dilemmas of the human condition. They are content with their role as mediators, interpreters, consultants, and therapists who can meet their professional responsibility by helping to provide directly and indirectly, some relief for some avoidable suffering of some individuals and by helping some persons to attain what growth, as persons, they are capable of. Their professional role is inextricably linked with medical training and practice.[75] It contains, the author would predict, some essential elements of the training, interests, attitudes, and activities of the psychiatrists of tomorrow.

REFERENCES

1. Arnhoff FN, Kumbar AH: The Nation's Psychiatrists—1970 Survey. Washington, D.C., American Psychiatric Association, 1973
2. Caplan G: The Theory and Practice of Mental Health Consultation. New York, Basic Books, 1970, pp 19–34
3. Jahoda M: Current Concepts of Positive Mental Health. New York, Basic Books, 1958
4. Lipowski ZJ: Psychiatry of somatic diseases: Epidemiology, pathogenesis, classification. Compr Psychiatry 16:105–124, 1975
5. Kaufman MR, (ed): The Psychiatric Unit in a General Hospital. New York, International Universities Press, 1965
6. Guze SB, Matarazzo JD, Saslow G: A formulation of principles of comprehensive medicine with special reference to learning theory. J Clin Psychol 9:127–136, 1953
7. Sweeney GH: Pioneering general hospital psychiatry. Psychiatr Q 36:209–268, 1962
8. Kanno C: Personal communication. March 21, 1974
9. Henry GW: Some modern aspects of psychiatry in general hospital practice. Am J Psychiatry 9:481–499, 1929–1930
10. Billings EG: The psychiatric liaison department of the University of Colorado Medical School and hospitals. Am J Psychiatry 122 (12, Suppl.):28–33, 1966
11. Dunbar FH, Wolfe TP, Rioch JMcK: Psychiatric aspects of medical problems. Am J Psychiatry. 93:649–679, 1936
12. Kaufman MR: A psychiatric unit in a general hospital. J M Sinai Hospital 24:572–579, 1957
13. Bernstein S, Kaufman MR: The psychiatrist in a general hosptial. J Mount Sinai Hospital 29:385–394, 1962

14. Kaufman MR, Margolin SG: Theory and practice of psychosomatic medicine in a general hospital. Medical Clin North Am 32:611–616, 1948
15. Mendel WM: Psychiatric consultation education—1966. Am J Psychiatry 123:150–155, 1966
16. Lipowski ZJ: Review of consultation psychiatry and psychosomatic medicine. I, II, III. Psychosom Med 29:153–171, 1967; 29:201–224, 1967; 30:395–422, 1968
17. Schwab JJ: Handbook of Psychiatric Consultation. New York, Appleton-Century-Crofts, 1968
18. Mannino FV: Consultation in Mental Health and Related Fields. Chevy Chase, Md, National Institute of Mental Health, 1969
19. Mannino FV, Shore MF: Consultation Research in Mental Health and Related Fields. Washington, DC, US Department of Health, Education and Welfare, Public Health Monograph No. 79
20. Bibring GL: Psychiatry and medical practice in a general hospital. N Eng J Med 154:366–372, 1956
21. Meyer E, Mendelson M: Psychiatric consultations with patients on medical and surgical wards: Patterns and processes. Psychiatry 24:197–220, 1961
22. Miller WB: Psychiatric consultation. I. A general systems approach. Psychiatry Med 4:135–145, 1973
23. Miller WB: Psychiatric consultation. II. Conceptual and pragmatic issues of formulation. Psychiatry Med 4:251–271, 1973
24. Sandt JJ, Leifer R: The psychiatric consultation. Compr Psychiatry 5:409–418, 1964
25. Mental Health Services and the General Hospital. Chicago, American Hospital Association, 1970
26. Issacharoff A, Redinger R, Schneider D: The psychiatric consultation as an experience in group process. Contemp Psychoanalysis 8:260–275, 1972
27. Brodsky CM: A social view of the psychiatric consultation. Psychosomatics 8:61–68, 1967
28. Lipowski ZJ: Physical illness, the patient and his environment: Psychosocial foundations of medicine, in Arieti S (ed): American Handbook of Psychiatry (ed 2), vol. 4. New York, Basic Books (in press)
29. Livsey CG: Physical illness and family dynamics, in Lipowski, ZJ (ed): Psychosocial Aspects of Physical Illness. Basel, Switz., Karger, 1972, pp 237–251
30. Engel GL: Is psychiatry failing in its responsibility to medicine? Am J Psychiatry 128:1561–1563, 1972
31. Psychiatric News, Nov. 21, 1973, p 13
32. Lipowski ZJ (ed): Current Trends in Psychosomatic Medicine. Int J Psychiatr Med, special issue, parts 1–2, in press.
33. Lipowski ZJ: Psychosomatic medicine in a changing society: Some current trends in theory and research. Compr Psychiatry 14:203–215, 1973
34. Alexander F: Psychosomatic Medicine. New York, Norton, 1950
35. Alexander F: The next ten years in psychiatry. Am J Psychother 12:438–442, 1958

36. West LJ: The future of psychiatric education. Am J Psychiatry 130:521–528, 1973
37. Barton D, Kelso MT: The nurse as a psychiatric consultation team member. Psychiatry Med 2:108–115, 1971
38. Abrahams D, Golden JS: Psychiatric consultations on a medical ward. Arch Intern Med 112:766–774, 1963
39. Baudry F, Wiener A: Initiation of a psychiatric teaching program for surgeons. Am J Psychiatry 125:1192–1197, 1969
40. Rothenberg MB: Child psychiatry-pediatrics liaison. A history and commentary. J Am Acad Child Psychiatry 7:492–509, 1968
41. Lipowski ZJ: Psychiatric liaison with neurology and neurosurgery. Am J Psychiatry 129:136–140, 1972
42. Cassem NH, Hackett TP: Psychiatric consultation in a coronary care unit. Annals Intern Med 75:9–14, 1971
43. Janes RG, Weisz AE: Psychiatric liaison with a cancer research center. Compr Psychiatry 11:336–345, 1970
44. Kaplan-DeNour A: Role and reactions of psychiatrists in chronic hemodialysis programs. Psychiatry Med 4:63–76, 1973
45. Bartolucci G, Drayer CS: An overview of crisis intervention in the emergency rooms of general hospitals. Am J Psychiatry 130:953–960, 1973
46. Lipowski ZJ, Ramsay RA, Villard HP: Psychiatric consultations in medical and surgical outpatient clinics. Can Psychiatr Assoc J 14:239–245, 1969
47. Gunther MS: Psychiatric consultation in a rehabilitation hospital. Compr Psychiatry 12:572–585, 1971
48. Mendelson M, Meyer E: Countertransference problems of the liaison psychiatrist. Psychosom Med 23:115–122, 1961
49. Abram HS: Interpersonal aspects of psychiatric consultations in a general hospital. Psychiatry Med 2:321–326, 1971
50. Hale ML, Abram HS: Patients' attitudes toward psychiatric consultations in the general hospital. Va Med Mon 94:342–347, 1967
51. Goodwin DW: Psychiatry and the mysterious medical complaint. JAMA 209:1884–1888, 1969
52. Peterson HW, Martin MJ: Organic disease presenting as a psychiatric syndrome. Postgrad Med 54:78–83, 1973
53. Goshen CE: Functional versus organic diagnostic problems. NY State J Med 69:2332–2338, 1969
54. Stein EH, Murdaugh J, Macleod JA: Brief psychotherapy of psychiatric reactions to physical illness. Am J Psychiatry 125:1040–1047, 1969
55. Paris J: Psychiatric practice in Canada pre- and post-medicare. Can Med Assoc J 109:469–470, 1973
56. Rahe RH, Tuffli CF, Suchor RJ, et al: Group therapy in the outpatient management of post-myocardial infarction patients. Psychiatry Med 4:77–88, 1973
57. McKegney PF: Consultation-liaison teaching of psychosomatic medicine: Opportunities and obstacles. J Nerv Ment Dis 154:198–205, 1972
58. Engel GL, Greene WA, Reichsman F, et al: A graduate and undergraduate teaching program on the psychological aspects of medicine. J Med Educ 32:859–

870, 1957

59. Small IF, Foster LG, Small JG, et al: Teaching the art and skill of psychiatric consultation. Dis Nerv Syst 29:817–822, 1968

60. Engel GL: Fainting: Physiologic and Psychologic Considerations. Springfield, Ill, Thomas, 1962

61. Engel GL, Ferris EB, Logan M: Hyperventilation: Analysis of clinical symptomatology. Annals Intern Med 27:683–704, 1947

62. Engel GL: "Psychogenic" pain and the pain-prone patient. Amer J Med 26:899–918, 1959

63. Engel GL: Studies of ulcerative colitis. V. Psychological aspects and their implications for treatment. Amer J Digest Dis 3:315–337, 1958

64. Schmale AH, Engel GL: The giving up-given up complex illustrated on film. Arch Gen Psychiat 17:135–145, 1967

65. Hughson B, Lyons R: Patient response to psychiatric consultation in a general hospital. Austr and N Zeal J Psychiat 7:279–282, 1973

66. Moses R, Barzilay S: The influence of psychiatric consultation on the course of illness of the general hospital patient. Compr Psychiatry 8:16–26, 1967

67. Schwab JJ: Evaluating psychiatric consultation work. Psychosomatics 8:309–317, 1967

68. Schwab JJ, Clemmons RS, Valder MJ, Raulerson JD: Medical patients' reactions to referring physicians after psychiatric consultation. JAMA 195:1120–1122, 1966

69. Corney RT: The efficacy of a liaison psychiatric consultation programme. Med Care 4:133–138, 1966

70. Lipowski ZJ, Kiriakos RZ: Borderlands between neurology and psychiatry: Observations in a neurological hospital. Psychiatry Med 3:131–147, 1972

71. Payson HE, Davis JM: The psychosocial adjustment of medical inpatients after discharge: A follow-up study. Amer J Psychiat 123:1220–1225, 1967

72. Whybrow PC, Spencer RF: Changing characteristics of psychiatric consultation in a university hospital. Canad Psychiat Ass J 14:259–266, 1969.

73. Noy P, De Nour AK, Moses R: Discrepancy between expectations and service in psychiatric consultation. Arch Gen Psychiat 14:651–657, 1966

74. Arthur RJ: Social psychiatry: An overview. Am J Psychiatry 130:841–849, 1973

75. Romano J: Psychiatry and medicine, 1973. Ann Intern Med 79:582–588, 1973

PART I

Psychosomatic Medicine and Liaison Psychiatry

Robert O. Pasnau

Introduction

In the preceding chapter Lipowski has clearly described the relationship that exists between liaison psychiatry and psychosomatic medicine. In the following chapters integration of knowledge about psychosomatic medicine in its various aspects is the key theme. Both Engel and Lipowski have called for this integration of knowledge as fundamental to contemporary psychosomatic medicine. Consultation-liaison psychiatry, viewed in this way, can be considered the clinical application of the growing body of psycho-socio-somatic knowledge called "psychosomatic medicine."

In the first chapter Kaplan presents a brief historical review of psychosomatic medicine which, from a psychodynamic viewpoint, is the history of the holistic approach to medicine. He reviews the modern development of psychosomatic medicine arising from the psychological theories based on psychoanalysis and touches upon the roles of some of the psychosomatic pioneers of the past and present. This chapter serves as a useful beginning for the student and practitioner alike and puts the chapters that follow into greater perspective. Kaplan's excellent bibliography can be used as the basis for a reading list of the "classics" in psychosomatic medicine. Psychiatric educators could well use this bibliography in developing a "Psychosomatic Journal Club."

The second chapter, by Rahe, presents with clarity a model for the relationship between life stress and illness of all kinds. Rahe gives the example of the clinical research that has led him and others to draw the conclusions about life changes that can be quantified in certain populations as units of stress. What makes this chapter particularly valuable is the integration of his earlier work in life change with psychodynamic, coping, and genetic factors. The bibliography in this chapter as well provides a rich resource for the student or practitioner who may wish to become more knowledgeable in this area of research.

In his chapter on cognitive aspects of illness, Yager considers the relationship between the cognitive processes by which we perceive, evaluate, and process information and psychological events, the sources of belief about illness, the patient's attitudes and behavior, and the implications for the physician–patient relationship. These long overlooked personal, social, and cultural dimensions of illness are becoming most important basic considerations for the consultation-liaison psychiatrist. Yager refers to the work in coping behavior of Lazarus and Hamburg. Once again this chapter is an example of the integration of work from many disciplines.

A further example of the integration of knowledge in contemporary psychosomatic medicine is found in the next chapter by Rubin. Rubin traces the development of psychosomatic medicine, neurochemistry, and neurophysiology with special emphasis on psychophysiological interactions and biological rhythms. His conclusion that it is necessary to direct mutually supportive treatments to the mind, brain, and body in many illnesses is a restatement of the underlying principle of liaison medicine.

Perhaps no research area in psychosomatic medicine in recent years has provoked more interest and controversy than biofeedback. In his scholarly chapter Shapiro has performed a great service to the field with his clear statements on its history and current research—particularly in the section on clinical aspects. As has been the case in the preceding chapters, the excellent bibliography provides an intriguing opportunity for further study.

Hoppe's wide-ranging and thoughtful chapter on liaison psychiatry and psychoanalysis concludes the section. In my original plan I included this chapter in the section on liaison psychiatry and medical education. While it is true that Hoppe touches on some educational aspects, I believe his chapter belongs in this section for two reasons. First, he presents some interesting current developments in psychoanalytic theory and practice that have direct relevance for liaison psychiatry, including the work of Balint, Kohut, Marty, de M'Uzan, Nemiah, and Sifneos, as well as his own important studies of patients with commissurotomies. Secondly, it seems most appropriate to complete the full cycle of this section by ending with an integration of psychoanalytic and liaison psychiatry. Hoppe's chapter answers his own opening question, ''Why after all, still psychoanalysis?'', most convincingly.

It is an axiom in medicine that the knowledge of medicine is most of value when it is translated into clinical application. It is also known that the consultation-liaison psychiatrist is most successful when he is able to convey useful information to the consultee. It is my belief that the information contained in this section provides a base of knowledge which will help to prepare the consultation-liaison psychiatrist for his difficult task.

Harold I. Kaplan

2

Current Psychodynamic Concepts in Psychosomatic Medicine

In reviewing current theoretical approaches in psychosomatic medicine, one should note that a definite causal relationship between psychological factors and true organic disease is even today merely an assumption. Psychogenesis in physical illness has never been proved. The assumption of a significant psychosomatic relationship rests a great deal on what appears to be solid circumstantial evidence; furthermore, such a relationship is very attractive from a theoretical standpoint. Psychosomatic investigators, therefore, agree in assuming that psychic factors play a significant causal role in many disorders. There is, however, little agreement about the mechanisms by which psychological and physical factors interact to produce disease. There is currently no one theory or construct adequate to explain the observed and assumed relationship between psychological difficulty and physical disease. In fact, even the definition and limitation of what constitutes a psychosomatic disease is controversial. For example, some workers consider every disease psychosomatic in that psychic and somatic phenomena are different aspects of the same process, and since all diseases are multicausal, psychic factors must play some role in every pathological process. Other workers think that the definition should be limited to those disease processes in which psychic factors are assumed to play a major causal role; the latter assumption is the one in this chapter.

DEFINITION

In the second edition of the American Psychiatric Association's *Diagnostic and Statistical Manual of Mental Disorders* (DSM-II) psychosomatic disorders are designated as psychophysiologic disorders (physical disorders of presumably psychogenic origin). DSM-II further states:

> This group of disorders is characterized by physical symptoms that are caused by emotional factors and involve a single organ system, usually under autonomic nervous system innervation. The physiological changes involved are those that normally accompany certain emotional states, but in these disorders the changes are more intense and sustained. The individual may not be consciously aware of his emotional state.

Included in this grouping are such diseases as bronchial asthma, hypertension, peptic ulcer, and ulcerative colitis.

HISTORY OF PSYCHOSOMATIC MEDICINE AND THEORY

"As it is not proper to cure the eyes without the head, nor the head without the body, so neither is it proper to cure the body without the soul." These words of a Greek king, quoted by Socrates, reflect the Greek recognition of a cause-and-effect relationship between the health of mind and the health of body. Before the Greeks a mind–body unity had developed in a context in which illness was thought to be of magical or religious origin. Later, the idea of a religious cause and cure for disease returned, ousting the ideas of a natural origin for disease that the Greeks had adopted.

During the European Renaissance, with its emphasis on examination of the visible and palpable world, the study of human health divided; the investigation of the body's visible structures flourished, and comment on the emotions ceased. As a result of this trend, it eventually became the practice to treat the disease and not the patient. Only since the development of psychiatry during the twentieth century and the increased understanding of psychological determinism as defined by Freud has the patient once again been viewed wholly, with his psychic and somatic symptoms considered as different expressions of the process.

The history of psychosomatic medicine is characterized by shifts back and forth from unity of psyche and soma within a religious framework to unity or duality within a natural system. This history is summarized in Table 2–1.

Early Societies

Among many primitive peoples the frightening spiritual powers controlling a threatening environment were thought to be responsible for the onset of illness. A patient fell ill because of the influences of another human being, who had solicited spiritual powers to bewitch him, or because of a demon, who had gained control of his body and actions. There is evidence that some Neolithic societies, after the introduction of polished stone tools (ca. 10,000 B.C.),

Table 2–1

History of Psychosomatic Medicine

Date	Historical Period	Psychosomatic Orientation
10,000 B.C.	Primitive society	Disease is caused by spiritual powers and must be fought by spiritual means; the evil spirit that enters and affects the total being must be liberated through exorcism, trephination, etc.
2500–500 B.C.	Babylonian-Assyrian civilization	Medicine is dominated by religion, and suggestion is the major tool of treatment. Sigerist: "Mesopotamian medicine was psychosomatic in all its aspects."
400 B.C.	Greek civilization	Socrates: "As it is not proper to cure the eyes without the head, nor the head without the body, so neither is it proper to cure the body without the soul." Hippocrates: "In order to cure human body, it is necessary to have knowledge of the whole of things."
100 B.C. 400 A.D.	Late Greek–early Roman civilization	Galen's humoral theory postulates that disease is caused by disturbance in the fluids of the body. Medicine adopts a holistic approach to disease.
500–1500 A.D.	Middle Ages	Mysticism and religion dominate medicine. Sinning is the cause of mental and somatic illness.
1500–1800 A.D.	Renaissance and Enlightenment	There is renewed interest in the natural sciences and their application to medicine; advances in anatomy (Vesalius), autopsy (Morgagni), microscopy (Leeuwenhoek). Psychic influences on soma are rejected as unscientific; the study of the mind is relegated to religion and philosophy.
1800–1900 A.D.	19th century	Modern laboratory-based medicine of Pasteur and Virchow comes to the fore: "Disease has its origin in disease of the cell." Psychosomatic approach discarded since all disease must be associated with structural cell change. The disease is treated, not the patient.
1900–present	20th century	Freud's early psyhoanalytic formulations emphasize the role of psychic determinism in somatic conversion reactions (Dora case). These early concepts are limited to major hysterical conversions; subsequently, Alexander differentiates conversion reactions from psychosomatic disorders.

Table by Harold I. Kaplan. Adapted with permission from *Comprehensive Textbook of Psychiatry*. 2nd Edition, edited by A.M. Freedman, H.I. Kaplan, B.J. Sadock, Baltimore, Williams & Wilkins, 1975.

practiced trephination. The hole bored in the skull was only the exit for the evil spirit; the effective work came in the rituals of the shaman, who exorcised the spirit from the afflicted body. The shaman by the power of his personality, psychological suggestion, and threat of punishment worked within a modern doctor-patient therapeutic framework to oust the spirit (so-called operant conditioning). If the patient recovered, it was probably because of the strength derived from a beneficent doctor-patient relationship.

Egyptians, Babylonian-Assyrians, and Jews

The Egyptians tried to take some medical cures out of the realm of magic and religion, reserving that older treatment for diseases accepted as incurable. Like other early doctors, the Egyptians considered the heart to be the center of intellectual activity; Ptahhotep (ca. 3200 B.C.) thought the emotions were controlled by the heart, by which he meant the intellectual capacities of a human being.

The doctors of the conglomerate Babylonian-Assyrian civilization (ca. 2500 B.C.) relied on a sophisticated magical and religious therapy, as had their Sumerian predecessors. Sin caused bodily suffering; therefore, a patient was encouraged to search his soul or to mediate on his sins until the incantations and rites of the priests released him from sickness. Such an approach, as Sigerist notes, was "psychosomatic in all its aspects."[20]

The Jews considered sickness to be a punishment for forsaking the law of Jehovah. Demons and spirits were not the effective agents of illness; rather, the patient, by disobedience to the omnipotent deity, brought on himself either mental or physical sickness. A restored relationship with that deity was the path back to health. An understanding of a pervasive interrelationship between psyche and soma occurs in a number of passages in the Book of Proverbs.

Greek Civilization

The Greeks (ca. 400 B.C.) were the first to consider disease to be caused by a disturbance within the natural body itself, specifically by an imbalance among the various humors or fluids circulating in the body. A number of clinicians think that the Hippocratic theory of humors is a simplified statement of what we now know about the endocrine system. According to Hippocrates, the four humors should be properly mixed to maintain a healthy body: too much yellow bile leads to anxiety and irritability, too much black bile to sadness, too much phlegm to apathy, and too much blood to an exaggerated hopefulness. Although the focus was on natural rather than religious causes of illness, the psyche and the soma were regarded as a unity. Hippocrates is said to have cured a king of an intestinal lesion by analyzing a dream. He connected sweating with fear, and he connected palpitations of the heart with shame. He was careful to advise young physicians to look at their patients with sympathetic expressions, never with impatience, in order to encourage the return to health.

Plato noted in the *Timaeus* that a defect in the soul brings trouble to the body and vice versa. Aristotle remarked that the emotions, such as anger, fear, courage, and joy, have an effect on the body. Aretaeus identified disturbances of the emotions as one of the six causes of paralysis, a correlation followed in the standard nomenclature of the 1952 edition of DSM-I under the listing of conversion hysteria.

Later, Greeks and Romans returned to the holistic approach to medicine; however, the incursion of the barbaric tribesmen with their slighter tradition of medical observation brought the return of superstition and fear. Nevertheless, years before the barbarian overthrow the Greek physician Galen (ca. A.D. 130–200) incroporated Hippocrates' humoral theory of disease into a sophisticated system of explaining the workings of the human body, a system that would stand for more than a thousand years as the foundation of standard medicine. Galen considered the brain to be the center of the senses and of emotional disorders. After autopsies on monkeys, he concluded that human nerves are hollow conduits for animal spirits flowing outward from the brain to produce movement and thought. The animal spirits had started out as natural spirits, products of digestive and reproductive functions produced in the liver and picked up there by venous blood. Taken to the heart, they were transformed into vital spirits and flowed through the arteries from there to the brain. Galen prescribed herbals, such as opium-containing theriaca, for both emotional and physical disturbances.

Middle Ages

In the period of the Middle Ages (A.D. 500–1500), the medicine of the Greeks was retained only within the Christian church, but it was drastically altered according to the church's culture. Once again, spiritual powers, demons, and witches were often implicated in the generation of disease, and, once again, healing became, in part, a function of faith. Healing resulted from an exchange of sinfulness on the part of the sick person for physical or mental health on the part of God or a spiritual power. Since this exchange took place with the assistance of a priest rather than within the doctor-patient relationship, the physician's status fell during this period.

Renaissance and Modern Times

After a thousand years of renewed religious dominance within medical theory, attention turned again during the Renaissance (1500–1700) to natural causes and cures of disease. First came a renewed interest in the study of mathematics, chemistry, and physics; then the information gained in those areas was applied to medicine in biochemistry, bacteriology, and pathology. Leeuwenhoek's work with the microscope invented by Janssen provided a spectacularly accurate tool for collecting new kinds of information. Morgagni in the eighteenth century showed by autopsy that a disturbance within an organ, rather than simply in the balance of the humors, could cause disease. His published findings correlated certain symptoms with the diseases of certain organs and proved that the circulating fluids could not be the only cause of illness. As new knowledge regarding the soma increased, the psyche was gradually relegated to a separate province of study; the mind was discussed only by philosophers and the soul only by theologians. In this atmosphere the idea of psychic influences on the soma was rejected as unscientific, and psychosomatic theory regressed.

During the nineteenth century Virchow, the father of pathology, demonstrated that every disease is originally a disease of the cells. First, he said, comes a change toward pathology within the individual cells; this change is followed by a change in the structure of the cell; ultimately, physiological disorder appears in the cells that make up the tissue of an organ. At last, the humoral theory of Hippocrates and Galen was undone, after having been challenged but not dethroned by Morgagni's work. The new approach was immensely profitable in the information relevant to cell pathology procured within its framework. It was not, however, holistic; no longer was the patient treated—the disease was treated.

"Disease has its origin in disease of the cell," Virchow concluded, and in the same century Pasteur, the father of bacteriology, studied the single-cell bacteria isolated in his laboratory. The laboratory, Pasteur stated, was to be the "temple of the future." Other investigators, such as Heinroth, Jacobi, Feuchtensleben, and Beaumont working within a holistic tradition virtually abandoned by others, contributed to a quietly, surviving set of observations on the relationship between psyche and soma. But these observations produced no adequate generalizations in the context of laboratory-based medicine.

It was Sigmund Freud in the early 1900s who repaired the schism between mind and body in the study of disease. His discoveries of how important the emotions are in producing mental disorders and bodily disturbances reunited psyche and soma. Freud also reestablished the lost therapeutic tool of the doctor-patient relationship and gave it a quality different from that of religious faith. By his concepts of transference and countertransference he showed the dynamic value of a patient's understanding his feelings toward his doctor and a doctor's understanding of his feelings for a patient. Freud's early psychoanalytic formulations emphasized the role of psychic determinism in somatic conversion reactions—as in the Dora case and in his first book, *Studies on Hysteria*—but his initial studies were basically limited to hysterical reactions.

This theory was criticized because it was believed that specific conscious personality patterns may be a cover up for any type of unconscious conflict.

Expanding on Freud's work, Franz Alexander in the 1930s advanced the idea that conversion reactions are produced by the voluntary nervous system and are symbolic displays of repressed emotions, whereas psychosomatic symptoms develop through the autonomic nervous system. He applied Cannon's newly studied fight-flight reaction to psychosomatic disease. The stress of conflict activates the autonomic nervous system; if outer-directed action is curtailed, the inner organism remains alerted and tense in accord with either the aggressive and hostile responses of the sympathetic system or the vegetative responses of the parasympathetic system. Prolonged tension leads to physiologic disorder.

Twentieth-century endocrine studies demonstrated the action of the hormones in binding psyche to soma. Shell-shock cases during World War I aroused interest in the psychogenic causes of physical illness. The reunification of psyche and soma continues now within the naturalistic framework retained from the Renaissance and from the laboratory scientists who followed.

MAJOR PSYCHODYNAMIC THEORETICAL APPROACHES

Psychodynamic theories may be divided into three groups—the specificity theories, the nonspecific theories, and the multidisciplinary theories. The multidisciplinary theories emphasize a total psychosocial approach to the problem.

Specificity Theories

The theories of specificity suggest that specific psychological events cause specific psychosomatic diseases. These theories vary in their explanation of the mechanisms by which psychosomatic diseases are produced. Included in this group of theories are the historically important personality profiles of Flanders Dunbar,[4] first expounded in the 1930s, in which she suggested that various personality constellations are etiologically associated with specific diseases; for example, coronary occlusion is associated with the driving, ambitious man. This theory was criticized because it was believed that specific conscious personality patterns may be a cover up for any type of unconscious conflict.

Another specific approach derives from Freud's libido theory as applied to the cause of conversion hysteria. Freud suggested that various hysterical somatic afflictions, such as paralysis, may be caused by specific unconscious psychological conflicts that were defensively transformed into symbolically significant functional somatic symptoms involving organs innervated by the voluntary nervous system. Freud, incidentally, never applied his hysteria formulation clearly to visceral diseases, although other workers have. For example, Garma has suggested a libido theory formulation with some Kleinian overtones in his hypothesis about the causation of peptic ulcer, in which the ulcer is explained as the result of the symbolic bite of the patient's gastric mucosa by his introjected hostile mother.

Most of these specific approaches, which suffer from the uncritical application of inappropriate psychological concepts, have been displaced in acceptance and popularity by Alexander's much more sophisticated but still controversial specificity theory, which has its conceptual roots in the amalgamation of Freud's, Cushing's, and Cannon's work. Alexander suggests that specific typical unconscious conflict situations result in specific diseases by virtue of a mechanism.[1] His theory in a very simplified form follows:

A specific typical conflict situation arouses anxiety in a particular patient. The anxiety, which in psychoanalytic theory is regarded as a signal of danger to the patient's ego, then sets in motion a series of specific unconscious psychological reactions that involve characteristic psychological defenses (repression) and regressive phenomena. These specific emotional reactions have specific parasympathetic or sympathetic concomitants, which affect specific visceral organs. The excessive autonomic organ innervation caused by the chronic tension of repressed conflicts leads to a disturbance in physiologic function, which may eventually lead to organic pathological changes in genetically predisposed persons.

Thus, the blocking of dependency needs in adult life in a patient with a passive-dependent character structure causes anxiety, with a resultant specific defensive regression to an infantile oral state. The discharge of psychic energy through the parasympathetic nervous system is associated with increased gastric acid secretion. If chronically aroused, this concomitant vegetative dysfunction may lead to peptic ulcer if the patient is susceptible.

Alexander's studies have been criticized on theoretical and experimental grounds. Theoretically, Alexander discounts the role of the voluntary nervous system in the genesis of psychosomatic disease. He has assumed as fact certain hypothetical and questionable psychoanalytic concepts and has proposed a series of fixed unconscious conflictual constellations as causative factors in various diseases. He assumes that certain psychological conflicts or stresses have specific physiologic concomitants. This last point has been experimentally challenged and represents an example of the conceptual confusion that results from mixing concepts from two levels of description.

Although there is some validation of Alexander's studies, there has been considerable disagreement on whether it is possible to demonstrate the same specific conflicts in all cases of the same disease. It is also questionable whether the conflicts postulated for one disease differ from those associated with other diseases. In other words, it has not been possible thus far to predict disease from conflict or vice versa. In addition, it is highly doubtful whether specific psychological conflicts can be correlated clinically or experimentally with specific physiologic vegetative changes.

Alexander's views have received significant support from several hundred case histories reported in the literature and from Mirsky's studies. Mirsky demonstrated that gastric secretory activity is paralleled by the excretion of uropepsin in the urine; he has, therefore, been able to correlate stomach activity with a variety of psychological stimuli that have been interpreted psychoanalytically. He concluded from his studies that there was a positive relationship between augmentation of uropepsin excretion, and hence gastric activity, and the mobilization of oral dependency wishes in various persons.[20] If true, this conclusion supports Alexander's theoretical views, particularly in reference to peptic ulcer pathogenesis. However, there are many dissenting opinions about the interpretation of the psychological data presented by many supporting investigators.

Thus, even though Alexander's theory of the typical unconscious conflict is a major theoretical force in the psychosomatic field, it remains at this time a basically unvalidated hypothesis, resting on questionable underlying assumption.

During the past few years, new specificity theories resembling Dunbar's early concepts have come to the fore. Friedman and Rosenman have indentified as coronary-prone a type-A personality characterized by restlessness, aggression, competitiveness, and a strong sense of urgency about getting things done before time runs out.[5] Friedman and others later reported that type-A persons possess high plasma triglyceride and high cholesterol levels, present hyperinsulinemic response to glucose challenge, and have high levels of noradrenalin in their urine.[6] Persons with such physiologic characteristics can certainly be called coronary-prone, and the findings provide a laboratory support for the psychological hypothesis. The fact remains, however, that this theory is fundamentally a return to Dunbar's personality profiles of the 1930s.

Similarly, Bahnson and Bahnson have identified a specific personality type that is prone to cancer.[2] They described cancer patients as using projection for defense less frequently than other people do; instead, the cancer-prone person tends to repress and deny emotional stress. Booth found cancer patients to be people who have great trouble recovering from depression after personal loss and suggested that the depression may be somatized as a neoplasm.

Nonspecific Theories

The second genre of theorizing does not try to link personality types or specific emotional stimuli with specific pathology but focuses on the effects of heightened anxiety within the human system and the tendency for stress to be translated into somatic dysfunction. When presented with an anxiety-provoking situation, the person responds, in part, by alerting the sympathetic nervous system; at the same time parallel adjustments in the parasympathetic system occur.

The nonspecific theoretical approaches to psychosomatic medicine include the theories of Wolff and Wolf, Mahl, Selye, and various animal experimenters, such as Liddell and Gantt. In general, the work of this group is not rooted in psychoanalytic theory. Therefore, although the resultant formulations may suffer from a limited insight into some psychological complexities, they gain the advantage of being unhampered by unvalidated and often misleading psychological assumptions.

Among the outstanding experimenters in the nonspecific group were the late Harold Wolff and Stewart Wolf and their associates at the Cornell Medical College. Wolff's main contribution to the field of psychosomatic medicine is the application of the experimental method to the study of the physiological and pathological functioning of various bodily organs and the correlation of these functions with various types of psychological stimuli. Using laboratory and clinical experimental techniques, Wolff in conjunction with Wolf demonstrated physiological and pathological changes in various organs and systems, notably the stomach, the colon, and the nasal mucosa under emotional stress during ordinary life situations.[22] The changes that they described generally involve variations in the swelling, vascularity, and motility of various viscera, and it is assumed that these changes are the logical precursors of potentially permanent pathological changes that constitute psychosomatic disease. They described, for example, two variations of physiologic change in the gastrointestinal and respiratory mucosa—hyperfunction and hypofunction in the vascular and secretory activities. In general, emotions such as hostility are associated with physiologic overactivity; fear and sadness involving a feeling of withdrawal are accompanied by diminished physiologic function. The character of the conflict evoking these emotions, although not specific for any particular illness, is specific for the individual patient and has its roots in the events of his socio-psychological development.

Wolff and Wolf and associates concluded that psychosomatic disease is a result of attempts of the total organism to protect itself against psychogenic stress in the form of threatening symbols or situations. In interpreting their data, they suggested that many of the physiologic changes described, although originally unconditioned protective reaction patterns and responses to noxious physical stimuli, later become conditioned to noxious psychological stimuli. They further suggested that the resultant physiologic reactions ultimately acquired symbolic psychological meanings—for example, nasal hyperemia associated with nasal obstruction represents a shutting-out–shutting-in pattern of nonparticipation in stressful life situations.

Wolff and his collegues have been criticized as naive in their selection and interpretation of psychological data. Margolin, representing the psychoanalytic approach, thinks that Wolff has failed to take account of important unconscious psychological data and has dealt with the behavioral aspect of his correlations on too superficial a level.

Other workers in the nonspecific group have demonstrated various possible mechanisms by which psychologically induced stress may cause organic disease in humans and animals. Selye feels that the hypophyseal-adrenocortical axis responds to various types of physical and psychic stress with hormonal changes that can ultimately cause a variety of organic diseases, such as rheumatoid arthritis and peptic ulcer. Selye views such diseases as a by-product of the body's attempt to adapt to stress from any source. [19]

Mahl, an experimental psychologist with a learning theory conception of behavior, has studied the effects of chronic unrelieved anxiety in humans and animals and has found that gastric hydrochloric acid production increases under such circumstances. [15] Since such acidity is a precursor of peptic ulcer, he has concluded that chronic anxiety, derived from any source whatsoever, is the variable intervening between the behavioral and the physical events involved in psychosomatic illness.

Other animal experimenters, such as Gantt and Liddell, have successfully produced a variety of psychosomatic symptoms, such as certain respiratory conditions in animals, by experimentally creating stressful situations and inducing conflicts. [8, 13] Since it can be assumed that animals do not have a human being's capacity for symbolic thought but since they do demonstrate psychosomatic phenomena in response to psychogenic stress, one wonders whether it is necessary or practical to postulate the operation of specific psychological conflicts, which can hardly be meaningful to an animal, in the etiology of such disease.

Multidisciplinary Theories

If symbolization is not involved, why does one person become psychophysiologically ill within the respiratory system and another with the gastrointestinal system? Malmo has suggested that organ selection depends on *genetic* and constitutional factors.

To help answer some of the open questions in the area of psychophysiologic illness, Grinker proposed that a barrage of investigators from different disciplines focus on one psychosomatic disease. [9] Sociologists, physiologists, psychologists, and others would all bring their particular methodologies and data to bear on one specific psychophysiologic symptom. This large-scale *field approach* investigation offers an interesting new focus for investigation.

CORRELATING PHYSIOLOGIC AND SOCIAL CONCEPTS

New physiologic findings have yet to be traced through all of their medical and psychological ramifications. It has been found, for instance, that a person can consciously control what was once termed the involuntary nervous system. The autonomic nervous system responds to reward and punishment; patients can control alpha rhythm frequency. This effect is known as biofeedback. Verbal stimuli have produced changes in electroencephalographic patterns. A difference in the skin potential level of people who tend to conform to social pressure and those who do not has been reported, with the conformers displaying a lower level.

Laboratory conditions of crowding have produced increased blood pressure in mice. Mice receiving psychosocial stimulation show increased catecholamine-forming enzymes, adrenalin, and noradrenalin in their urine.

Social factors are assuming a new importance in research. Rahe and Holmes and their colleagues attempted to rank life crises in the order of their average subjective rating by various groups.[18] The death of a spouse emerged as the prime crisis in terms of emotional output and time needed to adjust. Studies have shown that life crises often precede illnesses, and Rahe and Holmes found some correlation between the intensity—that is, the high ranking—of the crisis and the duration and intensity of subsequent illness.

A University of Rochester study described a complex of giving up–given up. The person experiencing this set of feelings finds himself in an environment that is not encouraging, and he is helpless to change it; or he feels flaws within himself and is hopeless about changing them. Things are worse than ever expected, and the continuity between past and future is broken; without a sense of continuity there is little hope or confidence. The individual feels that there is no use trying; he cannot cope, cannot take it any more. A person caught in this complex either becomes mentally or physically ill, perhaps due to a physiologic process involving the immunological and neuroendocrine systems, or becomes socially deviant. He may recover after an improvement in his life situation lifts him out of the complex.

Other studies have given more social complexity to such specific theories as those linking personality types and certain diseases. The sociological shadow of the ambitious, hard-driving, coronary-prone man described by Dunbar and by Friedman and Rosenman is seen in a study of telephone employees by Hinkle; the workers who developed heart disease were more apt to be those with only a high school education.[10] In Caffrey's study of myocardial infarction among monks a higher incidence was reported for those men rising from a low socioeconomic status.[3]

Attention is now turning to the patient's attitude toward the very idea of sickness. Although it has been apparent to many laymen that one's attitude toward being sick affects the duration of the episode, scientific investigations of this phenomenon are only now being attempted. With new information being presented from many different directions, it may not be long before a unified theory of the nature and operation of psychophysiological illnesses is evolved.

REFERENCES

1. Alexander F: Psychosomatic Medicine. New York, Norton, 1950
2. Bahnson MB, Bahnson CB: Ego defenses in cancer patients. Ann N Y Acad Sci 164:546, 1969
3. Caffrey BA: Multivariate analysis of sociopsychological factors in monks with myocardial infarctions. J Public Health 60:452, 1970
4. Dunbar F: Emotions and Bodily Changes. New York, Columbia University Press, 1954
5. Friedman M, Rosenman RH: Association of specific overt behavior pattern with blood and cardiovascular findings: Blood cholesterol level, blood clotting time, incidence of arcus senilis, and clinical coronary artery disease. JAMA 169:1286, 1959
6. Friedman M, Byers S, Roseman RH, et al: Coronary-prone individuals (type A behavior pattern): Some biochemical characteristics. JAMA 212:1030, 1970
7. Freud S: Fragment of an analysis of a case of hysteria, in The Standard Edition of the Complete Psychological Works of Sigmund Freud, vol. 7. London, Hogarth, 1953 p 7
8. Gantt WH: Experimental Basis for Neurotic Behavior: Origin and Development of Artificially Produced Disturbances of Behavior in Dogs. New York, Hoeber, 1944
9. Grinker R: Psychosomatic Research. New York, Norton, 1953
10. Hinkle LE, Jr, Whitney, LH, Lehman EW, et al: Occupation, education and coronary heart disease. Science 161:238, 1968
11. Holmes TH: The Nose: An Experience. Springfield, Ill., Thomas, 1950
12. Kaplan HI, Kaplan HS: An historical survey of psychosomatic medicine. J Ner Ment Dis 124:546, 1956

13. Liddell H: The role of vigilance in the development of animal neuroses, in Hoch P, Zubin J (eds): Anxiety. New York, Grune & Stratton, 1950

14. Lipowski ZJ: New perspectives in psychosomatic medicine. Can Psychiatr Assoc J 15:515–525, 1970

15. Mahl GFA: Anxiety, HCL secretion, and peptic ulcer etiology. Psychosom Med 12:158, 1950

16. Mirsky IA: Psychoanalysis and the biological sciences, in Alexander F, Ross H (eds): Twenty Years of Psychoanalysis. New York, Norton, 1932

17. Rahe RH: Life crisis and health change, in May PR, Wittenborn JR (eds): Psychotropic Drug Response: Advances in Prediction. Springfield, Ill., Thomas, 1969

18. Rahe RH, Meyer M, Smith M: Social stress and illness onset. J Psychosom Res 8:35, 1964

19. Selye H: The Physiology and Pathology of Exposure to Stress. Montreal, Acta, 1950

20. Sigerist HE: A History of Medicine, vol 1. New York, Oxford, 1951

21. Stainbrook E: Psychosomatic medicine in the nineteenth century. Psychosom Med 14:211, 1952

22. Wolf S, Wolff HG: Human Gastric Function. New York, Oxford, 1943

Richard H. Rahe

3
Life Stress and Illness

Since the mid sixties our research laboratory at the Naval Health Research Center in San Diego has conducted numerous studies of subjects' recent life changes and their retrospective and prospective illness reports.[1-24] These studies have included such diverse populations as U.S. Navy men aboard ships at sea, U.S. Navy Underwater Demolition Team (UDT) trainees, U.S. Navy aviators, American and Scandinavian males encountering acute episodes of coronary heart disease, and enlisted men in the Norwegian Navy. Results from these several studies allow for the formulation of a life stress and illness model.

In Figure 3-1 a series of lenses and filters are employed to indicate the various steps along the pathway between a subject's exposure to recent life stress and his subsequent illness symptomatology and illness reports. When one goes from left to right in the figure, a subject's recent life stress exposure is indicated by "light rays" of various intensities. Dark solid lines represent highly significant events; thinner lines represent less significant events. In our system of stress measurement these light rays represent various intensities of recent life changes expressed in life change units or LCU.[1-10] A subject's past experience may alter certain of his perceptions of the various significances of his recent life changes, and this possibility is shown by the "polarizing filter" in step 1. Next, a subject may employ certain ego defense mechanisms, such as

Report No. 74-1, supported by the Bureau of Medicine and Surgery, Department of the Navy, under Research Work Unit MF51.524.002-5011DD5G. Opinions expressed are those of the author and are not to be construed as necessarily reflecting the official view or endorsement of the Department of the Navy.

Expanded version of the article "A Model for Life Changes and Illness Research" published in the *Archives of General Psychiatry*, 31: 172–177, 1974, and copyrighted by the American Medical Association 1974. Used with permission.

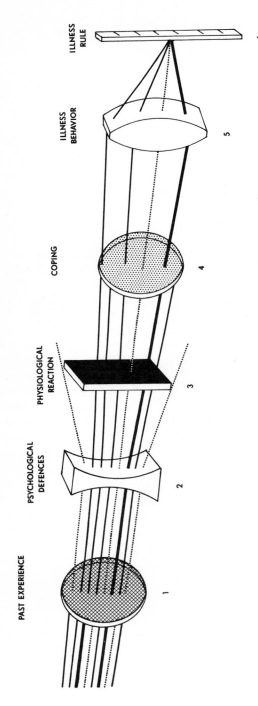

Fig. 3–1. A life stress and illness model. This model was drawn from current as well as previous studies of subjects' life changes data and their near-future illness studies of United States and Norwegian Navy men. These data indicate that the fewer the intervening variables and the less the time interval between the subjects' recent life changes and their near-future illness symptomatology, the higher is the correlation between these two parameters.

denial, that "diffract away" the impact of certain life change events. This possibility is shown in step 2 by the use of a negative lens. Life change events not diffracted away may be assumed to stimulate a multitude of physiological processes—as supported by the entire literature on psychophysiology. This assumption is symbolized in the figure by a physiological "black box" in step 3. Lines emerging from the black box now cease to represent recent life events and begin to represent various psychophysiological reactions, such as elevated blood pressure.

Once a subject's physiology is activated secondary to his perception of recent life events, the "color filter" shown in step 4 represents how the subject may or may not cope with and possibly "absorb" certain of his psychophysiological reactions. For example, by consciously relaxing large muscle groups he may achieve a lowering of an elevated blood pressure. The model goes on to assume that prolonged ("unabsorbed") psychophysiological activations will eventually lead to organ system dysfunction and bodily disease. Such psychophysiologic activations are frequently perceived by subjects as body symptoms, and once the subject has decided that they are significant, he may or may not report these symptoms to medical personnel. His tendency to report symptoms to medical personnel is indicated in the model by an "illness behavior" positive lens shown in step 5. This lens symbolizes a subject "focusing" his attention on his body symptoms in the presence of medical personnel and very likely receiving a diagnosis. Medical diagnoses are frequently recorded in health records, and such records are often used in research as a "measure" of illness—step 6.

Data presented in this chapter will be fit, where possible, to the model in Figure 3–1. These data suggest that the greater the number of intervening variables and/or the longer the time interval between any two steps in the model, the lower the correlation between these two steps.

SUBJECTS AND METHODS

Subjects

U.S. Navy subjects' recent life changes and near-future illness data were gathered on 2,485 enlisted men from the ship's companies of three U.S. Navy heavy cruisers. Demographic characteristics of the men, along with complete accounts of the ships' schedules of activities, have been previously reported.[6, 7, 8, 9] In brief, these men had a mean age of slightly over 22 years, over 90 percent were Caucasian, over 70 percent were married, and over 70 percent were Protestant. Their average educational level was between 11 and 12 years of school.

Norwegian Navy subjects were gathered in the following manner. In Norway, men reaching 19 years of age, approximately 30,000 per year, are called for screening examinations for military service. About 8.5 percent of this number are found to be unfit for service; the remainder are conscripted to serve 15 months' duty, starting at a time of their choosing over the next five years. Thus, the yearly input into Norway's military forces is about 27,450 men per year. The Norwegian Navy receives approximately 6000 of these men; 2000 enter the Coast Artillery and 4000 the general naval service. Approximately 2700, or 70 percent, of those entering the general naval service eventually qualify for sea duty. Of the men who qualify for sea duty, only the upper third of the group, following their recruit training, are sent to a specialty school in navigation, electronics, or communications. The sample of subjects utilized in this report was comprised of one year's input into these three specialty schools—1,058 men.

The Norwegian Navy subjects proved to be extremely homogeneous. Virtually all were Caucasian and Protestant. They ranged in age from 17 to 27, year, with a mean of 21 years. Nine out of 10 subjects were single. The modal subject had attained the equivalent of a high school education, although the educational system in Norway is not strictly comparable to that of the United States. When grouped according to their father's occupation, as an index of socioeconomic class, 20 percent reported their fathers to be either high-level managers or professional workers, 50 percent reported their fathers as skilled workers, and the remaining 30 percent reported their fathers as unskilled workmen (generally farmers).

Questionnaires—SRE and HOS

SRE

Both the U.S. and Norwegian Navy subjects' recent life changes were estimated by use of the Schedule of Recent Experience (SRE) questionnaire. This instrument, which has been described in previous reports, lists 42 life change events, and subjects may indicate which of these events they have experienced over the past two years.[1, 3, 4, 5] Subjects, in fact, mark their recent life change experience over each of the four six-month intervals comprising the recent two years. In an attempt to estimate the various significances of recent life events for the average subject, we used the life change unit (LCU) weighting system.[1-10] Each subject was thereby given four LCU total scores; one LCU total score for each of the four six-month intervals over the two years prior to the study.

HOS

A second questionnaire administered to both American and Norwegian Navy subjects was the Health Opinion Survey (HOS) originally devised by MacMillan.[25] This instrument contains 20 brief questions that primarily query a subject regarding his perception of body symptoms. For example, ''Are you ever bothered by your heart beating hard?'' ''Do you ever feel bothered by all sorts of pains or ailments in different parts of your body?'' Each HOS question was scored on a three-point continuum, except one dichotomously scored question. By this scoring system the higher a subject's total score, the greater was his adjudged body symptoms.

Illness Criterion Data

Health records were maintained on all U.S. Navy subjects during their six to eight months at sea.[6, 7, 8, 9] The collection of illness criterion data for Norwegian Navy subjects closely approximated that for the American subjects, except that the Norwegian subjects spent approximately 12 months cruising the coastline of Norway, and when they encountered an illness, they were referred to the closest civilian medical facility. Copies of Norwegian physicians' records for these men were subsequently sent to the Navy's central records department in Oslo. There the men's health records were reviewed by one of two Norwegian Navy physicians. As done in previous U.S. Navy studies, only illness reports where convincing symptomatology and generally objectifiable signs of tissue pathology were present were counted as a case. Only new illness reports were included; follow-up visits for the same complaint were counted as a single illness episode. (As more than 100 Norwegian subjects elected to remain on active duty past their obligatory 15 months' service, their health records were not available in Oslo at the time of review. Therefore, these men could not be included in the present study.)

RESULTS

Retrospective Analysis of Subjects' LCU and HOS Scores—Step 1–Step 3

Subjects' body symptoms perceived at the time of the study, measured by their HOS scores, were distributed as follows: approximately one-third of the subjects claimed minimal symptoms (HOS scores 20–27); one-third reported mild symptomatology (HOS scores 28–32); and one-third reported moderate to high symptomatology (HOS scores 33–59).

Correlations between the men's HOS scores and their four six-month LCU

Table 3–1

Correlations between Norwegian and U.S. Navy Subjects'
Recent Life Changes Unit (LCU) Scores over 2 years Prior to
Study and Their Body Symptoms (HOS) Scores Registered at
the Time of the Study

LCU time intervals prior to study (mo)	Norwegian Navy (n=821)	U.S. Navy		
		U.S.S. St. Paul (n=785)	U.S.S. Canberra (n=893)	U.S.S. Galveston (n=746)
0–6	0.22**	0.35**	0.22**	0.36**
7–12	0.23**	0.25**	0.16**	0.28**
13–18	0.16**	0.21**	0.19**	0.20**
19–24	0.11**	0.18**	0.15**	0.24**

*p<0.01
**p<0.001

totals over the two years prior to study are presented in Table 3–1. Highest
correlations, 0.22 and 0.23 (p<0.001), were seen for the two six-month
intervals immediately prior to sudy for the Norwegian subjects. For the U.S.
Navy subjects aboard the three cruisers (U.S.S. *St. Paul,* U.S.S. *Canberra,*
and the U.S.S. *Galveston)* their LCU totals for the six-month period immediately prior to study consistently showed highest correlations 0.22 to 0.36
(p<0.001), with their HOS scores. Although statistically significant correlations were seen for both Norwegian and U.S. Navy subjects' more chronologi-
cally distant six-month LCU totals with their HOS scores, these correlations
steadily decreased the further back in time that the LCU data was reported to
have occurred.

Prospective Analysis of Subjects' LCU Scores with Their Near-Future Illness Reports—Step 1–Step 6

The distribution of the Norwegian subjects' illness reports over the
13-month follow-up period showed that 12 percent of the subjects reported no
illnesses over the follow-up interval; 36 percent reported 1 to 2 illnesses; 28
percent reported 3 to 4 illnesses; and 24 percent reported 5 to 14 illnesses. All
illness reports were categorized into the organ system classifications proposed
by Hinkle and his associates.[26] By and large, the Norwegian Navy subjects
showed similar organ system distribution of their illness reports as did the U.S.
Navy subjects.[7, 8] Notable exceptions were that the Norwegians had decidedly
more muscular illnesses, 14.4 percent of all illness reports, and appreciably less
genitourinary illnesses, 4.4 percent of all reports, and dermatologic disorders,
15.8 percent of all reports, than did the U.S. Navy men. The American subjects

Table 3–2

Diagnostic Categories and Numbers of Illness Reports within
Two Organ System Classifications of the Norwegian Navy
Illness Criterion Data

Respiratory	n*	Gastrointestinal	n
Rhinitis	164	Upset stomach	83
Pharyngitis	107	Gastroenteritis	26
Tonsilitis	106	Gastritis	18
Upper respiratory infection	106	Diarrhea	14
Sinusitis	59	Hemorrhoids	12
Bronchitis	44	Ulcer	10
Pneumonia	13	Constipation	5
Cough	6	Cramps	4
Laryngitis	4	Anal fistula	2
Chest pain	3	Appendicitis	2
Asthma	1	Spastic colon	1
Adenoiditis	1	Umbilical hernia	1
Asphyxia	1	Colitis	2
Hemoptysis	1	Surgery (hemmorhage)	1
		Peritonitis	1
TOTAL	616	TOTAL	182

*n = number of illness reports within the diagnostic category.

reported only 6.1 percent of their total number of illnesses to be of muscular origin, 14.1 percent genitourinary origin, and 24.5 percent of dermal origin.

Previous reports concerning the nature of the illnesses of U.S. Navy subjects have not emphasized the extensive variety of illnesses seen within each organ system classification. The Norwegian reports, however, do point up the variety; the 2430 separate illness reports of the Norwegian subjects fell into 152 specific diagnostic categories—all of which were subsumed under 15 different organ system classifications. Two common organ system classifications—respiratory and gastrointestinal—are presented in Table 3–2 along with the various diagnostic categories included in each classification.

Correlations between Norwegian Navy and U.S. Navy subjects' recent LCU data and their illness reports over the follow-up periods are summarized in Table 3–3. For both groups of subjects the men's recent life changes scores for the six months immediately prior to study showed highest correlations with their number of illness reports, per 1000 men, per day, over the follow-up intervals. Once again, correlations seen for both samples of subjects between their recent LCU scores and their near-future illness reports progressively diminished the further back in time the LCU data were reported to have occurred.

Norwegian and U.S. Navy subjects' ranges of LCU reporting and their near-future illness rates were examined for linearity by dividing subjects into

Table 3–3

Correlations between Norwegian and U.S. Navy Subjects'
Recent Life Changes Unit (LCU) Scores over 2 Years Prior to
Study and Their Number of Reported Illnesses over Prospective
Follow-up

LCU time intervals prior to study (mo)	Norwegian Navy (n=821)	U.S. Navy		
		U.S.S. *St. Paul* (n=802)	U.S.S. *Canberra* (n=892)	U.S.S. *Galveston* (n=747)
0–6	0.12**	0.10*	0.12**	0.16**
7–12	0.09*	0.08*	0.03	0.16**
13–18	0.08*	0.06	0.08*	0.13**
19–24	0.05	0.05	0.07	0.14**

*$p \leqslant 0.01$
**$p \leqslant 0.001$

deciles of men on the basis of their LCU data for the six months immediately prior to study. As seen in Table 3–4, deciles of men with the low ranges of LCU scores over the six-month period immediately prior to study reported low mean illness rates, while deciles of men with the high ranges of LCU scores reported high mean illness rates. The progression of illness rates from deciles 1 to 10 was roughly linear, especially for the larger U.S. Navy sample.

U.S. Navy subjects, compared by deciles to Norwegian Navy men, reported higher ranges of LCU scores and higher mean illness rates. However, when the men in both samples were grouped according to similar ranges of LCU totals (0–75, 76–150, and 151–300), men with comparable LCU ranges reported similar mean illness rates. (See Table 3–4.)

Subjects' HOS Scores and Their Follow-up Period Illness Rates, Step 3–Step 6

The correlation between Norwegian Navy subjects' HOS scores and their follow-up period illness rates was 0.25 (p<0.001). The correlation seen between U.S. Navy subjects' HOS scores and their follow-up period illness rates was 0.17 (p<0.001).

Subjects' Illness Behavior Characteristics and Their Near-Future Illness Reporting, Step 5–Step 6

Demographic and job characteristics of subjects tended to identify men likely to report illnesses during the follow-up intervals. Subjects more likely to

Table 3–4

Comparison of Mean Illnesses Rates for Norwegian and U.S.
Subjects by LCU Deciles and by Approximately Equal Ranges
of LCU Scores

	Norwegian Sample		
LCU Decile	No. of Men	LCU Range (6 mo)	Mean Illnesses/ 1000 men/day
1	88	0	6.4
2	92	1–20	7.1
3	79	21–39 (0–75)*	7.2 (7.1)*
4	91	40–57	7.8
5	91	58–76	6.8
6	79	77–98	7.8
7	79	99–128 (76–150)	9.7 (8.2)
8	76	129–156	7.1
9	76	157–217	7.8
10	70	218+ (151–300)	9.3 (8.5)

	U.S. Navy Samples		
LCU Decile	No. of Men	LCU Range (6 mo)	Mean Illnesses/ 1000 men/day
1	276	0–28	8.1
2	242	29–57 (0–75)*	7.7 (7.7)*
3	244	58–88	7.5
4	241	89–119	8.8 (8.5)
5	247	120–151 (76–150)	8.2
6	246	152–189	8.9
7	247	190–239 (151-300)	9.2 (9.2)
8	246	240–299	9.6
9	246	300–383	9.5
10	250	384+ (300+)	10.3

* Approximate LCU ranges and average illness rates are given in parentheses.

report illnesses proved to be young, unmarried, lacking completion of a high
school education, and relatively unsatisfied with their work. Also, these men
tended to work in the more hazardous areas of the ship.[7, 10, 11]

DISCUSSION

The data presented in this chapter helped formulate the model presented in Figure 3–1. It was a consistent finding in our American and Norwegian samples that the more proximal were two steps in the figure, the higher was the correlation between these two steps. Namely, correlations between step 1 and step 3 were consistently around 0.30; correlations between step 1 and step 6 were consistently around 0.12; correlations between step 3 and step 6 were generally around 0.20. Similar correlations between the subjects' LCU scores over six months prior to the study and body symptoms at the time of the study have been obtained by other investigators.[27, 28]

Not shown in Figure 3–1 is another important variable—time. It was consistently seen, for both samples of men, that the further back in time their life changes occurred, the less effect these life changes seemed to have on either their body symptoms at the time of study or on their near-future illness reports. Also, since the time interval between step 1 and step 6 in our model was as long as a year and a half in the case of the Norwegians, the relatively low correlations seen between these two steps seemed, in part, a result of the lengthy time interval required for such prospective investigations.

In our prospective investigations subjects had to seek medical care in order for investigators to learn of their illnesses. Thus, we lost illness criterion data from those men who became ill but failed to report it. In a prospective study of subjects' LCU and near-future illness, Cline and Chosey were able to make all subjects report periodically, over the follow-up year, for medical histories and physical examinations.[27] In so doing these researchers gathered follow-up illness criterion data for all of their subjects. They found a relatively high correlation of 0.37 between their subjects' LCU total for the six months immediately prior to study and the number of illnesses experienced over the follow-up year. This important methodologic procedure of being able to collect illness criterion data on all subjects might partially explain why our correlations were relatively low (0.10 to 0.16) between subjects' most recent six-month LCU totals and their number of follow-up period illness reports.

Illnesses developed by Norwegian sailors proved to be extremely similar in organ system distribution to those previously reported for American sailors. The exceptions to this finding may be explained in large measure by the substantial difference in ambient temperatures between the coastline of Norway and the Pacific and Mediterranean environments of the American ships. Warm temperatures brought about skin rashes, sunburns, and the like for United States ship crew members while the freezing temperature of the north facilitated muscle sprains and strains for the Norwegians as they slipped on icy decks and so forth. The higher incidence of genitourinary illnesses for American sailors was most likely accounted for by the higher exposure of these men to venereal disease in their ports of call than was the case for sailors in port in Norway. The average Norwegian sailor had fewer recent life changes and a lower follow-up period illness rate than did the average United States sailor.

As illustrated in Table 3–2, illness reports of the men were generally of minor severity. However, these illnesses represented the common medical problems generally seen by a medical practitioner. They were not "imaginary" illnesses. They were not simply "excuses" to get out of work. In all, these illnesses accounted for thousands of man-hours lost from duty.

Much of our previous work has focused upon step 1 in our model—attempts to quantify subjects' recent life changes exposure. We have found in our studies of young sailors that the LCU scoring system adds very little over and above a simple unit scoring system where every life change event is counted equally.[23] This is primarily due to the fact that these young men are generally unmarried and tend to report recent life events of low and quite similar LCU values. In studies of older men and women, however, it has been found that the LCU scoring system significantly improves the discrimination of recent life events patterns of patients from control samples.[29]

Studies conducted in Sweden and Finland utilized the life changes questionnaire with samples of middle-aged men and women who developed acute myocardial infarction and with samples of spouses of subjects who had died sudden coronary deaths.[15, 16, 17, 18, 19] Results from these studies indicated subjects show an elevation in their baseline LCU levels of approximately 100 percent over the six months immediately prior to infarction. In the samples of spouses whose mates had abruptly died from their coronary heart disease, the subjects recalled an LCU build-up of nearly 200 percent over baseline values during the six months prior to death. In 1975, prospective studies were being carried out in these two countries that will assess the potential of subjects' recent LCU increases as a possible "risk factor" for coronary heart disease.

At the Naval Health Research Center in San Diego, we are assessing the nature of the associations between other steps in our model not previously the focus of our studies. For example, Theorell has found that Swedish subjects' weekly LCU totals significantly correlated with their urinary output of epinephrine (0.32, $p < 0.01$) and norepinephrine (0.23, $p < 0.05$) on the last day of the week.[29] This represents another approach to studying correlations between step 1 and step 3 in our model. Studies by Wolff, and his associates demonstrated the effects of certain psychological defenses (step 2 in our model) on subjects' abilities to maintain normal levels of serum cortisol concentration (step 3 in our model) in the face of severe life stress.[31] Lastly, subjects' coping styles, such as those mentioned by Lazarus (step 4 in our model), may well help us to understand how some subjects with high stress—and even high symptom levels—nonetheless, manage to remain in good health.[32]

REFERENCES

1. Rahe RH: Life crisis and health change, in May PR, A Wittenbornd R (eds): Psychotropic Drug Response: Advances in Prediction. Springfield, Ill., Thomas, 1969, p 92
2. Rahe RH, Arthur RJ: Biochemical correlates of behavior. (A digest of selected studies.) Dis Nerv Syst 29:114–117, 1968
3. Rahe RH, McKean J, Arthur RJ: A longitudinal study of life change and illness patterns. J Psychosom Res 10:355–366, 1967
4. Rahe RH, Arthur RJ: Life change patterns surrounding illness experience. J Psychosom Res 11:341–345, 1968
5. Rahe RH: Life change measurement as a predictor of illnesses. Proc R Soc Med 61:1124–1126, 1968
6. Rahe RH, Mahan JL, Arthur RJ, et al: The epidemiology of illness in naval environments. I. Illness types distribution, severities and relationship to life change. Milit Med 135:443–452, 1970
7. Gunderson EK, Rahe RH, Arthur RJ: The epidemiology of illness in naval environments. II. Demographic, social background, and occupational factors. Milit Med 135:453–463, 1970
8. Rahe RH, Gunderson EK, Arthur RJ: Medical and psychiatric epidemiology in the reporting of acute illness. J Chronic Dis 23:245–255, 1970
9. Rahe RH, Mahan JL, Arthur RJ: Prediction of near-future health change from subjects' preceding life changes. J Psychosom Res 14:401–406, 1970
10. Pugh WM, Gunderson EK, Erickson JM, et al: Variations of illness incidence in Navy populations. Milit Med 137:224–227, 1972
11. Rahe RH, Gunderson EK, Pugh WM, et al: Illness prediction studies. Use of psychosocial and occupational characteristics as predictors. Arch Envirn Health 25:192–197, 1972
12. Rahe RH: Subjects' recent life changes and their near-future illness susceptibility, in Advances in Psychosomatic Medicine, vol VIII. Basel, Switz., Karger, 1972, p 2
13. Rahe RH: Subjects' recent life changes and their near-future illness reports. Ann Clin Res 4:250–265, 1972
14. Rahe RH, Biersner RJ, Ryman DH, et al: Psychosocial predictors of illness behavior and failure in stressful training. J Health Soc Behav 13:393–397, 1972
15. Theorell T, Rahe RH: Behavior and life satisfactions characteristics of Swedish subjects with myocardial infarction. J Chronic Dis 25:139–147, 1972
16. Theorell T, Rahe RH: Psychosocial factors and myocardial infarction. I. An inpatient study in Sweden. J Psychosom Res 15:25–32, 1971
17. Rahe RH, Paasikivi J: Psychosocial factors and myocardial infarction. II. An outpatient study in Sweden. J Psychosom Res 15:33–39, 1971
18. Rahe RH, Lind E: Psychosocial factors and sudden cardiac death. A pilot study. J Psychosom Res 15:19–24, 1971
19. Rahe RH, Bennett LK, Romo M, et al: Subjects' recent life changes and coronary heart disease. An epidemiologic study in Helsinki. Am J Psychiatry 130:1222–1226, 1973

20. Rahe RH, Pugh WM, Erickson JM et al: Cluster analysis of life changes. I. Consistency of clusters across large Navy samples. Arch Gen Psychiatry 25:330–332, 1971

21. Pugh WM, Erickson JM, Rubin RT, et al: Cluster analysis of life changes. II. Method and replication in Navy subpopulations. Arch Gen Psychiatry 25:333 –340, 1971

22. Rubin RT, Gunderson EK, Arthur, RJ: Life stress and illness patterns in the U.S. Navy. VI. Environmental, demographic, and prior life change variables in relation to illness onset in naval aviators during a combat cruise. Psychosom Med 34:533–547, 1972

23. Rahe RH (ed): The pathway between subjects' recent life changes and their near-future illness reports: Representative results and methodologic issues, in Recent Life Events: Their Nature and Effects. New York, Appleton-Century-Crofts, 1974, p 73

24. Gunderson EK, Rahe RH (ed): Life Stress and Illness. Springfield, Ill., Thomas, 1974

25. MacMillan A: The health opinion survey: Technique for estimating prevalence of psychoneurotic and related types of disorder in communities. Psychol Rep 2:325, 1957

26. Hinkle LE, Jr, Redmont R, Plummer N, et al: II. An examination of the relation between symptoms disability, and serious illness, in two homogeneous groups of men and women. Am J Public Health 50:1327–1336, 1960

27. Cline D, Chosey J: A prospective study of life changes and subsequent health changes. Arch Gen Psychiatry 27:51–53, 1972

28. Dohrenwend, B: Life events as stressors: A methodological inquiry. J Health Soc Behav 14:167–175, 1973

29. Theorell T: Psychosocial Factors in Relation to the Onset of Myocardial Infarction and to Some Metabolic Variables: A Pilot Study. Stockholm, Karolinska Institutet, 1970

30. Rahe RH, Romo M, Bennett LK, et al: Recent life changes, myocardial infarction, and abrupt coronary death: Studies in Helsinki. Arch Intern Med 133:221–228, 1974

31. Wolff CT, Friedman SB, Hofer MA, et al: Relationships between psychological defenses and mean urinary 17-hydroycorticosteroid excretion rates. I. A predictive study of parents of children with leukemia. Psychosom Med 26:576–591, 1964

32. Lazarus RS: Psychological Stress and the Coping Process. New York, McGraw-Hill, 1966

Joel Yager

4

Cognitive Aspects of Illness

Cognitive processes are the means by which we perceive, evaluate, organize, comprehend, and make use of information; they help to orient us and give purpose to our behavior.[1] Our cognitive processes constantly attempt to structure and make meaning of our experiences, especially those of great personal relevance. Illness is an important experience; every person confronted with an illness tries to understand the situation and makes plans for dealing with the illness in relation to this understanding.

Such cognitive aspects are part of every illness. Patients possess an infinite variety of ideas, assumptions, attitudes, expectations, information, and misinformation about their illnesses and the implications of the illnesses for them. These notions not only influence how patients process new information presented to them by physicians, but also create possibilities for distortion and misunderstanding. By attending to the patient's views, concerns, and understandings of his illness, the physician may become aware of misconceptions, unrealistic expectations, or countertherapeutic attitudes. Such attention by the physician may increase the likelihood that therapeutic efforts will alleviate the patient's problems.

This chapter will consider the nature of cognitive processes and their relation to other psychological events, the sources of belief and information concerning illness, the relationship between the patient's attitudes about illness and the patient's behavior, and, finally, the implications of these issues for the physician-patient relationship.

COGNITION

We process information on multiple levels. Bits of information are related to one another in complex arrangements, according to rules we know little about. Information is organized symbolically, in memories and fantasies, by

61

means of images, thought, and language.[2, 3, 4] The concepts of "endocepts"[2] (preverbal tendencies to feel, think, or act) and "enactions"[3] (information-laden body movements) have been introduced to describe additional types of cognitive forms. These elements may or may not be within awareness, and they may or may not accurately reflect past experiences or current "reality."[5]

Cognitive elements are linked to affects, to motivations, and to coping and defense mechanisms. They are influenced by events in the external world and internal milieu. They may be related according to the rules of primary process (as in dreaming or schizophrenic thought), where confusion between similarity and identity exists, *or* according to the rules of secondary process, where logical relationships hold. In illness, as with other major stress, some regression in the mode of thinking may occur.

Through association with one another cognitive elements may be linked into multiple complex hierarchies that have been called *schema*.[4, 6] Schema have been viewed as quasi-permanent frameworks that serve as tools for the organization of cognitive processes. They may consist of very basic premises, assumptions, expectations, and dispositions (for example, a person's basic tendency toward trust or distrust), and they serve to screen, code, and evaluate incoming stimuli. In this way schema provide a framework for making sense of things; at the same time they bias our perceptions. How an individual cognizes an illness experience may be strongly influenced by self-concepts (schema), such as (1) how vulnerable versus indestructible one perceives oneself to be and (2) how powerful versus impotent one imagines oneself to be to influence through personal action major external events such as illness.[7, 8]

Cognitive elements have been characterized by a variety of qualities: flexibility-inflexibility, openness-closedness, abstractness-concreteness, and clarity-ambiguity. They vary in complexity and the degree to which they are differentiated from and interconnected with other cognitive elements.[6, 9] Ideas about illness in general, or about one illness in particular, may be vague or certain, fixed or subject to change through influence. Also, cognitive elements differ in the ease with which they will be triggered into awareness by environmental cues.[9] In general, most of our "internal models of reality"—the schema—can be evoked by very few "key" outside stimuli.[10] In this way one brief pain can call to mind a vivid and complex image of a disease.

How we think is partly determined by our individual cognitive styles. These are the characteristic modes of our handling information: alerting to, scanning, and screening input.[11, 12, 13] These styles may be related to specific individual neurophysiological patterns.[14] Cognitive styles may also be related to the individual's characteristic modes of coping and defense, for example, a general tendency to be vigilant about or to avoid dealing with stressful situations.[15]

Generally, coping may be considered bound to reality while defense mechanisms may be considered attempts to distort reality to some extent. Either may ultimately be adaptive or maladaptive.[16] An individual's characteristic coping and defense patterns may be determined by constitutional factors as well as by experience. Nevertheless, while individuals may be grossly classified according to basic coping styles (such as "deniers," who consistently minimize the experience of heart disease[17]), such labels may be too general to permit us to predict how that individual will behave in any specific future situation. Yet, while coping and defense patterns may be situation-specific, determined in part by the unique characteristics of the events, characteristic cognitive styles and coping and defense patterns may themselves determine how the unique events are perceived in the first place.

Cognition is closely related to affect.[1, 6, 16, 18, 19] Some affects may serve as systems to signal the differences between what we expect or would like to see in a situation and what we actually perceive—to let us know "how we're doing".[20] The feeling states associated with illness may be partly determined by our assumptions and expectations about the illness and its implications. However, while cognition may determine affect, it is conceivable that at times affect greatly influences cognition. This may occur in mania, where characteristic cognitive schema seem to reappear with each manic episode.[21] Also, excessive affective arousal may disrupt the ongoing cognition; great anxiety may prevent a patient from being able to think clearly about his illness or from being able to receive and process communications from the physician.[22]

Both cognition and affect may be influenced by basic physiological events, such as delerium or conditions of food or water deprivation. Cognition may also be subject to influence by the normal 90-minute basic rest and activity cycles (BRACs) that occur throughout the day.[23] Similarly, cognition may influence basic physiological systems, as in the physiological component of anxiety. The full implications of these relationships for psychosomatic events, presumably mediated by neural and neurohumeral mechanisms, are poorly understood.

Cognitive elements have value components—"good-bad" or "desirable-undesirable" associations—tied to hopes, preferences, and aspirations,[1] and these associations determine whether or not a perceived event is experienced as a threat.[18] Each cognitive element has value relative to others. For example, the attitude "taking care of health is important" may be positively regarded; yet, it may assume a negative value when associated with the attitude "submitting to a physician's painful procedures is bad."

Finally, our goals—determined by our experiences, values, and motivations—are, broadly, the schema that guide our plans for ongoing behavior.[24] These schema contain our ideas of how things "ought to be," and in this way they serve as internal reference signals that orient our actions. We constantly attempt to bring our perceptions ("what is") into accord with what we think *should be*.[25] What we want and how important each goal is in relation to others influence how we perceive, comprehend, and behave. For some individuals the goals of personal health are preeminent; for others different goals (such as not wanting to be a financial burden to one's family) may be most important.

SOURCES OF BELIEFS AND KNOWLEDGE ABOUT ILLNESS

The Macroculture

Each culture contains broad systems of belief about health and disease. These beliefs constitute the basic assumptions of the culture that act "like a map or blueprint that provides the outline of what members of a culture accept as real."[26] They are the filters through which members of a culture experience and understand their own illnesses. To illustrate, some Puerto Rican patients adhere to the "hot-cold" theory of disease, a system of beliefs derived from Hippocratic and Galenic views that was transmitted by Spanish conquerors, distorted, modified, and passed down through time. Through the years the system has continued to grow, incorporating elements of modern medicine along the way.[27] According to this theory, some illnesses, conditions, and treatments are considered "hot" (for example, rashes, ulcers, diarrhea, constipation, and penicillin, which may cause rashes); others are considered "cold" (for example, the common cold, arthritis, and drugs that may cause muscle spasms). "Hot" diseases require "cold" treatment and vice versa. A category of "neutral" treatments exists as well. The important point is that patients may not accept a "hot" treatment, prescribed by an unsuspecting physician, for a "hot" disease. Even the physician who is alert to this theory cannot easily alter his patients' beliefs; he must learn to work effectively within the system to render treatment acceptable.

The holistic psychosomatic views of the Ladino-Mestizo populations of the Chiapas highlands of Mexico, and the implications of these views for care seeking and care delivery have been described.[26] These beliefs encompass bodily, psychological, social, and environmental contributions to illness. "Helpers" who are impersonal, and mechanistically–technologically oriented with respect to disease—that is, who don't give proper attention to the noxiousness of certain emotions and interpersonal interactions—may not be trusted.

Mystical and demonic beliefs about illness still persist even in the United States. Some Mexican-American populations believe in such conditions as *mal ojo* (evil eye),[28] and one can still see the power of voodoo hexes.[29] Afflicted individuals may attribute symptoms caused by organic processes to folk diseases and follow folk treatments rather than seek modern medical care.

Beliefs about health, the experience of disease, and care seeking may be related to social class. Arthritis is attributed more to dampness and other environmental causes by lower-class than by upper-class individuals; similarly, populations who believe arthritis to be a natural consequence of the aging process may fail to seek help for remediable problems.[30]

The experience of symptoms, and underlying concerns and attitudes about those symptoms, varies among ethnic subcultures in the mainstream of our culture. Individuals of some groups tend to react stoically to pain; others are more demonstrative. Some are predominantly concerned that the present pain be adequately dealt with; others have "future-oriented anxiety" related to the underlying causes of the pain.[31]

Much of the information that people have about diseases comes through "lay authorities," word of mouth, and the popular press; the medical profession is certainly not the only, nor necessarily the most important, source for many prevalent health beliefs.[30, 32]

The Microculture

Within the broad cultural and subcultural framework of beliefs and attitudes each individual's cognitive world of health and disease is shaped by experiences within the immediate social network—among family and friends. While growing up, the child observes sick or dying individuals and overhears snatches of conversation; all the attendant distortions and elaborations influence his perception of his own and others' illnesses.[33] Each family has its own set of attitudes and responses to illness in the family. For example, it has been suggested that pain-prone patients may have been preferentially reinforced by their parents to couch their expressions of distress in terms of body pain rather than in terms of other feelings.[34] The significance that we mistakenly attribute to the mild symptoms that we all experience may be greatly influenced by the illness experiences of our family and other persons whom we have seen—as in the "medical student syndrome."[35] Undoubtedly, even sophisticated physicians hold idiosyncratic views about the nature and implications of their own individual symptoms.[36]

Within the microculture the individual's cognitive, coping, and defensive styles influence the construction of self-concepts that relate to illness, such as "sick role" and "personal control over illness outcome."[7]

Finally, persons may develop incorrect ideas about illness and its treatment because of not being provided correct information or because of simple misunderstanding.[37] Physicians frequently assume and act as if their patients know more than they do, and patients are often too anxious or embarrassed to ask too many questions.[38, 39] Even groups of sophisticated patients will demonstrate impressive variability in how they interpret what most physicians would consider to be straightforward instructions. To some "every four hours" means only during waking hours; to others, around the clock. A pill ''for fluid retention'' means to some that it will cause a diuresis; to others, that it will cause fluid to be retained.[40] Not infrequently patients will attribute new symptoms (incorrectly) to treatment side effects and stop taking their medications.[41]

COGNITION AND COMPLIANCE

Patient compliance with medication regimens is generally poor; from 30 percent to 75 percent of patients with a wide assortment of conditions do not adequately follow instructions in taking medication for B hemolytic streptococca infections, tuberculosis, pregnancy, cardiac disease, epilepsy, and psychiatric conditions, to name only a few.[42, 43, 44] Usually, the more careful the compliance study, the lower the degree of compliance that is found. Most physicians would hardly tolerate so high a margin of error in other aspects of their work (in the accuracy of laboratory determinations, for instance), yet, whereas presumably the outcome of all the physician's efforts hinge on the patient's carrying out the recommendation, physicians usually spend little effort in assuring that this occurs. Physicians tend to overestimate the compliance of their patients and are usually very poor at guessing which of their patients are compliant and which are not. Even when a patient unfailingly keeps all clinic appointments, this cannot be taken as assurance that the patient has been taking medication as prescribed.

Among the many factors associated with poor compliance are failure to understand the purpose of treatment, lower socioeconomic and poor educational background, problems in relating to authorities, complacency, and boredom—in short, a variety of factors with strong cognitive components: information, values, and attitudes. According to Blackwell, ''the most important contribution to compliance is the understanding a patient has of the illness, the need for treatment, and the likely consequence of both.''[43]

While the amount of actual knowledge a person has about his disease and its treatment may be an important factor contributing to compliance, there is no simple relationship between the amount of knowledge and compliance with the treatment.[41, 45, 46] Self-concepts of ''sick'' and ''ability to control illness through action'' are at times more potent predictors of patient compliance with continuing clinic appointments than is the amount of knowledge per se. While knowledge about illness may *add* to motivation for health-seeking action or compliance, it cannot by itself account for such motivation. It is not knowledge per se but, rather, personal knowledge that is related to action.

The patient's own perception of the severity of an illness may be more important than the physician's perception of severity in determining compliance, as illustrated by a study of mothers giving oral penicillin to their children.[47] Moreover, when patients' expectations for a visit with a physician are not met (for example, for x-rays or "shots") or when the patients' personal concerns about the illness are not discussed, patient satisfaction is low and compliance suffers. In the studies by Korsch and her associates attention to these issues by physicians was associated with patients having the experience of "being understood," and the office visits for these patients did not necessarily require more time than did the office visits for patients where these issues were ignored.[38, 39] Too, specific attention by the physician to patients' perceptions of the medication and possible side effects (misattributions) may increase compliance.[41]

Patients' cognitive, coping, and defensive styles, self-concepts, attitudes, and prejudices have been reported to influence care seeking and treatment compliance in a large number of conditions, including cancer,[48] heart disease,[17, 41] chronic renal failure,[49] and diabetes mellitus.[50, 51] In addition to operating directly to influence outcome through cooperation with specific components of a treatment plan, such cognitive factors may also influence the general process of healing and recovery through indirect, poorly understood ways. Attitudes such as hope may influence neurophysiological and neuroendocrine events and, consequently, events at the periphery. Less obscure cognitive factors may influence the amount of pain medication required and the patient's motivation and behavior with regard to self-care (such as, attending to dressings, pulmonary exercises).[15]

IMPLICATIONS FOR THE PHYSICIAN-PATIENT RELATIONSHIP

Clearly, persons experiencing illness have accomplished a great deal of cognitive work before seeking the expert help of the physician. They have perceived symptoms, scanned their memories and attitudes, and have sought additional information and advice from family and friends. Although they may remain open-minded, by the time most patients set foot in the physician's office they have conjured up visions about what their illness is, what it is due to, what can be done about it, and what they can expect the illness to do to them with or without treatment; in short, they have developed their own ideas about diagnosis, etiology and pathogenesis, treatment, and prognosis—the same assessment that the physician will carry out. The very act of seeking out the physician is a coping maneuver; for the patient the physician is a coping tool.

Therefore, physicians who expect that a patient will simply and without bias report his symptoms ("the facts") and then automatically follow the physician's instructions are apt to be disappointed frequently. Instead, attention to the patient's own ideas and concerns will *at least* impart to the patient a sense of being listened to and may increase compliance. In practice, the physician needs to explore the contents, sources, and tenacity of the patient's beliefs. Even when culturally, socioeconomically, and ethnically similar to the physician, each person is a unique "subculture" and may view his illness and its treatment quite differently from the physician. These differences may be disruptive to treatment by interfering with the patient's ability to assimilate what the physician has to say—and with compliance.[36]

What does the patient think that the problem is? What does he worry about? Has the patient ever known or heard of any people with similar problems? What did they turn out to have? How were they treated? How did it turn out? When a patient's concerns go undiscussed, the patient may be so preoccupied with these as not to be able to attend to what the physician has to say to him.[38, 39] Therefore, by first learning about the patient's perceptions and concerns, the physician is better able to provide information, opinion, and instruction.

Patients expect to be informed and educated by their physicians; they will acquire expectations whether or not their physicians say anything.[8] Uninstructed patients may develop unrealistic expectations that may be frightening or overly optimistic; they may overinterpret casual remarks or the physician's body language, sometimes confirming their worst fears or best hopes. If unchecked and unnoticed, these may interfere with treatment.

While simple education cannot guarantee compliance, it may help. Also, preparation of patients in what they might expect may favorably alter their perceptions and experiences, as with postoperative pain and childbirth.[52, 53] However, providing information is not simple; a good deal of what physicians say to patients may be quickly distorted, misinterpreted, or forgotten. Patients may recall best what they are told first by physicians. Diagnostic statements may be recalled better than information and advice.[21]

The physician is obliged, therefore, to enter a dialogue with the patient. He must share the patient's concerns and perceptions, allowing himself to enter the patient's cognitive world and thereby to experience empathy. His communications to the patient must be based upon his awareness of the patient's position vis-à-vis the illness. Since the patient may not correctly hear or recall what the physician says, clear, nontechnical written instructions that the patient can read over after the visit may be helpful, especially when accompanied by an explicit invitation to raise questions about ambiguities during subsequent visits or by phone.

The physician needs to close a feedback loop: a patient should be invited to reexplain what he *thinks* that the physician said and to discuss his revised concepts, attitudes, and expectations following his interactions with the physician, during both the initial and subsequent visits.

Attention to cognitive aspects of illness may enhance the quality of the physician–patient interaction and may increase the likelihood that the physician's efforts are successful—through increasing the patient's understanding in a personally relevant way and thereby the patient's cooperation with therapy.

REFERENCES

1. Harvey OJ: Cognitive aspects of affective arousal, in Tomkins SS, Izard CE (eds): Affect, Cognition and Personality: Empirical Studies. London, Tavistock, 1966, pp 242–262
2. Arieti S: The role of cognition in the development of inner reality, in Hellmuth J (ed): Cognitive Studies, vol 1. New York, Brunner/Mazel, 1970, pp 91–110
3. Horowitz MJ: Image Formation and Cognition. New York, Appleton-Century-Crofts, 1970, p 80
4. Rapaport D: Cognitive structures, in Bruner JS, et al: Contemporary Approaches to Cognition. Cambridge, Harvard University Press, 1957, pp 157–200
5. Lazarus RS: Cognitive and personality factors underlying threat and coping, in Appley MH, Trumbull R (eds): Psychological Stress: Issues in Research. New York, Appleton-Century-Crofts, 1967, pp 151–169
6. Beck AT: Depression: Clinical, Experimental and Theoretical Aspects. New York, Harper & Row, 1967
7. Gochman DS: The organizing role of motivation in health beliefs and intentions. J Health Soc Behav 13:285–293, 1972
8. Mechanic D: Social psychological factors affecting the presentation of bodily complaints. N Engl J Med 286:1132–1139, 1972
9. Scott WA: Conceptualizing and measuring structural properties of cognition, in Harvey OJ (ed): Motivation and Social Interaction: Cognitive Determinants. New York, Ronald, 1963, pp 266–288
10. Gregory RL: On how little information controls so much behavior. Ergonomics 13:25–35, 1970
11. Witkin HA, Goodenough D, Karp S: Stability of cognitive style from childhood to young adulthood. J Pers Soc Psycho 7:291–300, 1967
12. Gardner RW: Differences in cognitive structures, in Warr PB (ed): Thought and Personality. Baltimore, Penguin, 1970, pp 223–236
13. Lazarus RS, Averill JR, Opton EM Jr: The psychology of coping: Issues of research and assessment, in Coelho GV, Hamburg DA, Adams JE (eds): Coping and Adaptation. New York, Basic Books, 1974, pp 249–315
14. Cohen SI: Central nervous system functioning in altered sensory environments, in Appley MH, Trumbull R (eds): Psychological Stress: Issues in Research. New York, Appleton-Century-Crofts, 1967, pp 77–112
15. Cohen F, Lazarus RS: Active coping processes, coping dispositions and recovery from surgery. Psychoso Med 35:375–389, 1973
16. Lazarus RS: Psychological Stress and the Coping Process. New York, McGraw-Hill, 1966
17. Croog SH, Shapiro DS, Levine S: Denial among male heart patients. Psychosom Med 33:385–397, 1971

18. Arnold MB: Stress and emotion, in Appley MH, Trumbull R (eds): Psychological Stress: Issues in Research. New York, Appleton-Century-Crofts, 1967, pp 123–150

19. Schacter S, Singer JE: Cognitive, social and physiological determinants of emotional state. Psychol Rev 69:379–399, 1962

20. Engel GL: Psychological Development in Health and Disease. Philadelphia, Saunders, 1962, p 128

21. Janowsky DS, El-Youseff MK, Davis J: Interpersonal maneuvers of manic patients. Am J Psychiatry 131:250–255, 1974

22. Ley P: Primacy, rated importance and the recall of medical statements. J Health Soc Behav 13:311–317, 1972

23. Kripke D, Sonnenheim D: A-90 Minute Fantasy Cycle (in preparation)

24. Miller GA, Galanter E. Pribram KH: Plans and the Structure of Behavior. New York, Holt, Rinehart and Winston, 1960

25. Powers WT: Feedback: Beyond behaviorism. Science 179:351–355, 1973

26. Fabrega H, Manning PK: An integrated theory of disease: Ladino-Mestizo views of disease in the Chiapas highlands. Psychosom Med 35:223–239, 1973

27. Harwood A: The hot-cold theory of disease: Implications for treatment of Puerto Rican patients. JAMA 216:1153–1158, 1971

28. Martinez C, Martin HW: Folk diseases among Mexican-Americans: Etiology, symptoms, treatment. JAMA 196:161–164, 1966

29. Tinling DC: Voodoo, root work and medicine. Psychosom Med 29:483–490, 1967

30. Elder RG: Social class and lay explanations of the etiology of arthritis. J Health Soc Behav 14:28–38, 1973

31. Zborowski M: Cultural components in responses to pain, in Jaco EG (ed): Patients, Physicians and Illness. New York, Free Press, 1958, pp 256–268

32. Yager J, Young RT: Non-hypoglycemia is an epidemic condition. New Engl J Med 291:907–908, 1974

33. Schmale AH, Meyerowitz S, Tinling DC: Current concepts of psychosomatic medicine, in Hill OW (ed): Modern Trends in Psychosomatic Medicine, vol 2. New York, Appleton-Century-Crofts, 1970, pp 1–25

34. Engel GL: "Psychogenic" pain and the pain prone patient. Am J Med 26:899–918, 1959

35. Hunter RCA, Lohrenz JG, Schwartzman AE: Nosophobia and hypochondriasis in medical students. J Ner Ment Dis 139:147–152, 1964

36. Engel GL: Personal theories of disease as determinates of patient-physician relationships. Psychosom Med 35:184–185, 1973

37. Ley P, Spelman M: Communication in an outpatient setting. Br J Soc Clin Psychol 4:114–116, 1965

38. Francis V, Korsch BM, Morris MJ: Gaps in doctor-patient communication: Patients response to medical advice. N Engl J Med 280:535–540, 1969

39. Korsch BM, Negrete VF: Doctor-patient communication. Sci Am 227:66–74, 1972

40. Mazzullo JM, Lasagna L, Griner PF: Variations in interpretation of prescription instructions. JAMA 227:929–931, 1974

41. Weintraub M, Au WYW, Lasagna L: Compliance as a determinant of serum digoxin concentration. JAMA 224:481–485, 1973

42. Harper DA: Patient follow-up of medical advice: A literature review. J Kans Med Soc 72:265–271, 1971

43. Blackwell B: Patient compliance. N Engl J Med 289:249–252, 1973

44. Gillum RF, Barsky AJ: Diagnosis and management of patient noncompliance. JAMA 228:1563–1567, 1974

45. Elling R, WhittemoreR, Green M: Patient participation in a pediatric program. J Health Human Behav 1:183–191, 1960

46. Taglicozzo DM, Ima K: Knowledge of illness as a predictor of patient behavior. J Chronic Dis 22:765–775, 1970

47. Charney E, Bynum R, Eldredge D, et al: How well do patients take oral penicillin? Collaborative study in private practice. Pediatrics 40:188–195, 1967

48. Hackett TP, Cassem NH, Raker JW: Patient delay in cancer. N Engl J Med 289:14–20, 1973

49. Kaplan-DeNour A, Czaczkes JW: Personality factors in chronic hemodialysis patients causing noncompliance with medical regimen. Psychosom Med 34:333–344, 1972

50. Swift CR, Seidman F, Stein H: Adjustment problems in juvenile diabetes. Psychosom Med 29:555–571, 1967

51. Koch MF, Molnar GD: Psychiatric aspects of patients with unstable diabetes mellitus. Psychosom Med 36:57–68, 1974

52. Egbert LD, Battit BE, Welch CE, Bartless MK: Reduction of postoperative pain by encouragement and instruction of patients. N Engl J Med 270:825–827, 1964

53. Davenport-Slack MS, Boylan CH: Psychological correlates of childbirth pain. Psychosom Med 36:215–223, 1974

Robert T. Rubin

5

Mind-Brain-Body Interaction: Elucidation of Psychosomatic Intervening Variables

The history of psychosomatic medicine is long and complex. Over the years many brilliant thinkers have developed carefully reasoned, sensible theories about the interaction of the mind, brain, and body, based on ample clinical data with great heuristic value.[1] These theories include the James-Lange theory of emotion, later refuted by Cannon, the homeostasis and *milieu interieur* theories of Cannon and Bernard, the personality theory of Dunbar, the conflict specificity theory of Alexander, and the physiological specificity theories of Lacey and Wolff and others. Other chapters in this book consider these theories in greater detail. Their relevance to the present discussion is that they all are an attempt to create a conceptual bridge—based on analogy, descriptive data, and inductive logic—between human psychologic functioning and human physiology including the pathophysiologic changes that result in disease.

Perhaps the most encompassing recent advance in this area has been the conceptual shift away from psychosomatic medicine as a discrete subspecialty of psychiatry that focuses on a few illnesses that most observers agree have a major psychologic component in their onset and course.[2] Now there is ample evidence that all illness has psychologic components—before, during, and after the illness episode—and that a multivariate approach is necessary to elucidate the relative contribution of the many components (genetic,

Supported by NIMH Research Scientist Development Award K01-MH 47363 and Office of Naval Research Contract N00014-73-C-0127.

epidemiologic and environmental, psychosocial, psychodynamic, neuro-physiologic, metabolic) that comprise a given specific illness or syndrome—the "psychosomatic viewpoint."[3] Epidemiologic studies of thousands of subjects clearly indicate that periods of increased life stress precede many disabilities, including physical illness, psychiatric illness, and accidents.[4, 5] No disease is exempt from psychologic factors, and, as a corollary, all diseases have psychologic repercussions.

Another area of recent understanding that also broadens our perspective is that of early brain development. It is now known that brain-environment interactions in the human occur at least as early as the first minutes after birth.[6] The actual morphological development of the brain has been shown to depend on environmental stimulation.[7] This is true not only for gross sensory deficits, such as the disturbed brain maturation following the blinding of experimental animals, but even for more subtle influences, such as the amount of dendritic branching in the developing brain of experimental animals being dependent upon the amount of psychosocial stimulation following birth.[8] Discrete time-limited changes in the chemical milieu of the brain can result in permanent alterations of brain function. The exposure of the developing brain to androgens or to estrogens may be a major determinant of "male" (tonic) or "female" (cyclic) hypothalamic function, at least with respect to the hypothalamo-pituitary-gonadal axis, as well as influencing more subtle long-term behavior patterns, even in the human.[9]

Given this broader conceptual framework for the "psychosomatic viewpoint" (that is, for mind-brain-body interaction), are the multiple components of any illness inextricably interwoven or can they be dissected? The answer is, of course, that for some illnesses the interplay of factors has been elucidated to a far greater degree than for others. For example, the influence of environmental stress on brain mechanisms that foster the development of hypertension, and, in turn, the mechanics of the response of the arterioles to these altered brain mechanisms, has been clarified considerably since the late 1960s.[10] On the other hand, similar schemata for ulcerative colitis (traditionally considered a "psychosomatic" disease) and for cancer have not advanced to any significant degree, in spite of considerable speculation about these illnesses from the psychosomatic viewpoint.[11, 12] We shall examine some of the underlying neurophysiologic mechanisms in greater detail.

NEUROTRANSMITTERS AND STRESS

Since the 1960s considerable research has focused on the effects of environmental stress on neurotransmitter function in the brain and the importance of neurotransmitters in brain-body mechanisms. The putative central

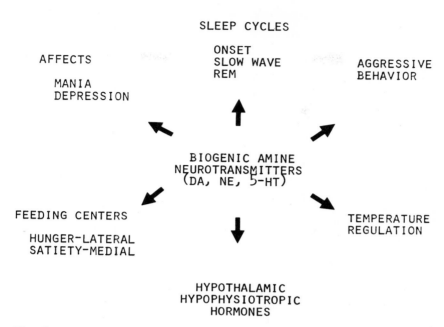

Fig. 5–1. Putative CNS biogenic amine neurotransmitters and some aspects of brain function that they may subserve.

nervous system (CNS) neurotransmitters that have been most extensively investigated are the catecholamines—dopamine and norephinephrine; the indoleamine—serotonin (5–HT); and acetylcholine. Other postulated neurotransmitters are receiving increasing attention, such as y-aminobutyric acid (GABA). To illustrate the key role of neurotransmitters in various aspects of CNS function, we shall concentrate on the three biogenic amine neurotransmitters—dopamine, norepinephrine, and serotonin. Figure 5–1 illustrates aspects of CNS function in which these neurotransmitters, on the basis of considerable evidence, are believed to be important.

Psychiatrists are most familiar with the postulated role of these neurotransmitters in the affective disorders of mania and depression.[13, 14] It has been suggested that in manic overactivity states there is a functional excess of one or more of these synaptic transmitters in the parts of the brain controlling activity levels, and, conversely, in depression there is a functional underactivity of these transmitters. The various drugs used to treat mania and depression may be partially understood from some of their effects on the neurochemistry of the synapse. For example, the tricyclic antidepressants decrease the reuptake of transmitters into the presynaptic nerve ending, thereby enhancing their concentration in the synaptic cleft. Conversely, lithium, an antimanic agent, has as one of its effects the enhancement of reuptake of neurotransmitters into the presynaptic nerve ending, thereby decreasing their concentration in the synaptic cleft. Other drugs, such as reserpine, the monoamine oxidase inhibitors, amphetamines, and the phenothiazine and butyrophenone antipsychotic agents, all can be partially understood at a neurochemical level by their effects on blocking or enhancing the action of these neurotransmitters.

In Figure 5–1 it is shown that sleep cycles also are influenced by these neurotransmitters. There is considerable evidence, primarily from work with the cat,[15] that a serotoninergic mechanism in the median raphe nuclei of the brain stem triggers the normal progression from wakefulness into sleep and the further progression into slow wave (stages 3 and 4) or deep sleep. Periodically, there is the well-known appearance of the rapid eye movement (REM) or dreaming sleep episode; this is believed to be triggered by cholinergic and noradrenergic mechanisms in the brain stem. There is conflicting evidence, from pharmacologic studies in humans, as to which neurotransmitters are important in the various stages of sleep in the human,[16] but the role of these transmitters in the orderly progression of sleep staging in the human, as well as in experimental animals, is generally accepted.

There is some evidence suggesting that these same neurotransmitters may mediate aggressive behavior, at least in experimental animals.[17] Placement of norepinephrine into the CNS of mice decreases fighting behavior, whereas placement of dopamine into the CNS enhances this behavior.[18] Extrapolation of these data to humans is tenuous at the present time because of the lack of comparative data. Furthermore, aggressive behavior appears to be a complexly intertwined process with inputs at psychosocial, hormonal, and neurochemical levels.

Let us continue clockwise in Figure 5–1. There is now ample evidence suggesting that the amine neurotransmitters are key elements in the function of the hypothalamus, a critical area between higher brain centers and general body physiology and metabolic function. Temperature regulation, the control of the hypothalamic releasing and inhibiting factors that affect the anterior pituitary hormones, and the function of the hypothalamic hunger and satiety centers all appear to be prominently regulated by neural pathways that utilize these synaptic transmitters.[19]

The concept that a common neurochemistry may underlie such diverse clinical imbalances as affective disorders, sleep disturbances, pituitary disorders, and feeding problems may provide a framework for the better understanding and more effective treatment of these diverse syndromes. As one example, it is known that the so-called endogenous depressions may have prominent physiologic components in addition to the affect disturbance, including fragmentation of sleep patterns (with early morning awakening), disturbances of anterior pituitary function (with elevated basal ACTH levels and nonsuppressibility by dexamethasone, blunted growth hormone responses to the usual challenges, disturbances of cyclic gonadotropin secretion in women resulting in amenorrhea), and anorexia.[20] These depressions respond fairly well to tricyclic antidepressants and to monoamine oxidase inhibitors, both of which, as pointed out earlier, tend to increase the functional levels of synaptic neurotransmitters.

There is another illness that has a similar constellation of symptoms but with a different order of prominence. Anorexia nervosa is primarily a disease of adolescent girls.[21] Therefore, it differs considerably in age group, with some difference in sex ratios, from the aforementioned endogenous depressive syndromes.[21] However, the schema illustrated in Figure 5–1 also can be applied to it. Considerable depression has been noted in anorexia nervosa patients.[22] They have a very characteristic hyperactivity, and may have disruption of sleep-wake cycles. Although they do not tend to exhibit enhanced aggressive behavior per se, their overactivity includes a tenacity and persistence of goal-oriented drives, particularly concerning food, such as hoarding, rough self-induced vomiting and purging, etc. There is frequently a lowered basal body temperature in these individuals. There also is a prominent disturbance of anterior pituitary function, including the cessation of menses (which may be the first presetting symptom), increased basal ACTH secretion, unusual patterns of growth hormone secretion, etc. Of course, the feeding disturbance of anorexia nervosa is the central issue.

The etiology of anorexia nervosa has been variously attributed to psychological and to somatic factors.[23] Some investigators have postulated a strictly psychodynamic explanation, such as the cessation of menses being a symbolic retreat from adult womanhood; others have attributed the various manifestations of this syndrome simply to the halting of food intake. Irrespective of the initial etiologic factors in this illness, one thing is clear: there is a disturbance of hypothalamic function in anorexia nervosa, and this disturbance may be at a neurotransmitter level. Furthermore, it is possible that such a neurotransmitter disturbance could be similar to that postulated for depression, for which there are known pharmacologic treatments. Therefore, could anorexia nervosa patients be treated with antidepressant agents? One study has already appeared in which tricyclic antidepressants were found to be useful for these patients.[22] Further research directed toward defining anorexia nervosa (and depression) at the neurotransmitter level will suggest more specific directions for therapy.

NEUROANATOMIC CONSIDERATIONS

It may be stated quite legitimately that the schema shown in Figure 5–1 offers nothing new, in that all of these phenomena take place within a single organ, the brain; therefore, these several neurotransmitters obviously must subserve the various functions of the brain. In this regard one of the links in the psychosomatic chain that has not been considered in sufficient detail is that of brain structure. There is a general belief that the limbic system, the structure and function of which have been carefully described, is the part of the brain that offers emotional coloration to cerebral cortical cognitive processes.[24] It is well known that the limbic system bears rich reciprocal functional relationships with lower brain centers, such as the hypothalamus, which, in turn, regulate the function of the autonomic nervous system, the anterior and posterior pituitary, etc.[25] From the psychosomatic viewpoint the limbic system should be a key CNS mediator in the translation of environmental stress and emotional distress into physiologic change. The postulated neurotransmitter functions discussed previously do not occur homogeneously within the CNS; rather they occur in discrete areas of the brain including the limbic system, hypothalamus, etc. If neurotransmitter dysfunction occurs in different structural and functional areas of the brain, then variable symptom complexes might be evident clinically. However, little is known about the regional areas of the brain that might be affected neurochemically by environmental stress, particularly in humans. Experimental animal evidence and some data in humans suggest that the turnover of neurotransmitters in the CNS is enhanced by exposure to stress.[26] This enhanced turnover would occur in those areas of the brain in which the concentration of these neurotransmitters is the greatest, namely, parts of the limbic system and the brain stem.

Nothing more definitive structurally, however, is known about this phenomenon that might help explain why environmental stress can lead to the pattern of sympathetic nervous system and adrenal medullary activation resulting in hypertension in one individual and the pattern of parasympathetic activation and gastric hypersecretion leading to the development of a duodenal ulcer in another individual.

SPECIFICITY OF STRESS RESPONSES

The more that is learned about the physiologic and metabolic ramifications of environmental stress, the more it appears that stress responses are quite specific.[27] Selye's general adaptation syndrome,[28] in which activation of the pituitary-adrenal cortical axis is the common result of many environmental stress situations,[29] is a major contribution to our knowledge of stress, but it is only the beginning of our understanding of the complexity of neural and endocrine responses to stress.

There is now evidence indicating that stress responses are adaptationally specific rather than general and that there is an overall organization of diverse biochemical and endocrine systems into coordinated patterns of response to many types of stimuli. Such stress responses are not limited to a single neuroendocrine axis, but rather they involve a host of hormonal responses.[30, 31] The hormones that show an immediate response to stress are generally catabolic and influential in promoting energy metabolism, whereas the hormones that tend to show a delayed response after the stress is finished are anabolic and therefore important in poststress rebuilding of tissues and energy stores. The continued study of the integrated patterns of endocrine and biochemical responses to stress must be paralleled by multivariate methodologies directed at individual neurophysiological or brain state patterns of functioning, including waking states at all levels of arousal and all stages of sleep. The techniques of surface and depth electrode EEG recordings, coupled with powerful computer analyses, may help elucidate the specific areas of the brain that are activated or inhibited during specific kinds of environmental stress situations, thereby furthering our understanding of the crucial role of the limbic system and other brain areas in the transduction of psychologic events into pathophysiology.[32]

BIOLOGICAL RHYTHMS

A particular area of great contemporary interest that relates directly to the importance of brain function is that of biological rhythms, or chronobiology.[33] It is now known that many hormones and other metabolites have periodic changes in their secretion rates and blood levels. These periodic changes may be on a 24-hour (circadian) basis, on a more frequent (ultradian) basis, on a monthly basis, as with the menstrual cycle, or even on a seasonal basis. A very useful paradigm for studying circadian and ultradian variations in hormone levels is the study of the sleep-wake cycle and the stages of sleep during the sleep period. Figure 5–2 represents a composite of many studies done on the blood levels of hormones in sleeping subjects.[34, 35] During a normal night's sleep there is an orderly progression of sleep stages, with slow wave (stage 3 and 4 sleep) being more prominent in the early hours and rapid eye movement (REM) episodes being more prominent in the later hours of the sleep period. Within the hours of sleep there is an alternation between non-REM sleep and REM sleep episodes, which is the sleep manifestation of a basic 90 minute rest-activity cycle that is detectable throughout the entire 24 hours in normal individuals.[36]

The hormone patterns shown in Figure 5–2 have several interesting aspects. The most striking is that all of the hormones shown, which include adrenocorticotrophic hormone (ACTH), growth hormone (GH), luteinizing hormone (LH), follicle-stimulating hormone (FSH), prolactin (PRL), testosterone (TESTO), antidiuretic hormone (ADH), and aldosterone (ALDO), are secreted in a pulsatile, episodic fashion rather than in a tonic, steady manner. The implication is that the bursts of hormone secretion, particularly the several pituitary hormones shown, are in response to bursts of neural activity within the

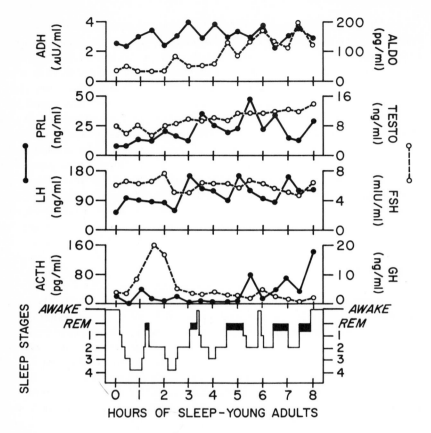

Fig. 5–2. Composite sleep-endocrine profile in a normal young adult male (see text for explanation).

CNS. Furthermore, many of these hormones show a prominent circadian rhythm, which is partially evident from the 8-hour block of data shown in Figure 5–2. For example, ACTH is lowest in the early hours of a normal night's sleep, but it rises rapidly between 3 and 8 A.M. to reach a maximum, which then declines gradually throughout the day. This rapid increase between 3 and 8 A.M. results from more rapidly occurring secretory episodes of higher amplitude, so that the average levels of ACTH in the blood increase.

The circadian rhythm of GH, on the other hand, is quite different from that of ACTH. The major release of GH during the entire 24-hour period in human adults occurs in the early hours of the night, in conjunction with slow-wave sleep. PRL also has a circadian rhythm, with highest blood levels occurring about 5 A.M., and this circadian rhythm is similar in both adult men and women.

The posterior pituitary hormone ADH and the adrenal cortical hormone ALDO, both of which are involved with water and electrolyte balance, also are secreted episodically. ALDO has a circadian rhythm similar to that for ACTH.

The metabolic importance of the episodic release patterns of these hormones, as well as the importance of their prominent and unique circadian rhythms, is quite unknown. The influence of all of these hormones on metabolic processes has been studied thoroughly, but the special significance of the dynamic aspects of their secretion patterns remains to be elucidated. As an example, as pointed out earlier, environmental stresses of all sorts, via brain mechanisms, result in the increased secretion of ACTH and the consequent release of glucocorticoids from the adrenal cortex.[29] The effects of prolonged stress and the consequent prolonged activation of the hypothalamo-pituitary-adrenal cortical axis on metabolic processes have been speculatively considered. For example, one psychosomatic theory of the pathogenesis of cancer states that prolonged stress results in chronic adrenal cortical hyperactivity, which suppresses immune mechanisms.[37] These immune mechanisms, which would be normally protective against foreign or altered proteins (including malignant cells), would be weakened to the point where a malignancy might flourish. Although many questions can be raised about the exact role of immune mechanisms in the retardation of malignant growth,[38] an interesting aspect is whether or not the time of day that the individual may be exposed to the environmental stress could have a differential effect on the suppression of immune mechanisms, based on the particular time of the circadian rhythm of ACTH upon which the environmental stress is superimposed. This is but one example of many chronobiological questions that must be raised about the physiologic and metabolic significance of these various hormonal and neurochemical rhythms.[39, 40]

SPECIFIC ILLNESSES

It is of interest to consider the recent advances made toward the understanding of mind-brain-body mechanisms in specific illnesses. With reference to hyperthyroidism, patients with thyroid "hot spots," that is, areas that take up radioactive iodine more strongly than other areas of the gland, have been followed prospectively for several years. It was found that changes in the hot spots are related to life strain, which, if prolonged and severe, may stimulate the hot spot to progress to clinical thyrotoxicosis.[41] It has been suggested that the sympathetic nervous system may have a direct influence on the secretion of thyroid hormone and may modulate the effects of this hormone.[42] An increased sympathetic activity thus might precipitate hyperthyroidism or enhance the symptoms of this illness.

Hypertension can be caused experimentally in animals by situations such as crowding that produce repeated arousal of the defense alarm response.[10] This response involves brain mechanisms that cause repeated discharge of the sympathetic nervous system and release of the vasoconstrictor, norepinephrine, from the adrenal medulla. The resultant hypertrophy of arteriolar musculature over time, in response to transiently elevated blood pressure, can produce a situation in which the same amount of vasoconstrictor stimulus will produce a considerably decreased arteriolar diameter, based on the ratio of the arteriolar wall to its lumen.[43]

With reference to bronchial asthma it has been suggested that asthmatics have a deficiency of epinephrine secretion by the adrenal medulla; therefore, they might have an imbalance of adrenergic influences on the bronchiolar musculature, resulting in bronchospasm.[44]

Illnesses not traditionally thought to have prominent psychological factors in their etiology have been reconsidered recently from the psychosomatic viewpoint. These include Cushing's disease,[45] hyperuricemia and gout,[46] and diabetes mellitus,[47] to name only a few. In contrast, the traditional psychosomatic disease of ulcerative colitis is less and less thought to be psychologically determined.[11]

CONCLUSION

It appears that any attempt to make a distinction between psychosomatic illness and other illness, or functional psychiatric disturbance as opposed to organic psychiatric disturbance, is artificial. Life stresses of many sorts can affect the course of any illness. One must investigate not only the specific illness, in terms of the magnitude of its psychologic components, but also the specific brain mechanisms whereby psychologic factors become translated into physiologic and metabolic changes. By such a multivariate approach to the understanding of any given disease a more potent therapeutic rationale can be developed. For example, Shapiro has pointed out the futility of trying to subdivide the large diagnostic group of essential hypertensives into specific etiologic categories.[48] Rather, he indicates the need to consider hypertension in its total functional and dynamic sense and to utilize any and all therapeutic modalities that might offer benefit. A patient with labile essential hypertension might simultaneously require antihypertensive drugs, antianxiety agents, and a regimen of psychotherapy directed at helping him resolve some of the stressful psychologic pressures in his life. In the future, then, mutually supportive treatments for many illnesses may be directed at several levels of psychobiologic functioning, from the psychologic factors inherent in "mind," to the neurochemical factors inherent in "brain" to the peripheral pathophysiologic factors inherent in "body."

REFERENCES

1. Alexander FG, Selesnick, ST: The History of Psychiatry. New York, Harper & Row, 1966, pp 388–401
2. Kimball CP: Conceptual developments in psychosomatic medicine: 1939–1969. Ann Intern Med 73:307–316, 1970
3. Knapp, PH: Revolution, relevance and psychosomatic medicine: Where the light is not. Psychosom Med 33:363–374, 1971
4. Rubin RT, Gunderson EK, Arthur RJ: Life stress and illness patterns in the U.S. Navy. VI. Environmental, demographic, and prior life change variables in relation to illness onset in naval aviators during a combat cruise. Psychosom Med 34:533–547, 1972
5. Rahe RH: Life change and subsequent illness reports, in Gunderson EK, Rahe RH (eds): Life Stress and Illness. Springfield, Ill., Thomas, 1974, pp 58–78
6. Condon WS, Sander LW: Neonate movement is synchronized with adult speech: Interactional participation and language acquisition. Science 181:99–101, 1974
7. Weiner H: Presidential address: Some comments on the transduction of experience by the brain: Implications for our understanding of the relationship of mind to body. Psychosom Med 34:355–380, 1972
8. Schapiro S, Vukovich KR: Early experience effects upon cortical dendrites: A proposed model for development. Science 167:292–294, 1970
9. Money J. Ehrhardt AA: Man and Woman: Boy and Girl. Baltimore, Johns Hopkins University Press, 1972
10. Henry JP, Cassel JC: Psychosocial factors in essential hypertension: Recent epidemiologic and animal experimental evidence. Am J Epidemiol 90:171–200, 1969
11. Mendeloff AI, Monk M, Siegel CI, et al: Illness experience and life stresses in patients with irritable colon and with ulcerative colitis. N Engl J Med 282:14–17, 1970
12. Crisp AH: Some psychosomatic aspects of neoplasia. Br J Med Psychol 43:313–331, 1970
13. Medical Research Council Brain Metabolism Unit: Modified amine hypothesis for the aetiology of affective illness. Lancet 2:573–577, 1972
14. Shopsin B, Wilk S, Sathananthan G, et al: Catecholamines and affective disorders revised: A critical assessment. J Nerv Ment Dis 158:369–383, 1974
15. Jouvet M: The role of monoamines and acetylcholine-containing neurons in the regulation of the sleep-waking cycle. Ergeb Physiol 64:166–307, 1972
16. Wyatt RJ: The serotonin-catecholamine-dream bicycle: A clinical study. Biol Psychiatry 5:33–64, 1972
17. Goldstein M: Brain research and violent behavior: A summary and evaluation of the status of biomedical research on brain and aggressive behavior. Arch Gen Psychiatry 30:1–35, 1974
18. Geyer MA, Segal DS: Shock-induced aggression: Opposite effects of intraventricularly infused dopamine and norepinephrine. J Behav Biol 10:99–104, 1974
19. Martini L, Motta M, Fraschini F (eds): The Hypothalamus. New York, Academic Press, 1970
20. Rubin RT, Gouin PR, Poland RE: Biogenic amine metabolism and neuroendo-

crine function in affective disorders, in de la Fuente R, Weisman MN (eds): Psychiatry (Part II), Proc V World Congr Psychiat 1971, Amsterdam, Excerpta Medica, 1973, pp 1036–1039

21. Crisp AH: Anorexia nervosa: Feeding disorder, nervous malnutrition, or weight phobia? World Rev Nutr Diet 12:452–504, 1970

22. Mills IH, Wilson RJ, Eden MAM, et al: Endocrine and social factors in self-starvation amenorrhea, in Symposium on Anorexia and Obesity. Edinburgh, Royal College of Physicians of Edinburgh, 1973, pp 31–43

23. Bruch H: Eating Disorders: Obesity, Anorexia Nervosa, and the Person Within. New York, Basic Books, 1973

24. Papez JW: A proposed mechanism of emotion. Arch Neurol Psychiatry 38:725–743, 1937

25. MacLean PD: The limbic system ("visceral brain") in relation to central gray and reticulum of the brain stem: Evidence of interdependence in emotional processes. Psychosom Med 17:355–366, 1955

26. Rubin RT, Miller RG, Clark BR, et al: The stress of aircraft carrier landings. II. 3-methoxy-4-hydroxy-phenylglycol excretion in naval aviators. Psychosom Med 32:589–597, 1970

27. Mason JW: A re-evaluation of the concept of "non-specificity" in stress theory. J Psychiatr Res 8:323–333, 1971

28. Selye H: The evolution of the stress concept. Am Sci 61:692–699, 1973

29. Rubin RT, Mandell AJ: Adrenal cortical activity in pathological emotional states: A review. Am J Psychiatry 123:387–400, 1966

30. Mason JW: Organization of psychoendocrine mechanisms. Psychosom Med 30:565–808, 1968

31. Levi L (ed): Stress and distress in response to psychosocial stimuli: Laboratory and real life studies on sympathoadrenomedullary and related reactions. Acta Med Scand 191 (suppl 528):1–166, 1972

32. Rubin RT: Biochemical and neuroendocrine responses to severe psychological stress, in Gunderson EK, Rahe RH (eds): Life Stress and Illness. Springfield, Ill., Thomas, 1974, pp 227–241

33. Halberg F: Chronobiology. Annu Rev Physiol 31:675–725, 1969

34. Rubin RT, Gouin PR, Poland RE: Neuroendocrine correlates of sleep stages in man, in Pharmacology and the Future of Man, Proc 5th Int Congr Pharmacology, vol. 4. Basel, Switz., Karger, 1972, pp 124–133

35. Rubin RT, Poland RE, Rubin, LE, et al: The neuroendocrinology of human sleep. Life Sci 14:1041–1052, 1974

36. Kleitman N: Basic rest-activity cycle in relation to sleep and wakefulness, in Kales A (ed): Sleep: Physiology and Pathology. Philadelphia, Lippincott, 1969, pp 33–38

37. Solomon GF: Emotion, stress, the central nervous system, and immunity. Ann NY Acad Sci 164:335–343, 1969

38. Prehn RT: The relationship of immunology to carcinogenesis. Ann NY Acad Sci 164:449–457, 1969

39. Curtis GC: Psychosomatics and chronobiology: Possible implications of neuroendocrine rhythms: A review. Psychosom Med 34:235–256, 1972

40. Lund R: Personality factors and desynchronization of circadian rhythms. Psychosom Med 36:224–228, 1974

41. Voth HM, Holzman PS, Katz JB, et al: Thyroid "hot spots": Their relationship to life stress. Psychosom Med 32:561–568, 1970

42. Melander A, Ericson LE, Sundler F: Sympathetic regulation of thyroid hormone secretion. Life Sci 14:237–246, 1974

43. Folkow B, Neil E: Circulation. London, Oxford University Press, 1971, pp 560–583

44. Mathe AA: Decreased circulating epinephrine, possibly secondary to decreased hypothalamic-adrenal medullary discharge: A supplementary hypothesis of bronchial asthma pathogenesis. J Psychosom Res 15:349–359, 1971

45. Gifford S, Gunderson JG: Cushing's disease as a psychosomatic disorder: A report of ten cases. Medicine 49:397–409, 1970

46. Katz JL, Weiner H: Psychosomatic considerations in hyperuricemia and gout. Psychosom Med 34:165–182, 1972

47. Hong KEM, Holmes TM: Transient diabetes mellitus associated with culture change. Arch Gen Psychiatry 29:683–687, 1973

48. Shapiro AP: Essential hypertension—why idiopathic? Am J Med 54:1–5, 1973

David Shapiro

6
Biofeedback

VISCERAL LEARNING AND BIOFEEDBACK: ANIMAL RESEARCH

In 1969 *Science* published Neal Miller's landmark article entitled "Learning of visceral and glandular responses."[1] Miller challenged the conventional position that the autonomic nervous system and the responses that it regulates are inferior in learning potential to the cerebrospinal system and the skeletal motor responses under its control. The prevailing view was that autonomically innervated functions, such as heart rate, peripheral blood flow, and palmar sweating, were not capable of being modified by experience in the same fashion as somatomotor functions. Miller presented the results of a series of experiments with dogs, rats, and cats showing that various visceral and neural activities could be increased or decreased in frequency by techniques of relatively straightforward instrumental learning (operant conditioning).

The experimental arrangement used is identical with that employed in studies of the modification of simple skeletal motor responses, such as the pecking of a disk by pigeons or the pulling of a lever by monkeys. The animal is placed in a controlled environment in which various responses can be measured, recorded, and counted. Whenever the specified response of interest occurs—for example, a decrease in blood pressure, an increase in skin temperature, or an increase in blood volume—the animal is *reinforced*, typically with food, water, or other needed substances that it has been deprived of or by

The author's research discussed in this paper was carried out at the Massachusetts Mental Health Center, Harvard Medical School, and supported by Office of Naval Research Contract N00014-67-A-0298-0024 and NIMH Research Grant MH-008853.

escaping from or avoiding electric shock or other noxious stimulation.

In many of the experiments reported by Miller rats were injected with d-tubocurarine chloride in order to block responses of skeletal muscles; the reinforcer used was either electrical stimulation of so-called rewarding areas of the brain (median forebrain bundle) or shock escape and shock avoidance. The purpose of muscular paralysis was to eliminate the influence of purely peripheral effects of muscular activity on the autonomic responses being conditioned. In both curarized and noncurarized animals clear-cut results were obtained with such physiological functions as salivation, heart rate, intestinal contractions, rate of urine formation, gastric vasomotor changes, stomach contractions, peripheral vasomotor changes, systolic blood pressure, and electroencephalogram voltage.

The findings reported were very dramatic. The changes, which were obtained quickly, were large in magnitude and bidirectional. That is, both large increases as well as large decreases were observed. Moreover, the effects obtained appeared to be precisely *specific* to the responses that were reinforced. A good example of specificity is an experiment by DiCara and Miller.[2] They placed photocells on both ears of curarized rats and rewarded the animals for differences in the vasomotor responses of the two ears. Six rats rewarded for relative dilatation of the left ear showed dilatation in that ear and little change in the other ear. Similarly, six rats rewarded for dilatation of the right ear showed dilatation in that ear and decreases in the other. The learned differences in vasomotor activity between the two ears were not correlated with vasomotor changes in the two paws of the rats. Nor were they related to heart rate, vasomotor activity in the tail, or body temperature. The fact that specific visceral responses can be selectively reinforced while others do not change differentially added strength to the use of an instrumental learning model as applied to visceral functions.

However, the significance of much of the animal research has been called into question by reported difficulties in reproducing results of earlier experiments on heart rate control in curarized rats.[3, 4] This failure has been attributed to certain uncontrolled peripheral autonomic and central nervous system effects of curare and to the problem of maintaining stable artificial respiration. Moreover, curare does not affect the central nervous system linkage between cardiovascular and somatomotor functions. That is, both somatomotor *and* autonomic changes can be simultaneously elicited by the brain, but the peripheral skeletal motor activity cannot be observed because the muscles are paralyzed. Therefore, visceral learning under curare does not provide a critical test of the role of *central* somatomotor neural processes in the learning.[5] Nevertheless, further basic research in animals using surgical lesions and paralytic and various biochemical agents is needed to elucidate neural and biochemical mechanisms of visceral learning.

VISCERAL LEARNING AND BIOFEEDBACK:
HUMAN RESEARCH

The 1969 Miller article came at a time when evidence had already been accumulating on the modification of visceral and neural activities in human subjects. It served to reinforce the determination of investigators to continue basic and clinical human investigation. A brief review of the highlights of human research, much of which preceded the more highly controlled animal research to follow, should begin with the work of Kamiya on the voluntary control of the alpha rhythm of the EEG. In a summary of his early work Kamiya outlined his research strategy.[6] He started with the question, ''Can people be trained to discern the comings or goings of brain rhythms, say the EEG alpha rhythm, just by using the standard learning procedures that have been developed for use with rats and pigeons?'' He proceeded to study the degree to which people could tell whether the alpha rhythm was present or not in their EEG. He found that subjects with training could improve in their ability to discriminate their own alpha rhythm. The training consisted of subjects making guesses as to the presence or absence of alpha waves in their EEG and of subjects being informed as to whether or not they were correct. Subjects trained in this fashion could also subsequently produce alpha or nonalpha waves on command. Kamiya also found later on that subjects could be trained either to enhance or to suppress their alpha rhythm without prior discrimination training. In these demonstrations instrumental learning procedures were used. An electronic device would turn on a tone whenever the alpha rhythm was present. The subjects were simply told to keep the tone on as much as possible or to keep the tone off as much as possible. In this experiment success in the task of turning the tone on or off may be regarded as the reinforcer.

My own involvement in research on the operant conditioning of autonomic responses was stimulated by Razran's article entitled ''The observable unconscious and the inferable conscious in current Soviet psychophysiology'' published in the *Psychological Review* in 1961.[7] In this article Razran digested and interpreted vast Russian literature in the areas of interoceptive conditioning, semantic conditioning, and the orienting reflex. ''One striking Russian experiment on psychic or cognitive control'' was described in which five subjects were given prolonged and moderately painful stimulations, while changes in the volume of blood vessels of the arm were recorded with a photoplethysmograph. The typical response to the noxious stimulation was vasoconstriction. The experimenter (Lisina) arranged it so that any instance of the opposite response tendency, vasodilatation, would terminate the stimulation. This avoidance procedure, however, was effective *only* when subjects were able to watch their blood volume recordings, and not otherwise. Razran's summary of the importance of this experiment follows:

In terms of current American psychology, the experiment offers two key findings: that contrary to assertions, autonomic reactions can be modified by subsequent reinforcement in operant fashion, and that such reinforcement is effective only when cognition is present.[7]

This particular emphasis on cognition in the development of physiological self-regulation (that is, on subjects being able to watch their own physiological responses as they are occurring in order to "voluntarily" control these very responses) is one of the earliest scientific recognitions of the concept of "biofeedback."

Biofeedback means biological feedback, and in this area of research it entails providing to the individual a visual, auditory, or other type of sensory display or analogue of his own physiological responses just as they are occurring in time. The direct and immediate link in time between actual physiological response and sensory analogue is critical to the feedback concept. Note that such externalized feedback is channeled back into the central nervous system through normal sensory channels. There is also afferent feedback of visceral responses into the central nervous system through direct interoceptive pathways. This interoceptive information serves to regulate the natural functioning of visceral organs. For example, changes in blood pressure are registered by pressure receptors in blood vessels. This information is relayed to the brain, resulting in compensatory alterations of heart rate in order to return pressure to a preset level. Such homeostatic mechanisms are feedback systems that operate reflexively and unconsciously. Biofeedback may be considered to "augment" inherent feedback processes through external sensory pathways of which the individual is aware.[8]

Biofeedback stimuli and reinforcers in experiments on the operant control of physiological responses are functionally equivalent. They *both* are presented in precisely the same defined relation to the ongoing physiological responses. Operant conditioning formulations of physiological regulation are basically atheoretical, while biofeedback formulations depend on theories of voluntary control,[8, 9] motor skill learning,[10] and biological control systems.[11]

The Lisina example prompted my colleagues and myself to begin research on the operant modification of fluctuations in electrodermal activity, commonly called the galvanic skin response or GSR. The electrodermal response is typically considered a reflexive, automatic or "involuntary" response, and there is much research showing how it is related to attentional, emotional, and motivational variables.[12] The electrodermal response also occurs spontaneously in the individual, without being correlated with external stimuli. Unlike continuously varying biological functions such as heart rate or skin temperature, the fact that it is discrete lends it readily to operant analysis and experimentation.

One of our early studies is cited because it exemplifies many of the critical methodological issues in biofeedback research.[13] In this study a spontaneous fluctuation of palmar skin potential of a given amplitude was selected as the response to be brought under control. All subjects were told that the purpose of the experiment was to study the effectiveness of various devices for measuring thought processes. The subjects were also told that each time that our apparatus detected an "emotional thought" they would hear a tone and also earn a monetary bonus, the latter as a further incentive to concentrate on the task. One group of subjects was given rewards each time the skin potential response occurred. A second group was given the same number of rewards but at times when the response was absent. The first group showed increases in response rate relative to the second group, which showed decreases in response rate over time. The fact that the same reward could either enhance *or* diminish autonomic responses eliminated the explanation that the eliciting effect of the reinforcer itself could account for the observed differences.

In a subsequent study even an aversive stimulus (a very loud tone) was found to have differential effects on electrodermal responding, depending on its relation in time to the occurrence of the response.[14] The contingent presentation of a punishing stimulus *suppressed* the electrodermal response, while randomly pairing the aversive stimulus with the response or its absence resulted in sustained electrodermal activity. In other words, a noxious stimulus that would be expected to *enhance* autonomic nervous system activity ("emotional" behavior), in this case could be used to *diminish* it. This result clearly indicates the importance of *contingency* between external stimulus and ongoing physiological responses of the individual as a means of regulating these responses.

Another significant result emerged from the analysis of the study by Shapiro and his associates.[13] Learned variations in electrodermal response rate were found *not* to be associated with other physiologically related functions such as skin potential level and heart rate. Nor were the variations associated with differences in breathing rate or breathing irregularities. Cognitive factors, as measured by blind ratings of recorded postsession interviews, were not relevant to the observed effects. In the two experimental groups, one rewarded for increasing and the other for decreasing electrodermal responses, subjects reported the same moderate relationship between the reinforcer (tone indicating bonus) and their thoughts or ideation. The level of involvement in the task was also about the same for the two groups.

The fact that a given autonomic function could be either increased or decreased while other presumably related functions (somatomotor, autonomic, cortical) did not appear to covary was to be given a more comprehensive evaluation. It was reasoned that if other concurrent functions were in reality independent of or only slightly interrelated with the function to be learned, under natural or preexperimental conditions, then the dissociation of one from the others through conditioning should not be surprising.

This line of reasoning was followed closely in research in our laboratory on the operant control of human blood pressure and its association with heart rate and other variables. Subjects rewarded for increases or decreases in systolic blood pressure showed relative pressure changes in the appropriate direction without differential changes in heart rate.[15, 16] Similarly, subjects could learn to increase or decrease their heart rate without corresponding changes in systolic blood pressure.[16] Starting with these reports, a model for research and theory on the control of "multiautonomic" functions was elaborated.[17] It was hypothesized that if two functions such as heart rate and systolic blood pressure are very highly correlated, then when one is reinforced and shows learning, the other should do the same. If they are uncorrelated, however, then reinforcing one should result in learned changes in that function but not in the other. Furthermore, if feedback and reward are given for a given function and it shows learning, the degree to which other concurrent functions also show learning is informative about the natural interrelations of the functions to begin with. This model of autonomic learning is based on the measurement and analysis of the commonality of responses comprising a complex set of functions.

In an empirical test of the model Schwartz found that when subjects were reinforced for a *pattern* of simultaneous change in *both* heart rate and systolic blood pressure, these two functions could either be deliberately associated (both going in the *same* direction) or deliberately dissociated (going in *opposite* directions). The degree of association or dissociation was further limited by certain biological and adaptive constraints. Changes in the two functions —systolic blood pressure and heart rate—tend to be unrelated in pre-experimental conditions, confirming the ability to shape their association in different directions with feedback and reward. On the other hand, changes in diastolic blood pressure and heart rate tend to covary from heart beat to heart beat. In this case conditioning one system, diastolic pressure, resulted in associated changes in the other, heart rate, a finding that was clearly predictable on the basis of the commonality model.[18] Furthermore, it was not possible to make these two highly integrated functions go in opposite directions by deliberately reinforcing differential patterns.[19]

These basic data obtained in systematic human experiments provide a framework for extending principles of instrumental learning to visceral and glandular responses and for examining associated mechanisms involved in developing learned control. Current research in biofeedback is being directed to the evaluation of patterns of change in physiological self-regulation. Concern is being directed to the interaction of somatomotor, visceral, neural, and biochemical processes in such learning. Some behavioral studies in this field are oriented to personality factors and individual differences, the role of various instructional and cognitive variables, persistence of learned control over time, and generalization of learning from the laboratory to the real world. It is hoped that this basic research in humans will help facilitate clinical applications of the procedures. Hundreds of studies have been published, and many have been reprinted. [20–24] A number of major reviews and position papers have also been published. [8, 25–33]

CLINICAL APPLICATIONS OF BIOFEEDBACK

Applications of biofeedback techniques have grown rapidly since 1969. It is not possible in this brief review to describe them all. The appetite for clinical relevance and the quest for dramatic cures of psychophysiological disorders have far outstripped the detailed examination of physiological, behavioral, and medical issues involved in any particular application. The burgeoning field of biofeedback seems to touch on almost every topic imaginable. This is understandable because the approach of biofeedback is direct and deceptively simple. All that one needs to do is define the physiological function or pattern of responses relevant to the disorder in question, acquire or develop the appropriate physiological instrumentation, and provide a suitable method of displaying the information to the patient. Then it is up to the patient to practice developing control of his symptoms with the aid of the feedback. To illustrate the range of feedback applications under consideration, the program of the Biofeedback Research Society in 1974 included papers on the following topics: subjective tension, relaxation, stress reaction, hypertension, insomnia, smoking, aging problems, obesity, migraine, anxiety, psychotherapy, epilepsy, orgasm, tension headache, pain, bruxism, menstrual distress, mental retardation, social behavior problems, cerebral palsy, alcoholism, muscular rehabilitation, Raynaud's disease, arthritis, depression, gastric acid secretion, penile erection, personality changes, and rehabilitation in prisons. Most applications of biofeedback are not as yet buttressed by a reasonable amount of objective evidence concerning their effectiveness. From a positive standpoint it should be said that biofeedback methods have generated enormous interest in the possibility of extending the techniques and principles of learning and behavior modification into many different areas of medicine. The term ''behavioral medicine'' has been proposed for this new area of research and treatment. [32] The approach of behavioral medicine refers not only to a concern for behavioral factors in the etiology and treatment of defined psychosomatic disorders, but also to behavioral factors in medical disorders in general.

The most extensive and systematic clinical research to date has been on hypertension, cardiac arrhythmias, epilepsy, and tension headache. In each area major recent reports or current review articles will be cited where available and a brief statement made about the status of the research.

Hypertension

A number of studies reported that patients with essential hypertension,[28, 34] can reduce their blood pressure (systolic and/or diastolic) by 10 to 20 percent with blood pressure feedback training or with feedback for reduction in muscle tension. The effectiveness of these biofeedback procedures has been compared with that of other behavioral procedures such as meditation,[35] yoga practices,[36] metronome-conditioned relaxation,[37] and autogenic training.[38] Comprehensive data have not as yet been obtained on nonspecific placebo effects of training, the generalization of laboratory effects to real-life conditions, the degree to which training can affect circulatory responses to stress, and the persistence of change in long-term follow-up studies.

Cardiac Arrhythmias

Engel and his associates have reported positive clinical findings in a number of different cardiac arrhythmias: premature ventricular contractions, atrial fibrillation, Wolff-Parkinson-White syndrome, sinus tachycardia, supraventricular tachycardia, paroxysmal atrial tachycardia, and third-degree heart block.[39] In this research patients typically practiced a number of different biofeedback procedures, including raising or lowering heart rate, depending on applicability to the particular syndrome and patient. Engel employed two procedures in order to enhance self-control and persistence of the beneficial effects of training: (1) patients were trained *both* to increase and to decrease frequency of the abnormal rhythm, and (2) feedback was gradually withdrawn, and patients practiced control without it. The reports of Engel and his associates, based on intensive case analyses, are among the most convincing in the biofeedback field.

Epilepsy

Sterman and his associates have worked successfully with patients having different epileptic disorders—including petit mal, grand mal, and major motor symptoms.[40] Feedback was given for 12–14 Hz activity of the EEG, which is called the sensory-motor rhythm (SMR). The SMR is known to be associated with voluntary suppression of movement. With extensive training patients showed clinical improvement with fewer seizure symptoms, a decrease in abnormal low-frequency discharges in the EEG, and positive behavioral side effects—increased general awareness, improved ability to sustain attention, and better sleep. Work is continuing in Sterman's laboratory and in other laboratories to reproduce these findings, to determine whether the training effects can be made to last, to consider alternative explanations of the obtained findings, and to examine the physiological mechanisms involved. Again, the clinical case evidence for the potential of biofeedback in epilepsy is positive and promising of further advances.

Tension Headache

Excessive sustained contractions of facial, scalp, and neck muscles characterize tension headache. The biofeedback technique used in the Budzynski study was to give information to patients of their frontalis muscle electromyographic (EMG) activity.[41] In one of the better controlled studies in this field it was shown that patients receiving EMG training lowered their frontalis muscle tension levels below that of controls, and they also showed a significantly reduced level of headache activity both during and in a follow-up study.

While only four areas of application have been mentioned specifically, biofeedback and related procedures have been used extensively in a number of other areas of clinical interest. Reports on these applications are not complete enough to warrant extensive coverage here. The topics are migraine headache,[42] Raynaud's disease,[43] muscular rehabilitation,[44] and chronic anxiety.[45] Blanchard and Young[29] and Shapiro and Surwit[46] provide additional information on systematic clinical biofeedback research, case studies, and anecdotal reports.

BIOFEEDBACK IN CLINICAL PERSPECTIVE

Biofeedback techniques have evolved at a time when concepts and methods of behavior modification have begun to take hold in psychiatry and medicine. In behavioral modification the emphasis is placed on the careful definition and observation of the specific maladaptive or unwanted behaviors in question and on an analysis of the social and behavioral context in which the behaviors occur. The design of a treatment program or a plan of behavioral management must also consider the complete behavioral pattern of the individual. Particular attention should be given to reinforcers and other factors in the social milieu of the individual that are effective in maintaining the behavioral pattern, including the undesired activities. To alter behavioral patterns, social contingencies reinforcing the maladaptive response can be changed or other behaviors that compete with or are antagonistic to the problem reaction can be strengthened. Other procedures used by behavioral therapists take their inspiration from the experimental analysis of behavior and processes of learning. In addition, constitutional, biological, cognitive, or other causative factors need to be considered in the analysis of any given problem.

The basic and clinical research on biofeedback and visceral learning discussed above supports the extension of concepts and techniques of behavior modification to the control of physiological symptoms (or physiological responses) in psychosomatic or other disorders. Thus, it has been argued that the findings of visceral learning remove the major basis for assuming that autonomically mediated symptoms are fundamentally different from hysterical or psychogenic manifestations.[1] To date, there has been little research on instrumental learning factors in the formation of physiological symptoms. In work with animals attempts are being made to induce sustained hypertension using operant procedures. The results have been promising. Maintained elevations of 20–30 mmHg in blood pressure have been reported in the baboon.[47] Whether or not such an approach will prove to be effective in developing a behavioral causation of psychophysiological disorders remains a problem for further research. Moreover, behavioral causes do not operate in isolation from other factors in illness, such as constitutional or organ vulnerability that may predispose the individual to excessive response or reactivity of the system in question, for example, lability of blood pressure. Use or misuse of various drugs, medicines, tobacco, alcohol, and food must also be put into the equation.

Regardless of the etiology of physiological symptoms, the clinical evidence reported above suggests that biofeedback offers a viable approach to their control. Ideally, the symptom should be observed and measured as it occurs under natural life conditions. If at all possible, physiological monitoring devices should be used in this evaluation. With the development of miniature electronic devices this possibility is not as remote as it appears right now. For example, portable automatic blood pressure recorders have been developed that can monitor pressure around the clock.[48] Verbal reports of the patient or of other relevant observers may facilitate this evaluation. Of course, clinical measurements of the symptom and other relevant physiological activities, obtained under controlled laboratory conditions, can be used to complete this evaluation. Following this evaluation, the following issues need to be considered in designing a treatment program for the individual:

1. What is the patient's symptomatology? What is the frequency of the target response? What other physiological changes are associated with that response?

2. What physiological or other biological constraints, if any, appear to limit the potential for change?

3. What features of the patient's environment (reinforcers) appear to control the occurrence of the symptom? Are the symptoms under strict stimulus control, or are they manifested under a variety of situations?

4. What alterations in the patient's social environment would help diminish or extinguish the symptom?
5. What alterations in the patient's behavioral–physiological patterns would facilitate a diminution in the symptom and positive readaptation?
6. Should biofeedback techniques be used in the clinic to facilitate physiological self-regulation? If so, what is the appropriate measure or pattern of response for which feedback should be given? For example, in the case of hypertension it is known that many factors can affect blood pressure, e.g., respiration, cardiac output, cognitive factors, vasoconstriction or vasodilation, and so on. In early or labile hypertension, cardiac output or heart rate would be a reasonable target response, but in fixed hypertension a better alteration would be pressure itself or functions correlated with peripheral resistance.
7. If biofeedback is used, what methods can be employed to help the patient maintain the effects over time and develop effective self-control?

As in all clinical practice, a variety of factors can influence the effectiveness of biofeedback methods of treatment, for example, patient motivation, clarity of instructions and explanations about the techniques and treatment process, beliefs and expectations of the patient concerning the effectiveness of the treatment, general relationship of patient and clinician, and cooperation of the patient in performing the required practice sessions. It should be added that biofeedback methods may be combined with other behavioral techniques and with other methods of medical treatment commonly in practice.[28, 30, 46]

CONCLUSION

Biofeedback and operant conditioning techniques have achieved wide recognition as a promising new approach to the regulation of visceral, neural, and somatomotor processes. Supporting basic research in man suggests that a wide variety of normal physiological responses or patterns of responses can be altered. The clinical data obtained thus far on the modification of physiological symptoms of psychosomatic disorders, if not completely convincing at this stage of development of the field, appears highly promising. The most substantial research has evolved in disorders for which medical and physiological factors are precisely defined. The symptoms are shown to vary as the treatment is varied, and long-term and follow-up data have been collected. The lack of controls for nonspecific effects leaves open the question as to what effects are unique to biofeedback and what are not. Suitable controlled outcome studies are needed so that biofeedback methods can take their place alongside other accepted practices in medicine.

From the standpoint of consultation-liaison psychiatry the importance of biofeedback does not depend solely on its potential for the control of symptoms of well-known psychosomatic disorders. As an approach to *physiological* behavior modification, biofeedback concepts may also be relevant to the understanding and possibly to the regulation of physiological functioning in medical disorders in general. It may be speculated that the methods and concepts described in this chapter will be useful in facilitating physiological adaptation in general—overcoming adverse side effects of medication or treatment, increasing the speed of action and effectiveness of medication, improving the probability of recovery from surgery, and enhancing recovery processes in physical illness.

The translation of biofeedback into a form of "behavioral medicine" calls attention to the significance of behavioral and environmental processes in maintaining health, in preventing illness, and in facilitating treatment and recovery. The clinical and research potential of biofeedback will provide a further means of integrating behavioral sciences, biology, and medicine.

REFERENCES

1. Miller NE: Learning of visceral and glandular responses. Science 163:434–445, 1969
2. DiCara LV, Miller NE: Instrumental learning of vasomotor responses by rats: Learning to respond differentially in the two ears. Science 159:1485–1486, 1968
3. Miller NE, Dworkin BR: Visceral learning: Recent difficulties with curarized rats and significant problems for human research, in Obrist PA, Black AH, Brener J, et al (eds): Cardiovascular Psychophysiology. Chicago, Aldine, 1974, p 312
4. Brener J, Eissenberg E, Middaugh S: Respiratory and somatomotor factors associated with operant conditioning of cardiovascular responses in curarized rats, in Obrist PA, Black AH, Brener J, et al (eds): Cardiovascular Psychophysiology. Chicago, Aldine, 1974, p 251
5. Obrist PA, Howard JL, Lawler JE, et al: The cardiac-somatic interaction, in Obrist PA, Black AH, Brener J, et al (eds): Cardiovascular Psychophysiology. Chicago, Aldine, 1974, p 136
6. Kamiya J: Operant control of the EEG alpha rhythm and some of its reported effects on consciousness, in Tart C (ed): Altered States of Consciousness. New York, Wiley, 1969, p 489
7. Razran G: The observable unconscious and the inferable conscious in current Soviet psychophysiology: Interoceptive conditioning, semantic conditioning and the orienting reflex. Psychol Rev 68:81–147, 1961
8. Brener J: A general model of voluntary control applied to the phenomena of learned cardiovascular change, in Obrist PA, Black AH, Brener J, et al (eds): Cardiovascular Psychophysiology. Chicago, Aldine, 1974, p 365
9. Schwartz GE: Toward a theory of voluntary control of response patterns in the cardiovascular system, in Obrist PA, Black AH, Brener J, et al (eds): Cardiovascular Psychophysiology. Chicago, Aldine, 1974, p 406

10. Lang PJ: Learned control of human heart rate in a computer directed environment, in Obrist PA, Black AH, Brener J, et al (eds): Cardiovascular Psychophysiology. Chicago, Aldine, 1974, p 392

11. Mulholland T: Feedback electroencephalography, in Kamiya J, Barber TX, DiCara LV, et al (eds): Biofeedback and Self-Control: An Aldine Reader on the Regulation of Bodily Processes and Consciousness. Chicago, Aldine, 1971, p 305

12. Edelberg R: Electrical activity of the skin: Its measurement and uses in psychophysiology, in Greenfield NS, Sternbach RA (eds): Handbook of Psychophysiology. New York, Holt, Rinehart and Winston, 1972, p 367

13. Shapiro D, Crider AB, Tursky B: Differentiation of an autonomic response through operant reinforcement. Psychonomic Sci 1:147–148, 1964

14. Crider A, Schwartz GE, Shapiro D: Operant suppression of electrodermal response rate as a function of punishment schedule. J Exp Psychol 83:333–334, 1970

15. Shapiro D, Tursky B, Gershon E, et al: Effects of feedback and reinforcement on the control of human systolic blood pressure. Science 163:588–590, 1969

16. Shapiro D, Tursky B, Schwartz GE: Differentiation of heart rate and systolic blood pressure in man by operant conditioning. Psychosom Med 32:417–423, 1970

17. Schwartz GE: Voluntary control of human cardiovascular integration and differentiation through feedback and reward. Science 175:90–93, 1972

18. Shapiro D, Schwartz GE, Tursky B: Control of diastolic blood pressure in man by feedback and reinforcement. Psychophysiology 9:296–304, 1972

19. Schwartz GE, Shapiro D, Tursky B: Self-control of patterns of human diastolic blood pressure and heart rate through feedback and reward. Phychophysiology 9:270, 1972 (abstract)

20. Kamiya J, Barber TX, DiCara LV, et al (eds): Biofeedback and Self-Control: An Aldine Reader on the Regulation of Bodily Processes and Consciousness. Chicago, Aldine, 1971

21. Barber TX, DiCara LV, Kamiya J, et al (eds): Biofeedback and Self-Control 1970: An Aldine Annual on the Regulation of Bodily Processes and Consciousness. Chicago, Aldine, 1971

22. Stoyva J, Barber TX, DiCara LV, et al (eds): Biofeedback and Self-Control 1971: An Aldine Annual on the Regulation of Bodily Processes and Consciousness. Chicago, Aldine, 1972

23. Shapiro D, Barber TX, DiCara LV, et al (eds): Biofeedback and Self-Control 1972: An Aldine Annual on the Regulation of Bodily Processes and Consciousness. Chicago, Aldine, 1973

24. Miller NE, Barber TX, DiCara LV, et al (eds): Biofeedback and Self-Control 1973: An Aldine Annual on the Regulation of Bodily Processes and Consciousness. Chicago, Aldine, 1974

25. Schwartz GE: Biofeedback as therapy: Some theoretical and practical issues. Am Psychol 28:666–673, 1973

26. Blanchard EB, Young LD: Self-control of cardiac functioning: A promise as yet unfulfilled. Psychol Bull 79:145–163, 1973

27. Shapiro D, Schwartz GE: Biofeedback and visceral learning: Clinical applications. Semin Psychiatry 4:171–184, 1972

28. Schwartz GE, Shapiro D: Biofeedback and essential hypertension: Current find-

ings and theoretical concerns. Semin Psychiatry 5:493–503, 1973

29. Blanchard EB, Young LD: Clinical applications of biofeedback training. A review of evidence. Arch Gen Psychiatry 30:573–589, 1974

30. Shapiro D: Operant-feedback control of human blood pressure: Some clinical issues, in Obrist PA, Black AH, Brener J, et al (eds): Cardiovascular Psychophysiology. Chicago, Aldine, 1974, p 441

31. Miller NE: Applications of learning and biofeedback to psychiatry and medicine, in Freedman AM, Kaplan HI, Sadock BJ (eds): Comprehensive Textbook of Psychiatry. II. Baltimore, Williams & Wilkins, 1975

32. Birk L (ed): Biofeedback: Behavioral Medicine. New York, Grune & Stratton, 1973

33. Kimmel HD: Instrumental conditioning of autonomically mediated responses in human beings. Am Psychol 29:325–335, 1974

34. Shapiro D, Surwit RS: Biofeedback in the behavioral regulation of normal and high blood pressure. Fifth International Symposium on Behavior Modification, Caracas, Venezuela, 1974

35. Benson H, Rosner BA, Marzetta BR, et al: Decreased blood-pressure in pharmacologically treated hypertensive patients who regularly elicited the relaxation response. Lancet 7852:289–291, 1974 (vol 1)

36. Patel CH: Yoga and biofeedback in the management of hypertension. Lancet 7837:1053–1055, 1973 (vol 2)

37. Brady JP, Luborsky L, Kron RE: Blood pressure reduction in patients with essential hypertension through metronome-conditioned relaxation: A preliminary report. Behav Ther 5:203–209, 1974

38. Luthe W, Schultz JH: Autogenic Therapy, Medical Applications, vol 2. New York, Grune & Stratton, 1969

39. Engel BT, Bleecker ER: Application of operant conditioning techniques to the control of the cardiac arrhythmias, in Obrist PA, Black AH, Brener J, et al (eds): Cardiovascular Psychophysiology. Chicago, Aldine, 1974, p 456

40. Sterman MB: Neurophysiologic and clinical studies of sensorimotor EEG biofeedback training: Some effects on epilepsy. Semin Psychiatry 5:507–525, 1973

41. Budzynski TH, Stoyva JM, Adler CS, et al: EMG biofeedback and tension headache: A controlled outcome study. Psychosom Med 35:484–496, 1973

42. Sargent JD, Walters ED, Green EE: Psychosomatic self-regulation of migraine headache. Semin Psychiatry 5:415–428, 1973

43. Surwit RS: Biofeedback: A possible treatment for Raynaud's disease. Semin Psychiatry 5:483–490, 1973

44. Marinacci AA: The basic principles unerlying neuromuscular re-education, in Shapiro D, Barber TX, DiCara LV, et al (eds): Biofeedback and Self-Control 1972: An Aldine Annual on the Regulation of Bodily Processes and Consciousness. Chicago, Aldine, 1973, p 286

45. Raskin M, Johnson G, Rondestvedt JW: Chronic anxiety treated by feedback-induced muscle relaxation. Arch Gen Psychiatry 28:263–267, 1973

46. Shapiro D, Surwit RS: Learned control of physiological function and disease, in

Leitenberg H (ed): Handbook of Behavior Modification and Behavior Therapy, New York, Prentice-Hall (in press)

47. Harris AH, Gilliam WJ, Findley JD, et al: Instrumental conditioning of large magnitude, daily, 12-hour blood pressure elevations in the baboon. Science 182:175–177, 1973

48. Herd JA: Personal communication, 1974

Klaus D. Hoppe

7

Liaison Psychiatry and Psychoanalysis

The information explosion and the new kinds of knowledge in psychiatry, ranging from biophysics, genetics, and neurophysiology to sociology and cultural anthropology, represent a challenge and a threat. It is thus not surprising that psychiatrists, teachers and students alike, raise the question: "Why, after all, still psychoanalysis?"

Bandler enumerates several reasons for its downgrading. However, he believes "that psychoanalysis is still the method par excellence for gaining understanding of one's self."[1] Along with Pattison, he proposes "the maximum of psychoanalytic understanding" for residency training in community psychiatry.[2] West, in his brilliant essay on "The future of psychiatric education," emphasizes that the new biosocial approach "must be accomplished without yielding the hard-won expertise in psychodynamics that psychiatry has accumulated in the past 90 years."[3]

Yet, there is some danger in confusing psychodynamic psychiatry with psychoanalysis, particularly all of psychoanalytic theory. Prominent psychoanalysts like Loewenstein are aware how harmful the psychoanalytic model might be if applied to all diagnostic assessments and psychotherapeutic situations.[4] According to Kubie, the term "dynamic" implies the transition from description to explanation. Dynamic psychiatry means "an effort to find explanations of psychological events in the interactions among prior psychological experiences and their after-images."[5]

Dynamics are predominantly preconscious processes; they should be taught to the student in the form of a "maturational" experience.[6] If we teach dynamic psychiatry as developmental psychology, we shall facilitate learning by positive transference and by an appeal to the intellect. For the medical student a partial and testing identification with the teacher may enhance his ability for introspection and empathy with the patient and for dealing with his peers or colleagues who may be hostile to psychiatry.[7] For the psychiatric resident in addition we can help him overcome his nostalgia for his old medical identity and transform it into a more inclusive professional identity.[8, 9, 10]

These goals can be particularly well achieved in the setting provided by the consultation-liaison service. Not only leading psychiatric educators as Kaufman, Romano, and West, but also progressive psychoanalysts as Wallerstein and Pollack ask for a "hospital and teaching psychoanalyst" as well as a "liaison with the community" and the "application of psychoanalytic knowledge to medicine."[3, 11, 12, 13, 14]

It is the purpose of this chapter to describe the methods that have been developed to include consultation-liaison psychiatry as a component experience in learning dynamic psychiatry by medical students and residents and to touch upon the new psychoanalytic concepts and therapeutic developments that are perhaps *best* learned in the context of the consultation-liaison setting.

LEARNING DYNAMIC PSYCHIATRY IN THE LIAISON SETTING

According to my own experiences, it is impossible to focus upon mind and body simultaneously with the same attention and intensity, the tenable holistic theory notwithstanding. I, therefore, use in the teaching process a step-by-step approach from the physiological to the psychological level that repeats the sequence of a physical and mental examination. A sound basic knowledge in physiology and psychology helps to counteract the distress of an "emotional double-vision," which students and residents complain of and suffer from in consultation-liaison psychiatry. Rather often this double-vision is used for rationalizing the reluctance to empathize with, accept, and understand the emotional disturbances of the patient. The student's resistance against psychodynamic explanations and interpretations is partly due to the double-vision. The teacher, on the other hand, may feel overwhelmed by the wealth of physiological and psychological findings and the difficulty of a valid synopsis. In order to avoid his double-vision, he rationalizes that the case is "too complex" and unattainable for dynamic interpretations. The teacher may also accuse the student of resistance and countertransference, or he may escape into wild speculations that shatter the already bruised confidence of the student.

Ekstein and Wallerstein describe these difficulties on both sides in the learning odyssey of the psychiatric resident Dr. W and in the not less stormy endeavor of his supervisor.[9] After having lost two patients with psychophysiological illnesses, Dr. W was able to hold and to work with a third patient who was suffering from obsessions and a severe torticollis. Dr. W could finally clarify "his problems about learning" by formulating his "learning problems" in supervision. The complex interplay of the component aspects of the supervisory relationship is more and more understood by both sides and leads, thus, from "work for love" to "love of work."[15] The beneficiary of this development is not for the least part the patient.

INTERACTION BETWEEN DYNAMIC AND
LIAISON PSYCHIATRY

The new psychoanalytic concepts and therapeutic approaches of Kohut and Balint, as well as the new findings concerning "split-brain" people, cogently substantiate the value of viable interaction between dynamic and liaison psychiatry.[16, 17, 18]

Kohut shows that one important pathological feature of narcissistic personality disorders lies in the psychosomatic sphere. These patients react to narcissistic injuries with vasoconstriction in skin and mucous membranes and are more susceptible to infections and common colds. In regular illness there occurs a preoccupation with one's own body as a manifestation of increased narcissism. If a person with strong prenarcissistic fixations becomes physically ill, then the increase in body narcissism may bring a further regression toward a stage of beginning body–self fragmentation, and the person will react with hypochondriacal anxiety.

Kohut describes further a specific treatment of narcissistic personality disorders that mainly consists of "idealizing transference" and "mirror transference." It seems to me to be of utmost importance to teach our students these therapeutic modalities since they are based on empathic understanding and acceptance of narcissistic personalities who are not rare in medical practice.[16]

Balint's treatment of the regressed patient in the area of "the basic fault" is also specifically applicable to psychosomatic disorders.[17] Furthermore, Balint has developed brief psychotherapies, the so-called focal therapy and the flash therapy. In the focal therapy the doctor, like a good detective, first elucidates and then focuses upon the crucial conflict of the patient. In the flash therapy he is "tuned in" and identifies with the patient, which creates a "flash" in the therapeutic situation.[18, 19] In another paper Balint asks for two kinds of diagnoses, a traditional one and an overall diagnosis, of which the latter should comprehend the whole patient with all of his problems. "The overall diagnosis and the therapy based upon it will constitute true psychosomatic medicine."[20]

New inroads in psychophysiology have been made in connection with commissurotomies, a surgical procedure disconnecting the two cerebral hemispheres via a sectioning of the corpus callosum and the anterior commissure. Therapeutically, such surgery is designed to bring an end to epileptic seizures in patients who suffered from them with extreme frequency. A windfall for psychophysiology was the discovery that the two cerebral hemispheres seem to fulfill different functions. In right-handed people the left hemisphere has been found to verbalize logical abstract thinking, while the right hemisphere specializes in the perception of the spatial aspect of the gestalt as a whole.[21] The right hemisphere senses the forest, so to speak, while the left one cannot see the woods for the trees.

In my own observations of ten patients following commissurotomy ("split-brain" people) I found a quantitative as well as a qualitative paucity of dreams, fantasies, and symbolization. Hypothetically, this might be due to the interruption of a preconscious stream between the two hemispheres and the predominance of a feedback–free primary process in the right hemisphere.[22]

The French psychoanalysts Marty and de M'Uzan have described a similar impoverishment of fantasies, dreams, and affects in psychosomatic patients. They named this kind of thinking *pensée opératoire*.[23] Their findings have been confirmed by Nemiah and Sifneos.[24]

The similarity of operational thinking in psychosomatically ill patients and split-brain people has led me to hypothesize a "functional commissurotomy" in cases of severe psychosomatic disturbances.[22] Such a functional commissurotomy might anchor in psychophysiological terms the model of biphasic defense advanced by Mitscherlich. According to this model, psychosomatic patients at first suffer from a neurotic conflict. In the second phase of defense they regress further to the psychosomatic level and exhibit resomatization of affect.[25]

Following my hypothesis, the first phase of a neurotic process engages both hemispheres with defenses being mainly intrahemispherical. The second phase of defense mechanisms involves the transcallosal interhemispheric system (i.e., functional commissurotomy), thus blocking all emotions and gestalt perceptions of the right hemisphere from being verbalized by the left hemisphere. Instead, these emotions are hypercathected in the right hemisphere, leading to a resomatization of affect.[22]

The neurophysiological aspects of psychoanalysis seem especially fit for a translation of the language "Psychological" into the language "Physical," the main concern of consultation-liaison psychiatry.[26] A discussion of the above discoveries, inferences, and hypotheses with medical students and psychiatric residents is a particularly rewarding task in view of their keen skepticism coupled with inquisitive enthusiasm. As partners on an equal level, one can communicate and debate with them—*sine ira et studio*—because the teacher-student gap no longer exists.

This brief review of old and new psychoanalytic approaches and possibilities in medical education demonstrates that psychoanalysis is not dead—especially not in consultation-liaison psychiatry.

REFERENCES

1. Bandler B: Current trends in psychiatric education. Am J Psychiatry 127:585–598, 1970
2. Pattison E: Residency training issues in community psychiatry. Am J Psychiatry 128:1097–1107, 1972
3. West L: The future of psychiatric education. Am J Psychiatry 130:521–528, 1973
4. Loewenstein R: Psychoanalytic theory and the teaching of dynamic psychiatry, in Bibring G (ed): The Teaching of Dynamic Psychiatry. New York, International Universities Press, 1968, pp 104–114
5. Kubie L: Invited discussion, in Bibring G (ed): The Teaching of Dynamic Psychiatry. New York, International Universities Press, 1968, pp 118–122
6. Zetzel E: Invited discussion, in Bibring G (ed): The Teaching of Dynamic Psychiatry, New York, International Universities Press, 1968, pp 126–131
7. Hamilton J: Some aspects of learning, supervision and identity formation in the psychiatric residency. Psychiatr Q 45:410–422, 1971
8. Erikson E: Invited discussion, in Bibring G (ed): The Teaching of Dynamic Psychiatry. New York, International Universities Press, 1968, pp 247–251
9. Ekstein R, Wallerstein R: The Teaching and Learning of Psychotherapy. New York, International Universities Press, 1972
10. Allen A: A note on the making of a psychiatrist: The transition from resident to private practitioner. Psychiatry 34:410–418, 1971
11. Kaufman M: Psychiatry and medical education from the vantage point of 45 years. Am J Psychiatry 126: 1155–1157, 1970
12. Romano J: The teaching of psychiatry to medical students: Past, present and future. Am J Psychiatry 126:1115–1126, 1970
13. Wallerstein R: The future of psychoanalytic education. J Am Psychoanal Assoc 20:591–606, 1972
14. Pollock G: What do we face and where can we go? Questions about future directions. J Am Psychoanal Assoc 20:574–590, 1972
15. Ekstein R: Psychoanalytic pedagogy. Paper presented at the joint meeting of the Psychoanalytical Societies of Los Angeles, La Costa, California, April 1973
16. Kohut H: The Analysis of the Self. A systematic Approach to the Psychoanalytic Treatment of Narcissistic Personality Disorders. New York, International Universities Press, 1971
17. Balint M: The Basic Fault. Therapeutic Aspects of Regression. London, Tavistock, 1968
18. Balint M: Psychotherapeutische Forschung und ihre Bedeutung für die Psychoanalyse. Psyche 26:1–9, 1972
19. Loch W: The doctor-patient relationship in general practice: Implications for diagnosis and treatment. Psychiatry Med 3:365–370, 1972
20. Balint M: Medicine and psychosomatic medicine—new possibilities in training and practice. Compr Psychiatry 9:267–274, 1968
21. Sperry RW, Gazzaniga MS, Bogen TE: Interhemispheric relationships: The neocortical commissures; syndromes of hemisphere disconnection, in PT Vinkon,

GW Bruyn (eds): Handbook of Clinical Neurology, vol 4. North-Holland Publishing Company, Amsterdam, 1969

22. Hoppe KD: Die Trennung der Gehirnhaelften. Ihre Bedeuntung für die Psychoanalyse. Psyche (in press)
23. Marty P, de M'Uzan M: La pensée opératoire. Rev Francaise Psychoanalyse, Numero Special 27, Suppl 1345:346–356, 1963
24. Nemiah J, Sifneos P: Affect and fantasy in patients with psychosomatic disorders, in Hill O (ed): Modern Trends in Psychoanalytic Medicine 2. Appleton-Century-Crofts, New York, 1970
25. Mitscherlich A: Krankheit als Konflikt. Studien zur Psychosomatischen Medizin 2. Frankfurt, Suhrkamp, 1969
26. Graham D: Health, disease, and the mind-body problem: Linguistic parallelism. Psychosom Med 29:52–71, 1967

PART II

Psychiatric Liaison: The Troubled Marriage of Psychiatry and Medicine

Norman Q. Brill

Introduction

Psychiatrists have traditionally pointed to their medical training and competence as the major feature that distinguishes them from other mental health professionals. In recent years, however, many psychiatrists have abandoned the medical model in their approach to the diagnosis and treatment of emotional disorders. They have focused on the role of sociologic, economic, political, and legal factors in human development and maladjustment; simultaneously they have lost interest in biochemistry, physiology, and organic illnesses. Behavioral science has replaced biological science as the foundation of their professional practice.

As their identity as physicians has faded, psychiatrists have begun to regard physical examinations as odious and beyond their competence. Medical colleagues in other specialties often have reacted to them with contempt and wondered about whether they were real doctors. In the minds of the public the psychiatrist has become, understandably, indistinguishable from nonmedical mental health professionals. Questions have arisen about the necessity of medical training for psychiatrists and about the viability of psychiatry as a medical specialty.

Fortunately, for the patient, there are psychiatrists who do not abandon their identity as physicians. They do not subscribe to the abandonment of the medical model because a disorder is psychogenic. They recognize that the practice of medicine involves disorders of all kinds—infectious, neoplastic, degenerative, toxic, nutritional, genetic, traumatic, endocrinological, *and* psychogenic—and that in the diagnosis and treatment of a patient it is impossible and regressive to separate psyche and soma.

Foremost among this group are liaison psychiatrists, such as those who in this section describe their roles, contributions, and opportunities on the medical, surgical, obstetrical, gynecological, neurological, and neurosurgical services. In addition, they discuss their problems and suggest ways of overcoming them.

The skill and competence of the psychiatrist is tried most when the success or failure of his work with patients is readily apparent to his non-psychiatric colleagues, who are more impressed by results than theories. Moreover, psychiatrists have frequently been unfairly critical of the surgeon or internist who has failed to interest himself in patients' emotional problems or has failed to deal with these problems while defending their own disinterest in maintaining basic skills in diagnosis and treating organic disorders. The liaison psychiatrist can afford no such luxury. He recognizes the need to be conversant with the problems with which his nonpsychiatric medical colleagues are confronted. He cannot pretend to be omniscient and sit in judgment. He is a physician who, through personal contact, must earn the confidence and respect of his colleagues. He is not entitled to them just because he is a psychiatrist.

All of the foregoing should not be taken to mean that the current preoccupation with the ills of society and the looking to their elimination as the solution to the problems of mental illness will not have a beneficial effect. But it will be disappointing as far as *eliminating* emotional disorders is concerned. Those psychiatrists who have worked intensively with psychiatric patients have had the opportunity to see how much personal friction, unhappiness, and conflict exist within families that are *not* underprivileged and to note the divorces, alcoholism, drug abuse, psychiatric and psychosomatic disorders that result from these conditions.

Clinical psychiatry must maintain its medical-biological orientation along with its psychosocial one. These interrelationships are the basis of psychosomatic medicine. There is much to be learned about the biochemistry and physiology of emotional disorders. And as the complexities of society increase, so does the incidence of psychosomatic disorders. Study of the interrelation of mind and body becomes more, rather than less, important and the role of the liaison psychiatrist more critical.

This was recognized a long time ago and expressed with impressive clarity by John Reid in 1821. Part of his essay on "The influence of the mind on the body" is relevant for the liaison psychiatrist of today:

> He, who, in the study or the treatment of the human machinery, overlooks the intellectual part of it, cannot but entertain very incorrect notions of its nature, and fall into gross and sometimes fatal blunders in the means which he adopts for its regulation or repair. Whilst he is directing his purblind skill to remove or relieve some more obvious and superficial symptom, the worm of mental malady may be gnawing inwardly and undetected at the root of the constitution. He may be in a situation like that of a surgeon, who at the time that he is occupied in tying up one artery, is not aware that his patient is bleeding to death at another. Intellect is not omnipotent; but its

actual power over the organized matter to which it is attached is much greater than is usually imagined. The anatomy of the *mind*, therefore, should be learnt, as well as that of the body; the study of its constitution in general, and its peculiarities, or what may be technically called its idiosyncrasies, in any individual case, ought to be regarded as one of the most essential branches of a medical education.

The savage, the rustic, the mechanical drudge, and the infant, whose faculties have not had time to unfold themselves, or which (to make use of physiological language) have not as yet been *secreted*, may, for the most part, be regarded as machines, regulated principally by physical agents. But man, matured, civilized, and by due culture raised to his proper level in the scale of being, partakes more of a moral than of an animal character, and is in consequence to be worked upon by remedies that apply themselves to his imagination, his passions, or his judgment, still more than by those that are directed immediately to the parts and functions of his material organization. Pharmacy is but a small part of physic; medical cannot be separated from moral science without reciprocal and essential mutilation.

Such observations are more particularly apt to occur to one whose station of professional experience is established in the midst of an intellectual, commercial and voluptuous metropolis, the inhabitants of which exist in a state of more exalted excitement and irritative perturbation, than can be occasioned by the comparatively monotonous circumstances of rural or provincial existence. Over a still and waveless lake a boat may move along steadily and securely, with scarcely any degree of skill or caution in the pilot who conducts it; whereas on the agitated and uncertain ocean, it requires an extraordinary degree of dexterity and science to insure the safety of the vesset, and the proper and regular direction of its destined course. Thus the practice of medicine is reduced to a few simple rules in the country, and in hospitals; but it is obliged to multiply, to vary, and to combine its resources, when applied to men of letters, to artists, and to all persons, whose lives are not devoted to mere manual labor.*

For the liaison psychiatrist the task is to reconcile the medical-biological approach with the psychosocial one and to somehow present this comprehensive psychiatric view in a practical and meaningful way in the medical setting.

It is not surprising that such marriages are often troublesome and that the skill and patience of the liaison psychiatrist may be the critical variable in determining whether the outcome will be wedded bliss or acrimonious divorce.

*Reid J: The influence of the mind on the body, in Essays on Hypochondriasis and Other Nervous Affections. London, Longman, Hurst, Rees, Orme and Brown, 1821

Richard H. Rahe

8

A Liaison Psychiatrist on the Coronary Care Unit

As the field of medicine becomes increasingly complex, areas of specialization naturally arise. This volume illustrates that the trend toward specialization is evident in the field of psychiatric consultation today. Traditionally, departments of psychiatry designated a few residents and a part-time staff member to cover requests for psychiatric consultations arising from the general hospital inpatient, outpatient, and emergency room services. These psychiatric consultants spent their time racing from one end of the hospital to the other to see patients in some type of crisis. The consultants generally obtained little longitudinal follow-up on the patients they saw. In contrast, a specialization of the psychiatrist's experience to a single hospital area allows him to develop interviewing skills and therapeutic programs for a restricted range of patients—and thus he soon develops expertise. In these specialized hospital settings opportunities for patient follow-up are excellent.

It is of some interest to note that the hospital areas that afford the liaison psychiatrist greatest opportunities for service and research are those areas of highly developed medical or surgical technology. Coronary care units, intensive (surgical) care units, renal dialysis centers, burn units, and rehabilitation services are all examples of such areas. It seems that in these centers of technological sophistication patients' human needs are apt to be ignored. In ad-

Report No. 75-6, supported by the Bureau of Medicine and Surgery, Department of the Navy, under Research Work Unit MR041.06.01-0020B5CG. Opinions are those of the author and are not to be construed as necessarily reflecting the official view or endorsement of the Department of the Navy.

115

dition, the variety of physiological measurements routinely made on patients in these centers provides the liaison psychiatrist a ready opportunity to study psychophysiological phenomena.

This chapter has two aims—first, to present some important guidelines for the novice liaison psychiatrist (if the psychiatrist gets off on the ''wrong foot'' in his liaison role, he will experience significant difficulties achieving his potential in service and research) and, second, to give some examples of useful contributions that can be made by the liaison psychiatrist in terms of patient care and research. Though the topic is the liaison psychiatrist on the coronary care unit (CCU), many of the guidelines presented are equally applicable to a liaison psychiatrist working in other specialized centers of care in the hospital.

GUIDELINES FOR THE FIRST DAYS ON THE UNIT

You Must Know All Aspects of The Service

Prior to starting his CCU service, the liaison psychiatrist should first meet with the medical director of the unit and request an introduction to the service much as would be done if he (the psychiatrist) were a third-year medical student. This approach allows the psychiatrist to be brought up to date on the technical advances that have occurred since he was last on a medical ward. In addition it allows him a few days of strict orientation without any expectations placed upon him to provide expert opinion.

During his orientation the psychiatrist should observe and note key interpersonal relationships with which he must subsequently deal. For example, the senior physician–junior nurse relationship is frequently a mutually satisfying one characterized by a technically knowledgeable, competent, and somewhat paternal cardiologist dealing in a kindly, teaching fashion with young, bright, receptive nurses. The senior nurse–junior physician relationship, however, can pose some problems. As the senior nurse is frequently a highly trained and extremely competent specialist (in contrast to her more administrative-minded senior nurse counterpart on the medical wards), she is frequently frustrated by the constant influx of interns and junior residents in need of training. To make matters worse, these junior physicians often spend but four to six weeks on the CCU before rotating to another service. Thus, the senior nurses may see these physicians as short-term intruders with an enormous potential for interfering with the smooth and competent functioning of the service.

It is extremely important that the liaison psychiatrist pay particular attention to the rounds schedule and other teaching sessions carried out on the CCU.

Early morning rounds are *the best time* for the psychiatrist to meet with the full medical ward staff, to become acquainted with newly admitted patients, and eventually to make pertinent suggestions regarding psychological aspects of patients with coronary heart disease (CHD). On occasion, the psychiatrist will identify problem-laden and/or potentially troublesome patients on the morning rounds. He can then interview these patients later that day, without waiting for a crisis to develop and formal psychiatric consultation to be requested.

In Order to Teach, You Must Be Prepared to Learn

A crucial question the liaison psychiatrist should ask himself before offering his services on a CCU is whether or not he is truly interested in what is being done there. Once the liaison psychiatrist shows an interest to learn, it is an easy step for him subsequently to offer to share his psychiatric knowledge with the CCU staff. A further reason that he should be conversant with the medical interests of personnel on the CCU is so that he can impart to the staff psychiatric concepts phrased in their "language." For example, rather than saying "I feel this patient's unresolved hostility may interfere with his treatment plan," the liaison psychiatrist might "translate" such a statement as follows: "Think of the effect on this patient's norepinephrine output if he continues to feel so angry."

To achieve acceptance by the CCU staff, the liaison psychiatrist does not need to have literally a stethoscope dangling from his pocket. However, he should consider the nonverbal communication implied by his appearance. The fact that many departments of psychiatry allow their residents to dress as if they were about to embark on a fishing trip has little bearing on how the liaison psychiatrist should appear on the CCU. If a shirt, tie, and a white lab coat are included in the standard of dress on the CCU, it is advisable to follow suit if the psychiatrist wishes to deal readily with staff, patients, and relatives.

See the CCU from the Patient's Perspective

Staff–patient interactions are largely influenced by how the patient perceives his illness. Patients with CHD have been described by several authors to show a notable capacity for minimizing, repressing, and otherwise ignoring the significance and limitations of their illness.[1, 2, 3, 4] Such patients are frequently labeled "uncooperative" by the nurses; they resist following orders, will not remain at bed rest during the early stages of their illness, and frequently wish to carry on their usual business and personal transactions while on the unit. In addition, patients on the CCU are generally males in their forties and fifties who receive close, daily, physical care from young, often attractive, female nurses. Problems related to patient or staff sexual tensions frequently occur.

Much of the patient's behavior is understandable once the psychiatrist views the CCU experience from the patient's point of view. Rather than being "uncooperative," patients are often trying to show self-sufficiency. Overt flirtations may serve to repress thoughts of their recent brush with death. Of major interest is the finding that this "denial" of illness by some patients is associated with lower morbidity rates than that seen for "nondeniers."[5]

Spending time with CCU patients during interviews opens the psychiatrist's eyes to the several inconveniences that patients experience—such as daily weighings, blood draws, medication schedules, rounds, and on and on. Many of these routines are timed for the convenience of the staff (like weighings at 5:00 A.M.) rather than for the patient. Reasons for daily blood draws and medication changes are often not given to the patient. For patients who like efficiency and explanation the CCU can be a very frustrating environment.

Beware of Nurses

The liaison psychiatrist should be alert in his dealings with the CCU nurses. To be an effective counselor when nurse–physician problems arise, the psychiatrist should strive to remain objective. Frequently nurses will invite the psychiatrist to attend nursing conferences where personnel problems are discussed. At first this seems a good chance for the psychiatrist to exercise his group therapy skills. Later, however, the nurses may ask him to carry their problems to the medical staff. Worse yet, he may find himself being "quoted" by senior nurses to younger, more independent-minded nurses, in order to keep them in line. On the other hand, the psychiatrist–nurse relationship is central to much of the success of the liaison psychiatrist. The nurses are the ones who generally have to deal with patients' psychological problems. They are also the ones who carry out the psychiatrist's suggestions on patient management. Thus, the psychiatrist should strive to develop rapport with the nurses, but he should beware of becoming their agent.

CONTRIBUTIONS TO PATIENT CARE AND RESEARCH

Patient Care

The psychiatrist will soon become engaged in the day-to-day problems of patient care. In the recent past a liaison psychiatrist had to deal with patients' psychological problems regarding their adjustment to the unusual surroundings of a CCU. Such problems of patient adjustment have undergone remarkable dimunition since 1960 with modernization of the CCU and with increased use of tranquilizing medications.

When coronary care units were first instituted in the general hospital, a few beds and a great deal of electronic cardiac monitoring equipment were frequently crowded into an out-of-the-way corner on a medical ward. Two to four patients shared the same room, and the proximity of patients and staff made the problems of one quickly apparent to the other. Cardiac emergencies were a frenzy of activity and patients were constantly reminded of the potential lethality of their disease.[5] Psychological problems of patients in these early CCUs have all but disappeared in the relatively spacious, modern CCUs of today. Patients frequently have private rooms and are relatively isolated from emergency medical procedures required by other CCU occupants. In addition, patients spend fewer days on the CCU prior to their transfer to the ward than was previously the case. Perhaps most important in reducing psychological problems of acute cardiac patients has been the trend for cardiologists to prescribe relatively high doses of tranquilizing medications. Thus, CCU patients spend their two to three days on the unit in a state of drowsiness very close to sleep. Patients medicated in this way are often amnesic for their CCU stay when later interviewed on the ward.

With some exceptions, the liaison psychiatrist will normally meet with cardiac patients after they have medically stabilized and are ready for transfer to the ward. Most of the patients will have suffered a myocardial infarction (MI), a disease entity about which these patients have little knowledge. The psychiatrist may find himself the recipient of several questions concerning this illness. For example, patients may wish an explanation in lay terms of "what is a heart attack." They may express concern about routine blood draws, emergency oxygen equipment, enforced bed rest, and so forth. To answer these questions systematically, it is best to assemble some type of a CHD information booklet. Anatomical illustrations of the heart and the coronary arteries can be included in order to talk meaningfully to the patient about his disease. Separate sections of the booklet should deal with CCU emergency equipment, diet, and smoking, the gradual resumption of physical activity following a MI, and so forth. The liaison psychiatrist could add a separate section dealing with persons' life stress and behavior characteristics associated with CHD.[4, 6, 7]

There are several benefits of such a CHD booklet. Patients receive a consistent, systematized presentation of information important for their rehabilitation. They can study the booklet at their own pace. The booklet encourages patient-staff interactions in terms of asking questions and assessing comprehension of the material. The booklet can also be given to the patient's spouse or near relative for his or her educational needs. Finally, the booklet tends to emphasize that several, rather than just one or two, physical and psychological adjustments are required for optimal rehabilitation from MI.

Research

Another attraction of the liaison psychiatrist experience in the CCU is the ample opportunities for the psychiatrist to become involved in research. Research problems that invite psychiatric attention are those of patient (and family) education and longitudinal studies of efforts toward rehabilitation. For example, on the CCU at the University of California Los Angeles University Hospital we wished to assess our patient education program, which utilized a CHD booklet. To accomplish this evaluation, a CHD teaching-evaluation questionnaire was created.[8] Questions were composed regarding what is a "heart attack," reasons for various CCU emergency equipment, potentially harmful dietary and smoking habits, resumption of physical activity following an MI, psychological factors important for persons with CHD, and problems related to returning home and to work following hospitalization. Patients were given the questionnaire immediately prior to receiving the CHD booklet—usually about the third hospital day. Analysis of the answers provided an estimate as to how much knowledge each patient had in these areas before receiving the booklet. The same questionnaire was readministered between the fourteenth and eighteenth hospital day, shortly prior to hospital discharge. These scores when compared to the scores for the first "test" helped us to evaluate how much had been learned from the booklet.[8]

When we analyzed the responses on both questionnaires for the first 25 patients, we discovered several areas where patient learning could be improved.[8] Despite a high degree of enthusiasm for the teaching program shown by both patients and staff, sections of the CHD booklet were not being read and/or understood. The results of this questionnaire study stimulated the staff to make several modifications in the patient education program. A dietition was invited to spend time on the ward and to hold occasional discussions with patients and their spouses. The liaison psychiatrist initiated patient and spouse group therapy discussions. A special rounds was started by the senior cardiologist and the nursing staff to discuss with the junior medical staff medical and psychological preparations of their patients for hospital discharge. A follow-up clinic was instituted where all discharged post-MI patients were scheduled to return for periodic checks on their understanding and compliance with rehabilitation schedules.

A second example of research inspired by work on CCUs was done at the U.S. Naval Hospital in San Diego.[7, 9] This experiment consisted of establishing two randomly composed groups of discharged post-MI patients. Both groups of patients received identical medical follow-up care, but one group received in addition a series of six group therapy sessions over the first three months following hospital discharge.[7]

During the first few group therapy meetings patients were encouraged to discuss their recent life stress and illness patterns as well as to assess whether or not they displayed various behaviors and attitudes reportedly associated with CHD.[4, 6] As the series of group therapy sessions progressed, patients having difficulties complying with their rehabilitation regimens frequently became the focus of discussion. In addition, since the patients were recuperating at home for a month or more following hospital discharge, their relationships with family members became a common theme of discussion. Toward the end of the group therapy sessions, a few patients had resumed work. Here, it was appropriate for the group to search out ways in which these patients might avoid or modify previously identified work stresses and/or difficulties with colleagues. Group therapy subjects completed the CHD teaching evaluation questionnaire after their series of sessions. These patients showed significantly greater knowledge about an MI and optimal rehabilitation than did members of the control group who completed the same form.[9]

Group therapy and control patients have now been followed since 1972.[9] Follow-up data have included patients' readmissions to hospital for all causes. Group therapy patients have returned to the hospital for episodes of coronary insufficiency at one-third the rate seen for control group patients. In terms of reinfarction, group therapy subjects have experienced one-fifth the reinfarction rate seen for control subjects. Follow-up interviews also evaluate various ''softer'' criteria for successful rehabilitation, such as incidence and prevalence rates for angina pectoris, medication usage, return to work percentages, and psychological adjustment.

IN CONCLUSION

This chapter presents examples of both initial difficulties and subsequent rewards peculiar to the liaison psychiatrist experience. If the psychiatrist can avoid early pitfalls inherent in this specialized experience, his potential for patient care and research experience greatly exceeds that which he might obtain through the conventional psychiatric consultant experience. As a specialized liaison psychiatrist, he rapidly develops diagnostic and therapeutic expertise that comes from seeing a restricted type of patient. Aside from soon making day-to-day contributions in patient care, the liaison psychiatrist may eventually help shape ward policy and design research investigations important in the longitudinal care of postinfarction patients.

REFERENCES

1. Rosenman RH, Friedman M: Behavior patterns, blood lipids, and coronary heart disease. JAMA 184:934–938, 1963
2. Hackett TP, Cassem NH: Factors contributing to delay in responding to signs and symptoms of acute MI. Am J Cardiol 24:651–658, 1969
3. Croog SH, Shapiro D, Levine S: Denial among male heart patients. Psychosom Med 33:385–397, 1971
4. Romo M, Siltanen P, Theorell T, et al: Work behavior, time urgency and life dissatisfactions in subjects with myocardial infarction: A cross-cultural study. J Psychosom Res 18:1–8, 1974
5. Hackett TP, Cassem NH, Wishnie, H: The coronary care unit: an appraisal of its psychological hazards. N Engl J Med 279:1365–1370, 1968
6. Rahe RH, Romo M, Bennett LK, et al: Recent life changes, myocardial infarction, and abrupt coronary death. Studies in Helsinki. Arch Intern Med 133:221–228, 1974
7. Rahe RH, Tuffli CR, Suchor RJ, et al: Group therapy in the outpatient management of post-myocardial infarction patients. Int J Psychiatr in Med 4:77–88, 1973
8. Rahe RH, Scalzi C, Shine K: A teaching evaluation questionnaire for post-myocardial infarction patients. Heart & Lung (in press)
9. Rahe RH, O'Neil T, Arthur RJ: Brief group therapy following myocardial infarction. Eighteen-month follow-up of a controlled trial. Int J Psychiatry in Med (in press)

Joshua S. Golden

9

The Surgeon and the Psychiatrist: Special Problems in Psychiatric Liaison

In the course of training psychiatrists to consult on the various wards and services of a general hospital, two observations were made repeatedly: the surgical services had a great need for psychiatrists, and psychiatric residents avoided those services with inspired ingenuity. The paradox is understandable in terms of the feelings of the resident psychiatrist. Although he has usually progressed far enough in his training to be able to recognize the fear, despair, and suffering of patients with surgical diseases, he is also far enough removed from any formal medical training to feel insecure and inadequate about his basic surgical knowledge. He may prefer a milieu like internal medicine or pediatrics where his area of competence, psychological medicine, is valued and respected.

Aware of the stereotyped attitudes that surgeons hold about psychiatrists, the latter expect and receive ridicule and neglect when they appear, unsolicited, on a surgical ward. When they persist in their efforts to establish liaison, they find their long hours on the wards are lonely. The surgeons are rarely there when the psychiatrists are. Surgical rounds begin traditionally very early, and then the staff is in the operating room until late in the day, by which time the psychiatrist is ready to leave. The nurses, patients, and supporting staff in the surgical service deal at first hand with the many psychiatric problems of patients, and they are eager to use the psychiatric consultant. But the consultant expects to be dealing on a peer level with surgical colleagues who will appreciate and esteem him. All too often he is disappointed. In addition, he grows resentful, both of his own rejection and of the neglect and insensitivity shown by the surgeons toward the psychiatric aspects of patient care.

For the psychiatric consultant, providing liaison to a surgical unit is one of the toughest assignments that he can face. The dying patient may create more anguish in the psychiatrist, but then it stems from identification with the problems of the patient. On a surgical unit the psychiatrist's main problems are his interactions with the physician, not with the patients. Surgery has made dramatic progress in recent decades. Open-heart operations are now common-place and organ transplants no novelty. However, the technical complexity of new procedures, based necessarily on new knowledge, has not narrowed the gulf between surgeon and psychiatrists. If anything, advances in surgical technology have led, for good reasons, to greater differences between them.

PSYCHODYNAMIC SOURCES OF CONFLICT
BETWEEN SURGEONS AND PSYCHIATRISTS

The psychiatrist usually feels unliked in a surgical setting. The raillery and banter that occur among physicians is an indication of the attitudes that they hold toward one another. Commonly, the surgeons view nonsurgeons with disdain. The most disdain is directed toward the "shrinks" or the "spooks," as the psychiatrists are called. The same processes occur among psychiatrists. Their own behaviors, adapted to make them feel worthy and secure, lead them to depreciate those who are unlike them.

Surgeons, as a group, are very unlike psychiatrists. In most areas the two specialties are different, for example, training involved, diseases treated, therapies employed. Their major common area of concern, of course, are the human beings with human problems of pain, suffering, and fear whom they both treat.

Not all their differences are due to the requirements of the specialty or the training that they receive after medical school. Study of the personality charac-teristics of medical specialists shows consistent differences among them, which can be identified before the first day of medical classes. Surgeons are assertive, active, not given to intellectual concerns. Psychiatrists are thoughtful, de-liberating, more inclined to intellectual and artistic interests.[1, 2] The two groups have different values, different interests, different tasks, and different ap-proaches to the solution of those tasks. The patient and his reactions to his illness and surgical treatment are their common concern. To be effective as a consultant to surgeons, a psychiatrist must first be able to understand the surgeon and himself. Then he can address himself to the problems of his patients.

Bigotry—whether it is prejudice involving a different religion, a different race, or different groups of medical specialists, has the same roots in all areas—ignorance. Ignorance of the other group's language and customs permits the bigoted person to attribute qualities and attitudes to the object of his prejudice that the latter may or may not have. The ubiquitous feelings of insecurity and inadequacy we all possess are projected onto the object of our bias. Surgeons suspect that psychiatrists can "read their minds." Psychiatric residents, uncertain of their knowledge generally—and knowledge of surgery particularly—are extremely sensitive to the hints of criticism that they feel from the surgeons. Both groups seek to enhance their self-esteem by beliefs and behaviors that demean the other group. The experience of being ridiculed and demeaned augments the feelings of inadequacy in the object of prejudice, who reacts with hostility and resentment toward his perceived antagonist. The result is to add fuel to a smoldering fire that destroys understanding and cooperation between the two parties. The patient, as usual, is the one who suffers most.

THE BASES OF SUCCESSFUL COLLABORATION

Another approach to understanding what is wrong between surgeons and psychiatrists is to examine the successful collaborations. On those rare occasions when a psychiatric resident has opted to consult on a surgical ward, one usually finds that the psychiatrist has previously established a friendship with someone on the surgical staff. Occasionally there will be a psychiatrist who once considered surgery as a career choice or, even less commonly, a psychiatrist who has had some prior surgical training. Previous experience indicates interest, surely, but also suggests a sense of competence with the field, which most psychiatrists have lost in direct proportion to their years out of medical school. Their familiarity with the field of surgery, and with surgeons, stands in clear contrast to the relative ignorance and resultant insecurity and defensiveness of most psychiatrists on surgery.

Some of the successful liaisons have resulted from consultants who, in effect, "brought the mountain to Mohammed." Rather than defensively withdrawing into pique because the surgeons did not request consultations or tender respect or friendship, some psychiatrists left the comfort of their own offices to seek out the surgeons. When they were not available on the wards, the psychiatrists would wait with them in the scrub rooms while surgeons were between cases. A particularly dedicated and enterprising resident scrubbed and assisted in the operating room regularly until he earned the interest, respect, and friendship of the surgical staff. Other successful liaison practices have included wearing the "white coats" and uniforms of surgeons rather than the more individualistic garb of the psychiatrist. Carrying a stethoscope, examining patients on rounds, and, in general, acting like a surgeon have been effective means of establishing a good liaison relationship.

The practices described point to certain principles that are fundamental to successful collaborations on any service. The ignorance of another person's language and customs and his unfamiliarity with yours can lead to prejudice, hostile projections, and ineffective liaison. By actions that make two groups familiar with one another, the ignorance necessary for the development of prejudice is diminished. The feelings of inadequacy surgeons feel toward psychiatrists are lessened by the behavior of psychiatrists who act as if they believe that what surgeons do is interesting and important. The opportunity to spend time together permits the development of a personal relationship. It is harder to project feelings of disinterest, ignorance, and hostility, even onto a psychiatric resident, if he does what you do, shows interest in you and your work, and demonstrates competence in doing it. The consultant should realize that he may need to establish a personal relationship that he may not want in order to establish a professional relationship that he desires. It is also important that the psychiatrist not react with anger and defensiveness when he meets with indifference or rejection from his professional associates. Often patients react toward psychiatrists with "transference" feelings of anger or frustration, which are more appropriately directed toward persons in their past life. The psychiatrist should learn to react with the same equanimity he shows to patients when he is treated in the same way by hostile colleagues.

Often one encounters a particularly vociferous antagonist on the surgical staff. He leads his fellows in denigrating psychiatry and psychiatrists. He would be the loudest critic of a nurse or medical student who might request a psychiatric consultation for a patient. Probably, he would be the surgeon most conspicuously insensitive to the emotional distress of his own patients, treating them coldly but, in surgical terms, efficiently. Such doctors are the most defensive. Should a liaison psychiatrist succeed in establishing a secure relationship with the surgical staff, and with his most vigorous prior antagonist, he may make an obvious discovery. The antagonistic surgeon may have been fearful that his personal emotional problems would have been apparent to the psychiatrist. His need to deny that patients have significant emotional problems is a need to deny his own. Frequently, the surgeon is well aware of his personal problems. He may be concerned that the psychiatrist, upon discovering his faults, would ridicule him or expose him to his surgical colleagues. Once he establishes a friendly relationship with a psychiatrist who accepts him with his faults, real and imagined, and who neither betrays nor humiliates him, he no longer needs to be as defensive. Once these essential conditions exist, true and effective liaison can follow.

WORKING CONDITIONS A BASIS FOR
ANTAGONISM

In what has been written to this point the psychodynamics of the surgeon and psychiatrist have been examined for sources of their mutual problems in establishing a comfortable working relationship. Not all of their problems are intrapsychic, however. Real, external difficulties exist also. The circumstances of their respective training programs and their respective professional practices also create differences. For example, the practice of psychiatry is generally predictable, with scheduled appointments, few emergencies, and rare nights and weekends on call, unless the psychiatrist chooses to work in an acute hospital setting with violent and suicidal patients. On the surgical services hours are long, emergencies are common, and one is never "off call." The surgeon sees his family rarely, spends his working hours under constant pressures, including, in many well-regarded training programs, a rigidly hierarchical system that treats junior trainees with aloofness and disrespect. Whether because of the conditions just described or merely as a consequence of being in a student's status for so many years, surgical residents (and psychiatrists too) develop substantial resentments. If the surgical neophytes were to express their feelings toward their residency program directors or toward their choice of a surgical career, per se, the consequences might be painful. They could either jeopardize their already vulnerable status in the program or face the painful decision to make a career change. Given this situation, the accumulated resentments are often displaced onto less dangerous objects. The psychiatric consultants serve admirably for such a purpose. They appear to be less overworked; their training programs are not usually so demanding or hierarchically structured; they spend more time away from the hospital, either with family or friends or in study; and—perhaps too frequently from the surgeon's standpoint—they do not look, talk, or act like doctors. As previously mentioned, they dress differently, talk in their own obscure jargon, and do not physically touch patients. The end result for the surgeons is envy, suspicion, and resentment directed toward psychiatrists. In addition there are displaced resentments accumulated from other sources, but not comfortably expressed.

The solution to this problem can be in making surgeons aware that psychiatrists are physicians too who can make positive contributions toward improved patient care. The more experienced and secure surgeons, i.e., senior residents and program directors, have come to know this. Unfortunately, except for the example of model that they provide for their younger trainees, their attitudes toward psychiatric consultation are not passed along to the surgical residents who have direct contact with the patients and psychiatric consultants. The liaison psychiatrist has to be highly motivated to succeed in a surgical service. He must be well prepared for the probable initial neglect and rejection that he will experience. He should realize that he must create an awareness of his potential usefulness and a receptive climate in order to be allowed to practice his tenuous skills in liaison on a surgical service. This can be accomplished, in part, by his zeal, interest in surgery and surgeons, and his outgoing, friendly nonthreatening and nondefensive behavior. To repeat what has been implicit in the previous discussion, the liaison psychiatrist should behave as much like a surgeon and as little like a psychiatrist as he can.

METHODS OF ESTABLISHING LIAISON

Most psychiatrists beginning their liaison training on a surgical service find this extremely difficult. Their personality characteristics, interests, training, and peer group values are all focused on supporting them in establishing an identity as a psychiatrist. To put these aside and take on a different image in order to struggle through to establish a liaison with surgeons who seem not to want it, is very hard for liaison psychiatrists to do, particularly the neophytes who are unsure of their own abilities and are trying to learn a job and do a job at the same time. It often seems easier to retire to the safer and more secure consulting rooms and conferences of the psychiatrists. The result is that liaison is not established. Both parties to the possible collaboration are successfully protecting themselves against imagined injury; nothing is learned, and patient care suffers.

One solution to this problem is for the psychiatrist, eagerly seeking acceptance of his role and his skills, to turn from the surgeons who may ignore him to the nurses who may adore him. Nurses have to deal, at firsthand, with the anxious, uncooperative, psychotic, depressed, addicted, or dying patients. They cannot delegate those responsibilities, as physicians do, to anyone below them on the pecking order. They need the psychiatrist—not only for his help, but also for his sympathetic ear in listening to their expressions of resentment about the surgeons they work with who treat them and their patients with neglect and insensitivity. The nurses and the psychiatric consultant offer one another what they lack, i.e., approval, acceptance, and assistance. The patients benefit too, but the surgeons are still excluded. Occasionally, the psychiatric consultant meets the ward staff, (i.e., nurses, attendants, technicians, and others), in a group to resolve interpersonal problems or to educate them about the common psychiatric problems encountered on a surgical service.

Another pattern that has become commonplace in the surgical unit is for the consultant to see patients on referral from the nursing staff, just as he would if the referral came from a surgeon. Unfortunately, this approach alone is rarely successful in gaining the support of the surgeons. Too often they feel excluded, conspired against, and resentful, even though patient care is enhanced.

Yet another approach is for an aspiring liaison psychiatrist to be introduced into a surgical service by a senior consultant who has established an effective liaison. The novice can tolerate the initial indifference of his surgical colleagues better if he has the support and, significantly, the advice and supervision of a more experienced colleague who knows the surgeons, relates well with them, and can teach the skills of liaison in a surgical milieu. Such an "apprenticeship" is quite successful; however, it is very expensive in time required of the two psychiatrists to establish a comfortable introduction for the new consultant. As a result it is not tried very often.

When circumstances permit, it is helpful for resident psychiatrists first to gain some confidence in their new identity in a liaison role before tackling the emotionally stressful territory of a surgical service. This can be accomplished by spending time on wards or in clinics that recognize the needs for psychiatric consultation and provide the acceptance so desperately sought after by the resident. If after a few weeks on service, such as Internal Medicine, the tyro consultant grows comfortable with his new skills, and renews his familiarity with his fading identity as "physician," he may gain the security that he needs to tolerate his initiation rites on the surgical services. Lacking such confidence in his identity as physician and his skills as psychiatric consultant, he may be vulnerable to the subtle rejection that he usually receives as he begins his surgical liaison. If the psychiatrist expects to share the fellowship, both professional and personal, of the surgical staff, he must be prepared to accept, and even approve of their values, life-styles, and practices. He is unlikely to be able to change the surgeons until he has first been accepted as being one of them, with the willingness to work hard and to be of genuine help to them personally and in turn to their patients. Once established, the liaison can work effectively without the psychiatrist needing to play the role of surgeon to the same extent. He can slip back into his more comfortable identity as psychiatrist because he no longer threatens his professional colleagues by being different; he has reassured them by establishing his likeness to them. Then the fundamental task of a liaison psychiatrist can begin—to teach the surgeons to manage the psychiatric problems that commonly occur in their patients.

PSYCHIATRIC PROBLEMS ON A SURGICAL UNIT

The range of psychiatric problems varies. Some are common to all surgical patients, indeed to patients of any sort, such as the fear and anxiety caused by being ill and having to consult a doctor or come to a hospital. Fears of disability, pain, and death are ubiquitous, but an illness brings them to the surface of our consciousness. Any physician should be aware of their presence. His sensitivity to the patient's needs permit him to reassure when indicated and assuage, generally, to the benefit of the patient and his concerned family. Other surgical problems are unique. If the patient will require an operation, that magical act forces him to submit, helplessly, to an anesthetic which he fears will tear away all his abilities to control his behavior, his inner thoughts, and his fantasies. Then there is the operative procedure itself with the anticipation of pain, mutilation, disability, and perhaps death. Most patients suffer these assaults on their psyches in silence. Surgical residents, the "warrior cult" of our medical social structure, are trained in stoicism in the face of suffering, and they are often annoyed or angry at patients who express their fears openly. Surgeons value independence, and in doing so they frequently deny the extent of their own dependent needs. The inevitable regression accompanying illness releases the expression of dependency in many patients. Surgeons commonly have difficulty in responding to such patients. Instead of offering reassurance and support, they withdraw from the patients, thereby aggravating the fears and anxieties that produced the regression initially. The shibboleth that some surgeons believe is that they must not gratify a patient's dependent needs (or their own) because the dependency will increase. No amount of discussion will dissuade them from this usually erroneous conclusion. A demonstration from the liaison psychiatrist is a more effective way of teaching that the dependency stems from fear and that alleviation of the fear with information and humane support minimizes the dependency.

There are a number of psychiatric problems that are prevalent in surgery. The phenomenon of a postoperative psychosis, occurring particularly following open-heart surgery, is a typical example. In addition to the psychological stresses of threatened death from high-risk surgery, there are physiologic stresses like oxygenation deprivation, hypotensive episodes, dehydration, and electrolyte imbalances, which contribute to the usually transient psychosis. There are also the adverse effects of insomnia due to pain and the frequent monitoring of vital functions that is required. Perhaps most significant is the sensory overload of an intensive care unit (ICU) with its lights, noise, emergencies, and other disorienting stimuli. Psychiatric consultants are frequently called for evaluation of patients with transient postoperative psychoses. Commonly, their precarious physical condition precludes the use of antipsychotic drugs or transfer to a psychiatric unit. The patients need to be treated, in situ, with attentive care, frequent orientation to their surroundings, and reassurance based upon an understanding of their fears and stresses. They do not improve with more quiet, more isolation, and being left alone among strange people in an unfamiliar place.

Another set of related problems concerns patients with chronic pain, often associated with burns, cancer, or postoperative complications leading to a prolonged hospital stay. The patients demand narcotics, often in increasing amounts and with ever greater stridency. Two crucial issues are involved in the assessment of chronic pain in such surgical patients. One is the attitudes of physicians toward prescribing narcotics. The other is the reaction of physicians, especially inexperienced ones, to a patient whose problems do not improve despite all the physician's efforts to help him. To state it succinctly, physicians are extremely uneasy in prescribing narcotics to a patient who demands them. One feels more comfortable prescribing to a patient who does not want them. Fears of addiction, perhaps based on reasonable evidence, seem to overwhelm all other considerations, including the presence of severe, chronic, and perhaps intolerable pain over weeks, months, or years. Doctors are taught that addiction is an evil, to be watched for and avoided. What they seldom recognize is that few patients who become addicted in the course of medical treatment remain addicted when the pain is eased or cured. What seems to be involved is a feeling that the patient may be malingering, exaggerating, or simulating pain in order to get narcotized. Such "undeserved" gratification of a patient's unacceptable wishes antagonizes most physicians, to a remarkable degree. At times the amount of anger and resentment the surgeon feels toward the potentially addictive patient makes him blind to the presence of real pain and suffering. What appears to be a cruel denial of analgesics to a suffering patient may be the outcome.

A related aspect of this common problem is the threat to the physician's self-esteem caused by the patient who does not get well. To a large extent, we physicians seek our professional satisfactions from making people better. There are other satisfactions of course (money, intellectual curiosity, pride in exercising one's skills optimally, and so on), but grateful patients who get well are the primary source of our self-esteem. Particularly for the younger physician in training, whose professional identity is forming and whose relative ignorance and ineptitude threatens his self-esteem, patients who do not improve are a serious problem. If the course of a patient's illness, for example, heart failure or cancer, is such that medical interventions are limited to prescribing drugs or relatively impersonal treatments, such as radiation therapy, the patient's failure to improve can be blamed largely on his disease. When surgery, particularly disabling, mutilating, and painful surgery, is used in treatment and the patient still fails to gain, the responsibility falls more certainly on the surgeon. He feels guilty. The guilt makes him uncomfortable, and the patient is blamed. The feelings of disappointment, failure, and guilt in the surgeon make him want to avoid the patient, if possible. If escape from the source of his discomfort is not possible, the surgeon may feel anger toward the patient and find fault with the patient for not improving. In this context the patient's need for narcotics is seen in distorted perspective. His problems are not seen as complications of surgical treatment or an incurable disease. They are addiction, malingering, and the like, which must be managed by denying the gratification of drugs to the patient.[3]

For the psychiatric consultant, management of problems like the one just described are difficult. One must be able to see the dynamics of the relationship between surgeon and patient. More importantly, one must be able to present the insights to the surgeon, tactfully, in order not to further alienate him from the patient, the consultant, or himself by adding to his guilt or embarrassment. A solid relationship with good rapport between surgeon and psychiatrist is necessary. Without it learning cannot occur because defenses against criticism are too high. When the liaison is comfortable and trust established, the surgeon can accept help from his consultant without feeling demeaned or blamed for the patient's failure to be cured.

There are many other psychiatric problems in surgery, such as the management of dying patients, organ transplants, and donor selection, that are very highly specialized and will not be considered in this chapter. One uncommon but unique set of problems, however, merits some discussion—that is the polysurgical patient who interferes with the healing of his surgical wound. It is fascinating to consider that some people will submit, willingly, to surgical procedures that are not indicated on the basis of surgical disease. The psychological forces impelling them to seek operations are obviously very powerful. Polysurgical patients are people who generally have severe personality disorders, diagnosable usually as hysterical character or passive-aggressive character disorders. They are most often women, and they have a history of going from surgeon to surgeon, simulating artfully the syndromes of surgical disorders. They tend to have several operations, occasionally leading to the development of true anatomical or physiological pathology, for example, adhesions, bowel obstructions, due to the surgical sequelae. They are ingratiating, compliant, and convincing, as long as they can have their way. Postoperatively they are slow to improve; old complaints reappear, or new ones arrive and they demand narcotics. They come to resemble the patients who factitiously interfere with the healing of their wounds, seeking to prolong, for whatever idiosyncratic reasons, the gratifications of being ill.[4]

For physicians, committed to the principle of making people well, and assuming that patients share their commitment, the behavior described is incomprehensible and infuriating. When once they begin to realize that they have been misled by the patients, they react with humiliation and anger. Objectivity is compromised. The powerful and relentless forces compelling a patient to act as he does, submitting to surgery and interfering with his recovery, are rarely considered. The patient, formerly seen as sick, and entitled to consideration as sick, is now seen as bad. The surgeons get angry, the patients get angry, and the psychiatric consultant gets little help from either camp. The patients, once discovered, rarely remain in treatment and even less commonly accept psychiatric care for the underlying psychiatric problems that motivate their behavior. The surgeons and psychiatrists may come to understand why they and the patients behave as they do, but little more can be done for the patients. They reject psychiatric care and usually resume their odyssey with new and unsuspecting surgeons. The surgeons with the help of the liaison psychiatrist can learn to recognize the polysurgical syndrome more skillfully. Perhaps they can come to react with greater objectivity and less sense of personal betrayal when confronted with someone who prefers not to get well. The most probable outcome is that they may at least be able to avoid contributing to the patient's self-destructive behavior by their unwitting acceptance of a plausible patient who seeks to be ill.

REWARDS OF A MEANINGFUL LIAISON

The description of the many problems in establishing a liaison between surgeons and psychiatrists has produced a bias. It might suggest that the task is difficult and the rewards are meagre. That would be only partially true. The task is usually substantial, but the rewards are too. The very fact of accomplishing a difficult task is often particularly meaningful to the liaison psychiatrist. There is more to it, however. Having once established a successful liaison, the psychiatrist will find his surgical colleagues immensely grateful to him and, therefore, gratifying to work with. The patients, of course benefit. For the psychiatrist there is a competence as a consultant, able to handle any situation, and often a sense of renewed identity as a physician that makes it all worthwhile.

REFERENCES

1. Myers I: The Myers-Briggs Type Indicator, Manual. Princeton, Educational Testing Service, 1962
2. Myers I: Relation of medical students' psychological type to their specialties twelve years later. A paper presented to the annual meeting of the American Psychological Association, Los Angeles, September 4–9, 1964
3. Golden JS, Nahum A: Emotional reactions to mutilating surgery; in Wahl CW (ed): New Dimensions in Psychosomatic Medicine. Boston, Little Brown, 1964
4. Wahl CW, Golden JS: The psychodynamics of the polysurgical patient: Report of sixteen patients. Psychosomatics 7:65–72, 1966

Robert O. Pasnau

10
Psychiatry and Obstetrics-Gynecology: Report of a Five-Year Experience in Psychiatric Liaison

Beginning with the early studies of Horney, Frank, and Benedek and Rubenstein in the 1920s and 1930s, a considerable literature has developed in the psychosomatic aspects of obstetrics-gynecology.[1, 2, 3] Although work in the field continues to be published and even to include at least two volumes devoted exclusively to psychiatric problems related to obstetrics-gynecology,[4, 5] surprisingly little has been written about the role of the liaison psychiatrist working specifically with obstetrics-gynecology. Lipowski, in his comprehensive reviews of consultation-liaison psychiatry, lists no references in this area of interest.[6, 7, 8] Furthermore, liaison psychiatrists, such as Mathis and Golden, both of whom spent many years working with departments of obstetrics-gynecology, touch only briefly in their writings on some of their personal experiences and focus mainly on the psychiatric aspects of the diagnostic problems and clinical services.[9, 10]

Perhaps this dearth of personal information can be explained by the authors' awareness that no individual should make generalizations about a whole field from any one experience in any one setting. This is the important *caveat* of Lipowski, which I respect.[6, 7, 8] Nonetheless, there is need for sharing with others the experiences that we have in our consultation-liaison work, leaving to the reader the responsibility of appropriate application of the information.

This chapter represents an attempt to share my personal experiences in a five-year period (1969–1974) as the liaison psychiatrist to the Department of Obstetrics-Gynecology at the University of California Los Angeles (UCLA)

135

School of Medicine. In this paper I shall describe the particular setting in which I have been working, something of the nature of the consultees and patients with whom I have worked, and some personal reflections on the nature of the specialty obstetrics-gynecology. In addition, I shall follow Lipowski's outline and briefly touch on the nature of the clinical problems encountered, sketch the teaching program developed, and describe some of the many opportunities for research. In conclusion I shall reveal what for me have been the very personal rewards of this effort.

THE CLINICAL SETTING

Obstetrics-gynecology is a unique specialty in many ways. From a practical standpoint perhaps the most unique is in the widely ranging nature of the clinical setting. It extends from the maternity ward–delivery room–prenatal and postnatal clinics to the intensive care unit–oncology wards of the gynecology services. No other clinical specialty, unless it be family practice, comes to mind as crossing so many clinical settings and systems of care.

Because of this, great emotional demands are made upon the obstetrician-gynecologist. He must function equally well in what Shneidman has described as the benign, the emergent, and the dire settings.[11] In the benign setting of the maternity ward where the anticipated product is a happy and healthy mother and newborn infant, death is always a shock, whether it be maternal or neonatal. In the emergent setting of the gynecology intensive care unit, one in which critical issues are dealt with on a moment-to-moment basis, there is little time for staff to become personally involved with their patients. In this setting death is at least anticipated in some of the cases, and in most cases the patient is transferred somewhere else for recuperation following the emergency situation. In the dire setting of the gynecology-oncology ward some patients spend many weeks or months, some intermittently hospitalized during a prolonged course of illness. In this setting staff has time to form meaningful personal relationships with the dying patients. Death, when it comes although anticipated, takes its toll in terms of the emotional reactions of the staff. The liaison psychiatrist must understand that, unlike psychiatry, obstetrics-gynecology functions in all three settings and that this is the day-to-day reality for the obstetrician-gynecologist and staff.

Another related problem of the obstetrics-gynecology services is simply geographical. While most other hospital-based specialties function in one or two clinics and wards, the obstetrician-gynecologist must be equally at home in the operating room, the delivery room, the intensive care unit, the labor room, the newborn nursery, the obstetrics clinic, the family planning clinic, the gynecology clinic, the emergency room, the maternity ward, and the gynecology and oncology wards, and he must be available to consult on any woman patient anywhere in the hospital, sometimes for the most minimal and trivial reasons. This role involves relating to many systems of supporting personnel, especially nurses, and makes it very difficult for a close doctor-nurse or even doctor-patient relationship to develop in these settings. It is small wonder that, as in psychiatry, subspecialization has become such a prominent trend in this specialty.

An additional real problem for obstetrician-gynecologists is ''sleep deprivation.'' Somehow, the other medical specialists have learned how to schedule their working days better than obstetrician-gynecologists. (I can remember as a medical student marveling at the seemingly indefatigable house staff in obstetrics. Only in the past five years have I learned when they sleep—in conferences!)

PSYCHOSOCIAL NATURE OF THE SPECIALTY
OBSTETRICS-GYNECOLOGY

There is something very special about the present era that is making considerable impact upon the obstetrician-gynecologist's image of his role. Perhaps only in psychiatry has there been a greater involvement in and controversy over the physician's role in social problems. The obstetrician-gynecologist can no longer concern himself only with advances in surgical and obstetrical techniques. He has been propelled into the problem areas of abortion, family planning, sterilization, and even sexual education and counseling. In almost no residency training program has he been prepared for this role, and even now such preparation takes a back seat to the training in the technical skills. Nonetheless, this social emphasis has brought about a growing awareness within the speicalty of the need for a close liaison with psychiatry. I do not believe that this pressure exists to the same extent in the other medical specialties.

There is also a growing recognition of the psychosocial problems of the special medical environments, including the oncology services, the intensive care unit, and even the delivery room, that has brought pressure on these services to develop close psychiatric liaison. This is an example of how the changing practice of medicine has made clearer the interdependence of all medical practitioners in providing comprehensive care.

In the final analysis, however, the same problems and needs for psychiatric liaison exist on obstetrics-gynecology services as for any of the other hospital-based services. These problems, which will be described later, often involve the difficult or demanding patient, the patient with chronic illness, or the mentally ill patient. In fact, it was a crisis over the management of a seriously ill diabetic woman in labor that led to my initial involvement as the liaison psychiatrist to the obstetrics-gynecology department.

THE OBSTETRICIAN-GYNECOLOGIST

In this section I am in the greatest danger of disregarding Lipowski's warning about generalizing from one's narrow experience. Obviously, the personality characteristics of obsterician-gynecologists are as varied as are those of other specialists, psychiatrists, internists and the like. Yet as Menninger and others have pointed out,[12] there are some characteristics that seem to apply to those physicians who choose obstetrics-gynecology for a specialty.

Obstetrician-gynecologists are often obsessional individuals who love "rules of thumb" and enjoy arguing minute points of clinical diagnosis and treatment. As a general rule, they are outgoing, and athletic and, like most surgeons enjoy doing things.[13] They are very hard-working individuals. As is the case with other physicians, they tend to be conservative in politics and religion. They often harbor the same attitudes toward psychiatry as described for most surgeons and, as with most physicians, often displace their anger to psychiatry and psychiatrists.[6, 7, 8, 13] Part of the task of a liaison psychiatrist is to try to understand and relate to a group of colleagues who view the world, the practice of medicine, and the role of psychiatry in a way different from most psychiatrists.

NURSING AND SOCIAL SERVICES IN OBSTETRICS-GYNECOLOGY

I have particularly enjoyed my work with the head nurse in obstetrics-gynecology and the social workers on the service. Without their support no liaison psychiatrist could function very long or well. At times my role has been to mediate, to cajole, to urge, and to tranquilize. Because of the settings in which they work, nurses often find themselves having difficulties with each other. Because they are in such close contact with the patients and because of the lack of presence of the physicians, the major responsibilities for minute-to-minute care fall upon them. They are in the "front line" in dealing with the emotional problems of the patients and of each other.

Sometimes the problems are of intergroup problems between the obstetrical nurses, the newborn nursery nurses, and the gynecology nurses. Sometimes the problems arise between the more highly educated registered nurses (usually white) and the licensed practical nurses (often minority group members). Occasionally, the problems center around conflicts with physicians—between the nurses and the physicians or the social worker and a physician over some aspect of management or disposition. Whatever the ostensible issue, it is clear that the feelings are often acted out to the detriment of patient care. Into such an arena the liaison psychiatrist comes unarmed and risks becoming the focus of the anger and resentment. If he can recognize that often at the bottom of the content issue lies the emotionally taxing nature of the work and responsibilities, complicated by the lack of support from the physicians due to their unavailability at crucial periods, he is better prepared to assist the staff at times of crisis. Nursing groups meeting on a weekly basis with a liaison psychiatrist are very helpful in preventing many of these problems, which are seemingly inherent in the medical care system in this specialty.

THE DOCTOR-PATIENT RELATIONSHIP IN OBSTETRICS-GYNECOLOGY

As Mathis, Golden, Kroger, and many others have described so well, what really makes obstetrics-gynecology unique is the patients.[9, 10, 15] They are all women. The problems for which they are seeking medical attention are all related in some way to the sexual and reproductive organs. In no other specialty does the clinical work de facto require a physician who understands the emotional process in relationship to the physical processes. That the attending physician so often does not possess this understanding is the most challenging problem of all for the liaison psychiatrist.

There are many reasons for this. Some are problems related to the time pressures associated with the practice of medicine. Usually, however, the chief obstacle is the resistance of the obstetrician-gynecologist to attempt to understand the emotions of his patient. Such resistance can only be explored once satisfactory personal liaison relationships have developed between the attending physician and the consultation-liaison psychiatrist. The following anecdote by Jones typifies the problem:

> Some years ago I was asked by the Chief of Obstetrics to help him with the case of a young woman who cried when she was informed that she was pregnant. He asked if there was anything he should do in such a situation. I replied that perhaps he ought to talk to her in order to discover if there was some problem in her life which was related to her being pregnant. If so, perhaps she would like to talk it over with him. He replied, "Why dammit, man, you know I can't sit still that long!"[16]

Even if one does not deal directly with the resistances of the obstetrician-gynecologist an appeal can be made to him that he *must* gather this kind of information in order to make a diagnosis, which is one of the requirements of the medical profession. As Mathis pointed out,

> Psychiatrists are not asking the obstetricians to do their work, but they are admitting that these specialists are frequently in the best position to do much of it, and that above all, they may be one of the few groups fitted to practice true preventive mental hygiene. And that, in the final analysis, must always be the aim of medicine: to prevent.[9]

Another way of dealing with the resistances can be by example. Rahe has taught that the liaison psychiatrist must be as willing to learn as much about the patient's physical processes as he asks the consultee to learn about the patient's mental processes.[17] This not only sets an example for the obstetrician-gynecologist, but it has the additional payoff for the liaison psychiatrist in that he becomes a better therapist for all of his women patients.

THE LIAISON PSYCHIATRIST

Thus far there has been no in-depth study of the personality characteristics of psychiatrists who specialize in consultation-liaison psychiatry. (Personally, I am convinced that they are a peculiar group, but to date I have only a few ideas about that.) Lipowski,[6, 7, 8] Rahe,[17] Mendelson and Meyer,[18] Abrams,[19] and many others have demonstrated the need to be free from disabling counter-transferences, critical comments, and confused jargon if one is to become an effective consultant. I would agree. I also find that the best consultation-liaison psychiatrists are those who have a good sense of humor, enjoy working with other people (as opposed to the solitude of the usual psychiatric setting), are more physically active than their professional colleagues, and have the ability to be very direct and even authoritarian at times when the situation demands it. The usual psychiatrist feels uncomfortable in the latter situation. Interestingly enough, it is the most promising liaison psychiatrist who needs the very quality of patience and perseverence that his more passive colleagues seem to possess in an unlimited amount. Work in obstetrics-gynecology requires the same degree of frustration tolerance that has been described for other liaison work.

In my experience, the sex, prior medical training or background, or theoretical orientation of the liaison psychiatrist are not factors in being a successful and effective liaison psychiatrist. Some of the best liaison psychia-trists in obstetrics-gynecology are women despite a commonly held belief to the contrary. Former internists or family practitioners are not per se suited for liaison work, despite the common belief that they are "naturals" in this field. Some of the best are psychoanalytically oriented. On the other hand, it is not uncommon to find a very effective liaison psychiatrist who has little interest or background in psychoanalysis. Whatever it is that liaison psychiatrists bring to their work, they must possess dedication, knowledge of psychiatry, and the ability to communicate both of these to their colleagues in a helpful and nonthreatening way.

CLINICAL PROBLEMS

Table 10–1 outlines the most frequently encountered clinical problems in psychiatric liaison to obstetrics-gynecology that I have encountered. Reflecting the social and legal changes, consultation requests for therapeutic abortion have significantly decreased, while consultations associated with family planning, sterilization, pelvic pain, and death and dying have increased. Part of the change is due to staff awareness and education. We are beginning to receive requests for assistance in areas that were not considered to be problems in 1969.

One of the most perplexing clinical problems for both the psychiatrist and the gynecologist is that of pelvic pain. We are still ineffective in distinguishing those very complex cases of organic pathology with overlying psychiatric illness from those with more clear-cut psychogenic components. However, we have been able to engage the gynecologists in a search for some of the answers and have not lost stature because we do not have all of them.

Hospital management problems, both in obstetrics and gynecology, continue to be the main service areas of psychiatric liaison. In this respect obstetrics-gynecology is not so very different from any other area of the hospital. The difficult patient, whether she be psychotic, infantile, frightened, uncooperative, or chronically ill, poses a very real problem for most hospital staffs. Often the liaison with the staff is the single most important factor in a successful outcome for the patient. An interloping, unfamiliar psychiatric consultant, no matter how experienced or knowledgeable, cannot provide the psychiatric help that is needed in these cases. The psychiatrist must be seen as a member of the team in order to have the cooperation of all concerned in managing these ''difficult'' patients.

TEACHING PROGRAM IN LIAISON PSYCHIATRY

The development of the teaching program can be sketched as follows:

1. During the first year I began weekly walking rounds with the Obstetrics-Gynecology house staff and one liaison psychiatry resident. We also began weekly meetings with the social workers and head nurses. The meetings were primarily case-oriented, and a good

Table 10–1

Five Year Summary of The Most Frequently
Encountered Clinical Problems in Psychiatric Liaison to
Obstetrics-Gynecology

OBSTETRICS

1. Hospital management problems associated with chronic diseases and pregnancy, including
   - A. diabetes
   - B. hypertension
   - C. sickle cell anemia
   - D. toxemia
   - E. personality disorder
   - F. psychosis
2. Assessment of the competency of mother to care for the infant
3. Postpartum reactions: Psychosis, depression
4. Stillbirth
5. The unwanted pregnancy—therapeutic abortion
6. The psychotic patient in labor
7. Infertility
8. Repeated spontaneous abortions
9. Sterilization: Family planning clinic problems
10. Problems related to father's presence in delivery room

GYNECOLOGY

1. Hospital management problems associated with
   - A. pelvic infection
   - B. narcotics addiction
   - C. personality disorder
   - D. psychosis
2. Pelvic pain, including dyspareunia, dysmenorrhea
3. Emotional reactions following pelvic surgery
4. Menstrual disorder, including menopausal syndromes
5. The dying patient and her family
6. Delirium
7. Sexual counseling

deal of teaching of psychiatry occurred. Consultation services for patients were offered as well for both in- and out-patients.

2. During the second year I began attending the Obstetrics-Gynecology departmental weekly conferences. In addition, special consultation projects were undertaken with the family planning clinic, especially around the areas of abortion and sterilization counseling. Weekly rounds with the social workers and nurses continued. Two liaison residents began making walking rounds with the housestaff. Several nursing discussion groups were started by the liaison residents.

3. During the third year several research projects were begun, primarily in the area of family planning. Several special medical education programs for clinical faculty were offered. Liaison residents began involvement in special projects, nursing groups, and special clinical problems. The weekly conferences led to several "grand round"

presentations on psychiatric aspects of obstetrics-gynecology. I continued to attend the weekly departmental conferences where I had become an accepted participant.

4. In the fourth year the Chairman of the department asked me to co-chair a special course for the faculty and staff on psychosocial aspects of obstetrics-gynecology. All other programs continued as in the previous year. Several papers were submitted for publication with joint Psychiatrist & Ob-Gynecologist authorship.

5. During the fifth year my task was to gradually replace my presence with the presence of other younger faculty and residents. During this year three faculty members and four psychiatric residents became involved in some aspects of the program, including the wards, clinics, rounds, conferences, and meetings. I continued to supervise the liaison residents and attend the weekly departmental meetings.

What should be obvious from this account, is that the "payoff" for the liaison psychiatrist in return for the clinical services that he provides is the request to develop a program for the service involving the psychiatric aspects of the service. In the weekly meetings with the staff and residents on obstetrics-gynecology the individual cases, with adequate references to the medical literature, provide the liaison consultant excellent content for teaching. Occasionally these meetings are of such interest or importance that they furnish the content for the department's "grand rounds." Particularly notable grand rounds in which I have participated have concerned still-birth, therapeutic abortion, and pelvic pain. Of course, the best place for teaching is during the weekly departmental clinical rounds and the morning and evening working rounds.

For me, the most rewarding opportunity for psychiatric education on the obstetrics-gynecology service came in the fourth year of my work when I was asked to co-chair a weekly seminar in the psychosocial aspects of obstetrics-gynecology. This meeting was part of the regular residency and medical student curriculum and was attended by the faculty as well. That this seminar took four years in gestation provides some idea of the time required to bring about complete acceptance on a service of liaison psychiatry. Table 10–2 outlines the topics discussed at this conference.

RESEARCH OPPORTUNITIES FOR THE LIAISON PSYCHIATRIST IN OBSTETRICS-GYNECOLOGY

Lipowski wisely lists research in third place in his outline of consultation-liaison psychiatry.[6, 7, 8] It is only after the clinical services and teaching programs have matured that the proper atmosphere for interdisiciplinary research can be created. Then the opportunities for research are limitless; only the time available sets limits.

Table 10–2
Topics Discussed at Psychosocial Aspects of Obstetrics
and Gynecology Conference

DIAGNOSTIC AND/OR THERAPEUTIC PROBLEMS
1. Psychiatric Sequelae of Hysterectomy: A review of the pertinent literature and a discussion of some illustrative cases
2. Psychiatric Aspects of Pelvic Pain: A review of the psychiatric literature on "pain-prone" patients, the symbolic nature of pelvic pain, and presentation of psychological data and psychiatric findings in selected cases
3. Psychiatric Sequelae of Abortion and/or Sterilization: A multidisciplinary approach to a review of current practices and individual cases, including
   a. The unmarried adolescent patient
   b. The physically disabled patient
   c. The mentally retarded patient
   d. The emotionally unstable or immature patient
   e. The psychotic patient
4. The Treatment of Human Sexual Dysfunctions: A multidisciplinary review of the physical, psychotherapeutic, and behavioral approaches to treatment and diagnosis
5. Stillbirth: The role of the staff and physician, the effect upon the family, the effect upon the staff, medical-legal aspects, and pathological grief reactions
6. Sterilization of the Never Pregnant, Never Married: A review of the practice of voluntary tubal-ligation in a special population
7. Sterilization of the Mentally Retarded: A discussion with a distinguished authority in the field of mental retardation about the changing climate of practice

SOCIAL PROBLEMS
1. Midlife Crises in Women: A new look at the "menopause" from the point of view of the psychoanalyst, with a review of current literature; guest discussant
2. The Psychiatric Implications of Adoption: A discussion of the effects of adoption upon the adoptees and their families; guest discussant
3. Rape: A discussion by a panel of women physicians, lawyers, and social workers on the treatment of women by the police, gynecologists, and the courts with a review of some of the pertinent social and legal issues involved
4. Death and Dying: A discussion with an authority on the problems of the dying patient and her family, with a review of the literature

Listed in the References are some of the research papers that resulted from the psychiatric liaison with the Department of Obstetrics-Gynecology at the UCLA School of Medicine. [20–25] These efforts have been directed at examining the psychiatric sequelae of therapeutic abortion, developing guidelines for the use of psychiatric consultation in cases where abortion is requested, comparing the emotional responses after amniocentesis abortion to those following first trimester curretage, and studying the counseling problems with adolescent, unmarried pregnant women. We have also begun an important study of the effects of sterilization upon young women who have never been pregnant and who request tubal ligation as a personal "right" or for ecological reasons. Other areas currently being evaluated for possible research projects are (1) the effects upon staff and nursing personnel of prolonged tours of duty on the oncology wards, (2) the prevention of pathological grief reactions following stillbirth or neonatal mortality, and (3) the impact of staff attitudes upon the course of illness in chronically hospitalized patients on the obstetrical wards. These are only some of the potential areas to be explored in this clinical specialty.

There is no doubt that much important work is yet to be done, and that this specialty represents a potential "gold mine" for the young liaison psychiatrist.

CONCLUSION

This chapter has highlighted the positive experiences that I have had in a five-year career in liaison psychiatry to obstetrics-gynecology. It has not been without serious problems at times. Sometimes, one of our group has been met with outright hostility or ridicule. At other times lip service and passive resistance have proven more difficult to deal with than overt expressions. However, as in work with psychiatric patients, these attitudes are all part of the "grist for the mill." As Wahl has quipped, "At times you can't give liaison psychiatry away with a set of dishes." On the other hand, there are many rewards, some very personal.

This has been a personal essay written about one liaison psychiatrist's experiences. The rewards are very personal too, and they reveal as much about the liaison psychiatrist as they do about consultation-liaison psychiatry. However, I shall make the attempt to reveal the rewards of working with obstetrician-gynecologists, faculty, residents, students from all disciplines, nurses, social workers, and patients over the five years:

Reward: The Chairman of the Department of Obstetrics-Gynecology announced to his incoming group of medical students that one of the outstanding aspects of his department was the "psychiatric orientation" of his program and the unique relationship that exists between his department and the Department of Psychiatry through the Psychiatric Liaison Service.

Reward: A second-year resident in obstetrics-gynecology requested to do a six-month research project in the psychiatric aspects of obstetrics.

Reward: A professor of obstetrics-gynecology asked for help in understanding a psychiatric case report from the nineteenth century while writing a paper on hysteroepilepsy.

Reward: I was asked to participate in a continuing education program for practicing obstetrician-gynecologists in which for many years previously no psychiatrist has participated.

Reward: Fathers were permitted to be present in the delivery room following the efforts of all members of the staff to have policy changed.

Reward: Patients are no longer scheduled for psychiatric evaluation of pelvic pain *after* being placed on the operating room schedule.

Reward: The chief resident in the delivery room announced that he wished to visit personally with every woman and her family following an unexpected neonatal death to help them "initiate the grief process."

Reward: I was asked to co-chair the seminar on psychosocial aspects of obstetrics-gynecology.

Reward: The vice-chairman of the Department of Obstetrics-Gynecology announced jokingly at a departmental meeting that because all of the house staff and faculty would be attending the annual house staff picnic, I would cover the delivery room and emergency room on the following Saturday. I made a reciprocal offer for the vice-chairman to cover the psychiatric emergency room, which he, as I had done, respectfully declined.

Reward: I was invited to spend a sabbatical six months in Germany studying the psychosomatic aspects of obstetrics and gynecology in Europe in the nineteenth century.

Reward: More than a dozen dedicated former psychiatric residents who worked with me over the past five years and are now practicing psychiatrists are all heavily involved in consultation-liaison psychiatry. Several work full time in this field, three primarily in liaison work with obstetrics-gynecology.

Reward: I have seen in consultation hundreds of women patients with every conceivable condition, complication, and complaint. The job is never done. There are always new patients, new staff, new residents, new faculty, and the opportunities and challenges are as great today as they were when I began.

REFERENCES

1. Horney K: Premenstrual tension (1931), in Kelman H (ed): Feminine Psychology. New York, Norton, 1967
2. Frank R: Hormonal causes of premenstrual tension. Arch Neurol Psychiatry 26:1053–1057, 1931
3. Benedek T, Rubenstein B: Correlations between ovarian activity and psychodynamic processes (1939), in Benedek T (ed): Studies in Psychosomatic Medicine: Psychosexual Functions in Women. New York, Roland, 1952

4. Norris M (ed): Psychosomatic Medicine in Obstetrics and Gynecology. Basel, Switz, Karger, 1972

5. Howells J (ed): Modern Perspectives in Psycho-Obstetrics. New York, Brunner/Mazel, 1972

6. Lipowski ZJ: Review of consultation psychiatry and psychosomatic medicine. I, II, III. Psychosom Med 29:153–171, 1967; 29:201–224, 1967; 30:395–422, 1968

7. Lipowski ZJ: Consultation-liaison psychiatry: An overview. Am J Psychiatry 131:623–630, 1974

8. Lipowski ZJ: Consultation-liaison psychiatry: Past, present, and future, in Pasnau RO (ed): Consultation-Liaison Psychiatry. Seminars in Psychiatry. New York, Grune & Stratton, 1975

9. Mathis J: Psychiatry and the obstetrician-gynecologist. Med Clin North Am 51:1375–1380, 1967

10. Golden JS: Psychosomatic problems in obstetric and gynecologic practice, in Wahl CW (ed): New Dimensions in Psychosomatic Medicine. Boston, Little Brown, 1964

11. Shneidman ES: Deaths of Man. New York, Penguin, 1974

12. Menninger K: Psychological factors in the choice of medicine as a profession. II. Bull Menninger Clin 21:99–106, 1957

13. Golden JS: The surgeon and the psychiatrist: Special problems in psychiatric liaison, in Pasnau RO (ed): Consultation-Liaison Psychiatry. Seminars in Psychiatry. New York, Grune & Stratton, 1975

14. Vaillant G, Sobowale A, McArthur C: Some psychologic vulnerabilities of physicians. N Engl J Med 287:372–375, 1972

15. Kroger W (ed): Psychosomatic Obstetrics, Gynecology, and Endocrinology. Springfield, Ill, Thomas, 1962

16. Jones R: Personal Communication, 1973

17. Rahe RH: A liaison psychiatrist on the coronary care unit, in Pasnau RO (ed): Consultation-Liaison Psychiatry. Seminars in Psychiatry. New York, Grune & Stratton, 1975

18. Mendelson M, Meyer E: Countertransference problems of the liaison psychiatrist. Psychosom Med 23:115–122, 1961

19. Abrams H: Interpersonal aspects of psychiatric consultations in a general hospital. Psychiatry Med 2:321–326, 1971

20. Pasnau RO: Psychiatric complications of therapeutic abortion. Obstet Gynecol 40:252–256, 1972

21. Marmer S, Pasnau RO, Cushner I: Is psychiatric consultation in therapeutic abortion obsolete? Int J Psychiatry 53:201–209, 1974

22. Glasser M, Pasnau RO: The unwanted pregnancy in adolescence. J Family Practice 2:91–94, 1975

23. Farash J, Pasnau RO: Loss and amniocentesis abortion (unpublished manuscript)

24. Crumley K, Pasnau RO: Sterilization of the never pregnant (in preparation)

25. Pasnau RO, Auerbach DB, Rahe RH, et al: Liaison psychiatry: A resident educative process. A panel discussion presented at the 126th Annual Meeting American Psychiatric Association at Honolulu, May 1973

Burton Roger

11

The Role of the Psychiatrist in the Renal Dialysis Unit

With the advent of chronic hemodialysis as a therapeutic procedure in the early 1960s, patients with anticipated or existent end-stage renal failure suddenly obtained hope for the prolongation of their lives. This technical discovery required physicians, communities, and governments to suddenly become aware of the need for close cooperation in understanding human response to stress and life support systems, the need for communities and governmental organizations to provide the means for acquiring sufficient facilities and staff to enable patients to benefit from the discovery, and the need to study the legal, moral, and ethical implications of medical practice and research.

It was rather inevitable that these demands upon medicine and society would not go overlooked by psychiatrists, who were often sought out by medical and surgical colleagues or community agencies to provide assistance in the selection of the patient for dialysis, and to apply their skills and expertise in arriving at an understanding of the patient's response and adaptation to his illness and its new treatment, as well as the reactions of the patient's family and professional caretakers. A great deal of the medical literature abounds with studies reporting on these areas of investigation, and it is hoped that the bibliography provided with allow the reader to further pursue his inquiries into areas of special interest.

The experiences and understandings of some two years work in consultation-liaison with a six-bed university hospital dialysis unit with an associated transplant program has provided me with numerous observations and opportunities to define the role of the psychiatrist in the dialysis unit. Psychiatric skills and consultations have been most often required in three areas:

1. The selection of patients for dialysis with attention to factors influencing outcome.
2. The evaluation, treatment, and understanding of the patient's response and adaptation to his illness and its treatment.
3. The consultation-liaison with the patient's family and his professional caretakers that permits the patient to relate to those around him in a fashion that preserves his independence and promotes his rehabilitation while simultaneously allowing his family and caretakers to express and understand their feelings and continue to function at their optimum.

SELECTION OF PATIENTS
AND FACTORS OBSERVED TO FACILITATE
ADJUSTMENT TO DIALYSIS

The development and implementation of federal and state aid plans for the funding of dialysis centers and trained personnel has now made hemodialysis readily available to most end-stage renal patients. What used to be an arduous process of selection, greatly influenced by the relative scarcity of equipment and personnel and often based on such imponderables as "social worth," etc., has now become more appropriately based on medical and psychiatric grounds. At present in many programs the only patients considered for exclusion for psychiatric reasons are those who are functioning on a psychotic level unrelated to uremia and whose psychosis is or has been unresponsive to psychotropic drugs, a structured environment, or a combination thereof and is severe enough to prevent him from adapting to a dialysis regimen. The development of the internal shunt and improved dialysis techniques, requiring lesser dietary restrictions, has reduced the likelihood of excluding patients who are mentally defective and incapable of comprehending what is expected of them.

The ready identification of those patients who present a higher risk of maladaptation to dialysis and who may require psychiatric intervention is of vital importance. Numerous investigators have studied groups of hemodialysis patients over varying lengths of time in an attempt to further elucidate what psychosocio-biological factors facilitate and enhance or impede the patient's adjustment to the dialysis situation. Sand et al. studied a group of 18 patients between 1962 and 1966.[1] They found that the more adaptive patients had higher intelligence, a less defensive attitude about admitting normal amounts of anxiety and difficulty in adjustment, less utilization of hypochrondiracal and hysterical somatic defenses, and more satisfactory emotional support from their family. Between 1969 and 1971, Foster et al. evaluated factors influencing survival in 21 patients on chronic hemodialysis.[2] Factors favoring survival in their group included affiliation with the Roman Catholic Church, continued presence of one or both parents, low BUN levels, and a marked indifference to fellow dialysis patients.

Starting in October, 1968, Hagberg studied 23 patients (aged 13 to 60).[3] He attempted to describe their intellectual and cognitive status as well as their dominant personality characteristics and the changes therein at times preceding the onset of dialysis and again 6 and 12 months after dialysis was begun. Importantly this most recent study seems to indicate that a higher general intelligence level and fewer marked signs of organicity before the onset of dialysis may result in a more rapid adjustment to dialysis but were of no predictive value after 12 months of dialysis. In addition, evidence of cerebral dysfunction similar to that found by Foster and Abram[4] was seen in all patients in Hagberg's study before the start of dialysis but was found to regress during the treatment period with no signs of organicity being present 12 months after the start of dialysis. The disappearance of all psychometric signs of cerebral dysfunction at 12 months is not consistent with earlier reporting by Short and Wilson who in 1969 reported progressive development of a cerebral dysfunction as dialysis continued.[5] Halberg also noted the presence of denial in dialysis patients as had been seen in studies by Kaplan de-Nour and Czaczkes and Wright et al.[3, 6, 7] Study techniques assessing repression, the less conscious counterpart of denial, were used by Hagberg, and he concluded that patients with a disposition to react with repressive defenses when exposed to a real threat adapted well while those with a habitual disposition to react with mere isolation had a less favorable prognosis.[3] Hagberg and Malmquist correlated psychiatric and psychological pretreatment variables in the rehabilitated (working) patient and found the favorable prognostic variables to be the patient's expecting rapid rehabilitation and having regular social contacts, an adequate reaction toward kidney disease, and other defense mechanisms rather than only isolative maneuvers.[8]

Identification of potential problems that may arise in the course of the patient's treatment can often be made by having the patient seen separately and individually by what may constitute the medical team comprised of the nephrologist, urologist, and transplant surgeon, the psychiatrist or his designated assistant, and a social worker or nurse with special training in renal disease and the emotional aspects of medical and surgical illness. Of importance in the psychiatric history are the patient's past exeriences with both medical and surgical illnesses, his responses to date in the acceptance and understanding of his disorder, and his capacity to tolerate symptoms and cooperate with treatment. Information regarding his vocational and recreational pursuits, the scope and quality of his relationships with friends and family, and any familial incidence of psychiatric problems or personal past psychiatric disturbance is sought after and utilized to understand the anticipate his response to his current illness. Interviews with the patient should be early in the course of his illness, often months before his disease requires hemodialysis, and the idea of his eventual need for dialysis is introduced as currently the natural course of his disease. Patients should be encouraged to visit the dialysis unit and observe and talk with other patients on dialysis prior to starting their treatment.

THE PATIENT'S RESPONSE
AND ADAPTATION TO DIALYSIS

On the subject of partial death, Shneidman has written

There are many alternatives in our lives that we can appropriately refer to as endings—conclusions of phases or aspects of our lives, the closing of episodes that irreversibly put a stop to habitually expected stimuli, psychological states, interpersonal relationships, and living patterns. The dying process itself (in, for example, cancer or leukemia) often seems, psychologically, to consits of a series of endings, in which the dying person successively, in the midst of incapacitating pain and discomfort, comes reluctantly to face increasingly constricting truncations and losses of his actual and potential competencies, in a lugubrious series of little deaths.[9]

Seeing numerous dialysis patients often prompts the realization that for these patients life is characterized by a long series of endings culminating in ultimate physical death. Usually throughout the course of dialysis the patient's medical state is often fragile and unpredictable, and there is a progressive deterioration of most organ systems with numerous complications. Feelings of general lassitude and weakness, changes in facial and bodily appearance, impotence, loss of libido, and all of the many medical complications of chronic uremia are seen as well as the primary complications of immunosupressive therapy for transplanted patients (infections, diabetes, cushingoid facies, glaucoma, cataracts, acne, osteoprois, capillary fragility). Each of these changes and complications soon allows the patient to see and experience the seriousness and relentlessness of his illness, often making him aware of the inevitability of its fatal conclusion. The patient frequently reacts to the fear of dying that often results with denial, anger, bargaining, envy, depression, regression, withdrawal, and apathy.[10, 11] I do not see these reactions as stages of the dying process occurring in any sequence but as a collection of intellectual, cognitive, and affective states with which the patient tries to relocate himself in relationships to significant others such as family and professional caretakers. His success in doing this is contingent on the nursing and technical staff, attending physicians, and family all becoming aware of the patient's struggle with ongoing loss and death and the simultaneous permission and assistance by these individuals in showing the patient how to tolerate and understand his illness and the treatment it requires.

Abram, in a paper that also refers to the early work of Baker and Knutson[12] and the more recent work of Schreiner and Maher,[13] describes the patient's adaptation to dialysis as occurring in four phases.[4] Phase I, or uremia, before any dialysis, is characterized by apathy, fatigue, drowsiness, poor concentration, and instability. In Phase II Abram notes a shift to physiological equilibrium in the first to third weeks (two to nine dialyses treatments), that he calls "The Return from the Dead." It is manifested as lessened apathy between the first and third dialyses and at times anxiety or euphoria with the patient's growing awareness of a reprieve from death. Phase III is referred to as "The Return to the Living" or a phase of equilibrium that usually begins by the third week (six to nine dialyses). Abram sees this phase as one where the patient begins to struggle with the new prospect of dealing with dialysis and its rigors and the beginnings of conflicts with dependency and interdependency, depression, and regression. In the third to twelfth months, Phase IV, that Abram calls "The Struggle for Normalcy—the Problem of Living Rather than Dying," the patient has made some adjustment to the routine of dialysis, may be back at work or prior activities, and will be dealing with and contemplating the arrival of new complications of his disease and treatment.

CONSULTATION-LIAISON
WITH THE PATIENT'S WORLD

Earlier I described the patient's responses to the fear of dying and his series of endings, unique to himself, that are mediated by renal failure, his disease, and dialysis, its treatment. Each patient is an individual with varying capabilities, needs, desires, and responsibilities. How does one bridge the gap of "what was" for the patient and "what is to be," with his world of family, friends, coworkers, and caretakers? It is a rather simple and straightforward statement yet one that requires constant reinforcement in the thinking of the patient, his family, and professional caretakers.

Much of the work that allows the patient to retain his individuality gets done in our unit in the time allocated for group meetings of both shifts of nurses and technicians, unit and staff secretaries, social worker, and unit nephrologists. This group of 12 to 15 people usually meets twice per week for one hour to discuss any and all problems relating to patient care. These may include the psychosocial, philosophical, ethical, medical, surgical, and rehabilitative aspects of patient care as well as any inter- or intrapersonal problems the staff is experiencing with themselves or the patients. At these meetings the patient's psychodynamics are correlated with social service history, the psychiatric interview, and total staff observations with the intent of enlightening all staff as to the meaning and appropriateness of the patient's cognitive and affective status and the associated behavior of the patient and his family. The goal is always to assist the patient in the maintenance of skills that foster independence and rehabilitation.

From time to time varying staff members have sought me out individually for assistance with attitudes or feelings they were experiencing in interactions with patients. At times they were representative of more general reactions the entire staff was having to some patients and when identified as such, often permitted an enhanced awareness of the entire staff and increased ability to relate appropriately to the patient.

Often the patient is losing ground and deterioration is progressive and evident to all. The permission by the staff for special care of this patient in the dialysis unit by a friend or relative and/or additional assistance by the staff is usually forthcoming after open and frank discussions with the patient regarding the change in his condition. All patients are encouraged to do whatever they can for self-care on the unit, which includes weighing themselves, preparation of the dialysis machine, self hook-up, and performing their own clotting times, blood pressures, charting, etc. To reduce time spent on the unit, most patients are now on the relatively new four-hour coil (three times per week), and scheduling for dialysis favors those patients with regular jobs.

Nursing staff has a great deal of autonomy in terms of their selection of variation in the dialysis procedure, the utilization of adjunctive medications, and the institution of emergency procedures. The weekly meetings have allowed attending physicians, nurses, technicians, and administrative staff to gain confidence in each other's judgment, skills, methods of treatment, and overall caring and concern for the patient.

It is not uncommon for many patients and their family members to become very close to the unit's personnel. The concepts of the dying patient, "an appropriate death,"[14] and "postvention" and the "survivor-victims"[9] are constantly being observed and carried out on the unit. Often nurses, technicians, or attending physicians find themselves talking with the patient or his family regarding their views on the patient's illness, what changes it is causing, and what should be done if all goes wrong. It is not unusual for staff members to visit with a recently deceased patient's family, attend the funeral, or see those survivors of the patient whose adjustments to the patient's illness were marginal or who displayed excessive feelings of guilt, anger, shame, or resentment. For the survivors these visitations often represent the beginning of the necessary work that still lies ahead of them in working through the loss that they have incurred.

By arranging meetings on a regular basis with the majority of the dialysis unit's staff, which allowed for the discussion of any and all subjects concerning the patients, their families, and their caretakers, the unit's personnel and consultants gained an understanding of the patient's and family's response and adaptation to renal failure and its treatment, an improved awareness and respect for different professional's skills and training, and a more mature acceptance of the limitations and finiteness of one's life and relationships with others.

SUMMARY

The psychiatrist who consults with a dialysis unit has an opportunity to formulate and coordinate ideas and plans for hospital and community health care of severly ill patients and to work with patients and families undergoing severe stress and adaptation to life-threatening illness. He also can provide consultation-liaison to numerous professionals that can foster the mutual sharing of multidisciplinary skills and educational values as well as the acquisition of further perspectives regarding the care and treatment of those involved in the process of dying and surviving. The dialysis unit thoroughly tests the psychiatrist's skills and resourcefulness and simultaneously provides a most unique experience (the growing awareness of one's own finiteness) felt by all individuals who treat the dialysis patient—an experience that is best able to be understood and tolerated with the psychiatrist's assistance.

REFERENCES

1. Sand P, Livingston G, Wright R: Psychological assessment of candidates for a hemodialysis program. Ann Int Med 3:602–610, 1966
2. Foster F, Cohn G, McKegney F: Psychobiologic factors and individual survival on chronic renal dialysis—a two year follow up. I. Psychosom Med 35:64–81, 1973
3. Hagberg B: A prospective study of patients in chronic hemodialysis. III. Predictive value of intelligence, congitive deficit, and ego defense structures in rehabilitation. J Psychosom Res 18:151–160, 1974
4. Abram H: The psychiatrist, the treatment of chronic renal failure, and the prolongation of life. II. Am J Psychiatry 126:157–167, 1969
5. Short M, Wilson W: Roles of denial in chronic hemodialysis. Arch Gen Psychiatry 20:433, 1969
6. Kaplan de Nour A, Czaczkes J: Professional team opinion and personal bias—a study of a chronic hemodialysis unit team. J Chron Dis 24:533–538, 1971
7. Wright R, Sand P, Livingston G: Psychological stress during hemodialysis for chronic renal failure. Ann Int Med 64:611, 1966
8. Hagberg B, Malmquist A: A prospective study of patients in chronic hemodialysis. IV. Pretreatment psychiatric and psychological variables predicting outcome. J Psychosom Res 18:315–319, 1974

9. Shneidman E: Deaths of Man. New York, Quadrangle, 1973
10. Beard B: Fear of death and fear of life. Arch Gen Psychiatry 21:373–380, 1969
11. Halper I: Psychiatric observations in a chronic hemodialysis program. Med Clin North Am 55:177–191, 1971
12. Baker A, Knutson J: Psychiatric aspects of uremia. Am J Psychiatry 102:683–687, 1946
13. Schreiner G, Maher J: Uremia: Biochemistry, Pathogenesis and Treatment. Springfield, Illinois, Thomas, 1961
14. Weisman A: Discussion of suicide and appropriate death. Internat J Psychiatry 2:190–193, 1966

Z. J. Lipowski

12
Psychiatric Liaison with Neurology and Neurosurgery

Psychiatry and neurology were once indivisible, or at least closely allied. This alliance was based on the shared belief that disorders of mental functioning and behavior were manifestations of dysfunction of the brain and would ultimately be explicated by the investigative methods and in the language of the neurosciences. Yet, as Woodger observed, it is a mistake to identify a *person* with his brain, that is, to put him into his own head.[1] Neurology has developed its own methodological approaches to the study of cerebral activity and a language to describe it and to formulate explanatory hypotheses about it. Similarly, psychology and psychopathology have evolved their distinct research strategies as well as descriptive and theoretical statements. These cannot be reduced to the methods, language, and statements of the neurosciences. This development has created a chasm between these two approaches to the study of man and an estrangement between neurology and psychiatry. Toulmin points out, however, that to give an adequate account of the mind-body problem involves a *parallel* pursuit of neuroscientific empirical studies of the cerebral substrate of mental functioning and an analysis of progressively more complex levels of human behavior.[2] This pursuit does not imply that either approach should be reduced to the other, but it does call for close collaboration and exhange of ideas between the neurosciences and the behavioral sciences. Such a rapprochement is particularly vital for neurology and psychiatry. The study of psychopathology presents neurologists and other neuroscientists with challenging questions about the neural substrate of deranged mental functioning and behavior of persons. At the same time psychiatrists cannot make progress in the study and treatment of mental disorders if they confine themselves to purely psychological and social investigative methods and explanatory systems. All three conceptual approaches, the neuroscientific, the psychological, and the

157

social, are indispensable for a unified science of human behavior and its disorders.

We do not need a revival of old-fashioned neuropsychiatry. We must eschew reductionism. We also need to build bridges between neurology and psychiatry for the purpose of exchange of knowledge, for collaborative research, and for improved care of both neurological and psychiatric patients whose needs transcend artificial interdisciplinary boundaries. A few neurologists and psychiatrists are keenly aware of the need for closer collaboration between our specialties both in clinical work and in the teaching of medical students and the training of residents.[3, 4] The author has reported on such liaison, developed over more than a decade, with neurologists and neurosurgeons at the Montreal Neurological Institute.[5, 6] The present chapter is based on that personal experience and outlines the problems at the interface between neurology and psychiatry from the viewpoint of a liaison psychiatrist working in a neurological hospital.

COMMON DIAGNOSTIC AND PSYCHOSOCIAL MANAGEMENT PROBLEMS

Each medical and surgical specialty presents the liaison psychiatrist with diagnostic and patient management problems that are in some degree unique to it. Neurological and neurosurgical patients commonly show some of the following features: First, many of them suffer from diseases of the central nervous system that affect their capacity for information processing, their experience and control of drives and emotions, their communicative and psychomotor skills, and their social judgment and overall competence.[6] This impairment of the highest integrative functions is particularly threatening to people for whom efficient intellectual functioning is essential for earning a living and for the maintenance of self-esteem. More generally, cognitive performance is vitally important for people living in today's complex society; hence its impairment constitutes a vital threat and/or loss to the patient with consequent arousal of anxiety, depression, and other dysphoric emotions. Furthermore, cerebral disease often brings about a personality change that for the patient may signify damage to his very self as well as interfere with his interpersonal relationships. Clearly, diseases of the central nervous system are liable to have both direct psychopathological and secondary adverse psychosocial effects and complications. Second, neurological diseases are frequently manifested by impairment or loss of such vital functions as locomotion, use of hands, control of elimination, sexual performance, sensation, and so forth, which are likely to have a disturbing personal meaning.[6] Third, some of the chronic diseases, such as multiple sclerosis, provoke uncertainty. The patient has to face and cope with the unpredictability of his prognosis, which makes adjustment far more difficult than in the case of a stable disability.

Fourth, a large proportion of patients suffer from chronic or intermittent pain, be it migraine, trigeminal neuralgia, or backache. There is invariably a psychological component in these painful conditions that may play a part in precipitating or aggravating the pain and at times makes it resistant to all forms of treatment because the pain has acquired a symbolic meaning of a just punishment, for example. Fifth, some of the disorders, such as epilepsy, evoke fearful and aversive responses in other people and thus carry a stigma that may affect the patient's self-image, chances for employment, and interpersonal relationships. Sixth, other diseases involve disfigurement, as facial paralysis, and are liable not only to change the patient's body image but also undermine his self-esteem. Seventh, disorders of the nervous system are notoriously used as models for conversion hysteria, that is, for unconsciously motivated expression and communication of personally repudiated impulses and needs (sexual, aggressive, and/or dependent) in the form of somatic symptoms.

The above list is incomplete, but it does serve to highlight the manifold psychosocial problems that arise in the course of neurological diseases and present the staff with diagnostic and management difficulties. A liaison psychiatrist may help to identify them and offer practical advice on their treatment. His role in this setting will be made explicit by a more detailed discussion of the clinical problems he encounters and by giving examples of specific cases.

Diagnostic and therapeutic problems will be discussed together. Both diagnosis and therapy are viewed in their comprehensive sense, one that comprises psychological and social aspects in addition to the strictly psychiatric ones.

PSYCHOLOGICAL PRESENTATION OF NEUROLOGIC DISEASE

A common diagnostic problem is the psychological presentation of neurologic disease. It refers to the patient's mode of verbal and nonverbal behavior creating the impression that he is suffering from a purely functional psychiatric disorder, that is, one that can be adequately explicated in psychodynamic and psychosocial terms. For example, a patient may complain of a change in his affective state, most often depression or anxiety, and implicitly or explicitly relate it to a social event, such as a recent loss of a loved person or a job, and imply that his symptoms, psychological and somatic, have been caused by his distressing social situation. In other cases the patient may be brought by a family member who has noticed a personality change in the patient, either in the sense of accentuation or alteration of his habitual mood, attitudes, and conduct. A third type of patient presents with more or less flagrant conversion symptoms and either displays affective indifference toward them—the la belle indifference—or, on the contrary, communicates his distress in dramatic and exaggerated language.

All of these types of patients are not likely to go first to a neurologist; rather they are usually referred to him by another physician who wishes to rule out possible neurological disease. The neurologist may find nothing suspicious and request a psychiatric consultation. The consultant's main diagnostic tool is a psychiatric interview, usually supplemented by information from the patient's family, employer, physician, and the like. The first task is a thorough psychiatric assessment of the patient. This involves not only taking a comprehensive history but also an appraisal of the patient's cognitive functioning. This may provide subtle clues to an underlying cerebral disorder, primary or secondary to systemic disease. If this inquiry reveals the recent onset of forgetfulness, inattention, perplexity on facing new or complex tasks, reduced efficiency in dealing with occupational and social situations that the patient used to handle well, unaccustomed impulsive behavior, and blunting of social judgment and finer emotional responses, then the index of suspicion of an underlying cerebral disorder must be high. This is especially so if the patient is over 40 years old, gives a history of an adequate coping with psychosocial stresses in the past, and shows relatively atypical psychopathology. Relatives may describe transient episodes of disorientation, irrational behavior, or general falling off of the patient's efficacy. In such a case the consultant should recommend a more thorough neurological and medical work-up, which may reveal a cerebral disease. From that point on the primary therapy, if such is currently available, has to be directed at the neurological disorder, but the consultant may still advise on the management of the patient's concurrent psychopathology or assume its treatment himself.

The diagnostic problem often involves identification of one of the organic brain syndromes[7] and its differentiation from depression, schizophrenia, paranoid psychosis, or a hysterical dissociative neurosis. If the patient presents what seem to be conversion hysterical symptoms, such as pseudoseizures,[8] the consultant has to be careful not to accept too readily a plausible cause-and-effect relationship between the patient's psychological conflicts and his somatic symptoms. Both a thorough neurological examination and an independent assessment of the patient's personality, psychodynamic patterns, and recent life changes preceding the onset of symptoms are necessary to establish if the latter are likely to be hysterical, organic, or both.[9] In the author's experience, hysterical fits often coexist with epilepsy and may create difficult diagnostic problems, especially when psychomotor seizures are involved.[6] In other cases conversion symptoms may mimic or mask multiple sclerosis,[10] myasthenia gravis,[11] paraplegia,[12] and virtually every neurological disease.

A few clinical vignettes may illustrate the above diagnostic dilemmas.

A 47-year-old single female librarian complained of forgetfulness, nervousness, palpitations, insomnia, irritability, and unaccustomed outbursts of temper. She saw her family physician. He felt that she suffered from anxiety neurosis and prescribed sedatives. She felt better for a few months but then developed some instability on walking and had a number of falls that she ascribed to osteoarthritis. She gradually started to feel tired and depressed, and her doctor recommended a psychiatric consultation. While waiting for her appointment, the patient had yet another bad fall and found it difficult to get up. At this point she decided to call a neurologist whom she knew, and he hospitalized her at once. A few days later she had surgery and an olfactory groove meningioma the size of a tangerine was removed. This took place about two years after the onset of her symptoms, which were considered psychiatric by the patient. She minimized and rationalized the significance of her leg weakness, repeated falls, and personality change. A liaison psychiatrist entered the picture only when the patient developed a postoperative psychosis: a mild delirium followed by a typical acute schizophrenic episode with auditory and olfactory hallucinations and delusions of persecution and influence. She heard voices calling her "masturbator," smelled gas, which she believed was pumped in to poison her, and insisted that the staff could both read her thoughts and put some obscene ones into her head by "distant means." She promptly recovered after treatment with Stelazine. The psychiatric consultant visited her daily, obtained the history of a transient schizophrenic episode 15 years before, and systematically helped the patient to improve her reality testing as well as to gain some insight into the causes and contents of her psychosis in the light of her personality dynamics, life-style, and subjective meaning of surgery.

A 46-year-old married man began to show apathy, general loss of interest, neglect of his business, lack of libido, somnolence, and forgetfulness. His family and his personal physician considered him depressed. A course of antidepressant drug therapy failed to change the picture. Some two years after the onset of symptoms the patient was referred to a neurologist, underwent suboccipital craniectomy, and was found to have stenosis of the upper fourth ventricle with chronic increase of intracranial pressure. Obstruction was released and cerebellar tonsillectomy performed. This man was referred to a psychiatric consultant a few months after surgery. His wife reported a "complete personality change." The patient became sexually demanding and morbidly jealous of his wife. He insisted on staying with her at all times and had frequent outbursts of rage. He attempted to run his small laundry business but could not remember prices or give proper change. In addition, he deterred customers by making sarcastic remarks and telling lewd jokes in their presence. The patient himself denied that he was ill and insisted that his wife was a changed person: forgetful, uncaring, and promiscuous. On examination the patient showed a marked, global intellectual impairment. The diagnosis was that of dementia with marked paranoid projection and depression. Psychiatric treatment was attempted to no avail. One might conjecture that had the patient been diagnosed earlier and treated surgically before brain damage occurred, he would have been spared his miserable fate. With his psychopathology evidently irreversible, the main effort was directed at helping his wife cope with his irrational, disinhibited, and incompetent conduct.

A 24-year-old single clerk consulted a neurologist about ''headaches,'' which he described vaguely as a funny warm and tight sensation that spread from his face to his whole head. He gave a history of close attachment to his mother, with whom he lived, shyness, and problems with workmates, who made jokes about his avoidance of girls and naivete. Neurological examination was negative: the patient was given the diagnosis of hysteria and referred to the psychiatric clinic. A resident at the clinic treated him for several months with psychotherapy and attempted to interpret his ''headaches'' as a symbolic expression of anger at his domineering mother. Finally, his mother arranged a consultation with another psychistrist since the patient continued to complain of his ''headaches.'' A diagnostic interview revealed that what the patient called headaches consisted of a sudden nausealike sensation rising from the epigastrium to his neck, followed first by a warm feeling in his face, and then by a visual hallucination that varied in content. Once he hallucinated a rabbi in a synagogue filled with yellow light, while on another occasion he saw the ''squashed'' face of a girl he knew. These symptoms always occured in this sequence, came on suddenly and unpredictably, lasted a few minutes, and were followed by an intense feeling of loneliness and dread that could last for some 10 or more minutes. Why the patient insisted on calling this experience a headache was not clear. The consultant suspected temporal-lobe seizures and referred him for an EEG, which showed a right temporal focus. Surgery resulted in the removal of a temporal-lobe astrocytoma.

These vignettes underscore the need for taking a detailed history of the presenting complaints regardless if the patient shows an affective disorder, neurotic symptoms, or a suggestive causal relationship between his psychiatric disturbance, on the one hand, and his psychodynamic profile and psychosocial stress, on the other.

PSYCHIATRIC COMPLICATIONS OF NEUROLOGICAL DISEASES

There are three broad classes of psychiatric complications of neurological diseases: first, the organic brain syndromes; second, psychotic, neurotic, and behavioral disorders reactive to the meaning of the illness and its consequences for the patient; and, third, deviant illness behavior, that is, conduct that jeopardizes the patient's chances for recovery and/or results in psychogenic invalidism.[13]

Organic Brain Syndromes

About 20 percent of psychiatric referrals in a neurological setting involve organic brain syndromes.[6] It is reasonable to assume that their incidence among neurological and neurosurgical patients is much higher. The author has proposed a new classification and presented a set of definitions of these syndromes elsewhere.[7, 13, 14] A liaison psychiatrist must be constantly alert to the subtle and early manifestations of these syndromes, which may be minimized or even concealed by the patient or masked by what seems to be an obvious functional psychiatric disorder. Furthermore, the consultant must be familiar with the numerous etiological factors causing organic brain syndromes and with the whole gamut of psychological reactions to and social influences on their course and manifestations. Finally, he should be conversant with symptomatic treatment and the overall management of these syndromes, both when they give rise to psychiatric emergencies and when they require prolonged psychosocial rehabilitation.

The most common reasons for referral of organic patients to a psychiatrist are diagnosis between dementia and depression; diagnosis between delirium and acute schizophrenia; management of a noisy, belligerent, overactive delirious patient; diagnosis between akinetic mutism and psychogenic stupor—depressive, catatonic, or hysterical; diagnosis between a hysterical fugue and delirium or psychomotor seizure; and diagnosis between hysterical amnesia and an amnestic syndrome. Of course, in most of these cases the consultant is not content with diagnostic labeling; but also tries to offer advice on management whenever psychological factors significantly contribute to the patient's predicament. It is particularly in this area that the liaison consultant's knowledge of psychopathology and of general medicine, including neurology, is put to an exacting test. The consultant must, for instance, counteract the common and deplorable tendency of inexperienced neurologists to dismiss every patient over the age of 50 who shows cognitive impairment as suffering from senile or arteriosclerotic dementia.

This diagnosis carries the implication of hopelessness and therapeutic nihilism, both of which are dangerously misleading. First, a whole range of eminently treatable conditions may give rise to a dementialike picture, which the author prefers to call a subacute amnestic-confusional syndrome. It may be caused by head injury, various endocrinopathies, a benign tumor, chronic drug intoxication, avitaminosis, a normal-pressure hydrocephalus, and so forth.[15] Second, the so-called arteriosclerotic dementia may be partly prevented by the adequate treatment of hypertension,[16] and often shows striking though partial remission. Third, any true dementia, that is, global cognitive impairment due to widespread brain damage, may be significantly compensated psychologically if the patient is actively rehabilitated, if he is protected against social isolation as well as information underload and overload, and if his commonly present affective disorder is adequately treated.[17, 18, 19, 20]

Reactive Syndromes

The whole spectrum of neuroses and functional psychoses are covered by the reactive syndromes. In a series of 200 neurological and neurosurgical patients referred for psychiatric consultation 50 percent had the diagnosis of neurosis, 54 percent of them depressive.[6] Functional psychoses accounted for

13 percent of the referrred sample. The reasons for the higher incidence of the depressive syndromes (30 percent of the series) in neurological patients can be gleaned from my initial remarks on the common characteristics of these patients. Ubiquity of loss of vital functions, chronicity and unpredictable course, social stigma, unemployability—these are only some of the salient features of many neurological disorders that can readily account for the frequency of depressive syndromes. It must be emphasized, however, that there is no evidence of a simple correlation between the nature and severity of disease-related disability, on the one hand, and the presence and intensity of the affective disorder, on the other.[21] Many, probably the majority, of neurological patients may experience some initial depression and/or anxiety, but they then channel their energy into rehabilitation and adaptation to persistent disability. This potential for successful adaptation and coping must be always looked for and deliberately fostered by the liaison psychiatrist.

Those neurological diseases that have a sudden and dramatic onset, such as stroke, head injury, paralysis of any etiology, epilepsy, Meniere's disease, and so on, may give rise to a traumatic neurosis ushered in by a sense of shock, disbelief, and, at times, denial of the full significance and likely long-term consequences of the catastrophic event. If the patient's consciousness is at first interrupted, he will go through a period of delirium whose duration is roughly proportionate to the duration of the initial coma. Once full awareness is regained, the person will appraise what has happened to him. During that period he may be particularly receptive to and in need of a psychiatric consultation aimed at discussion of the traumatic event and its likely consequences. Stress on the positive aspects of rehabilitation, on the patient's personality assets, and on his ability to cope is important at this stage and may help prevent psychological disorganization and deviant illness behavior. Assessment of the patient's personality and of his family and other interpersonal relationships is crucial if all available resources are to be brought to bear on his rehabilitation.[22]

Conversion and dissociative hysterical neurosis is at times precipitated by any type of neurological disorder. It may serve as a defense against anxiety and depression, or provide a means of accentuating the patient's sick role for the purpose of either avoiding conflict between incompatible strivings, or for evoking care-taking and nurturing attitudes in others, or both. In any case, these symptoms should be identified early and dealt with vigorously with psychotherapy, behavior modification, or both, before they become fixed and sometimes irreversible. Here again the liaison psychiatrist has a vital diagnostic, therapeutic and preventive role to play.

Deviant Illness Behavior

This connotes conduct that results in prolongation of disability or even death of the patient. It includes gross denial of illness in a state of clear consciousness, excessive dependence, noncompliance with medical treatment and advice, and suicidal attempts and other forms of deliberate self-injury in response to physical disease. Motivation for this type of behavior ranges from unconscious and explicitly disavowed to intentional. It may express a self-destructive or self-punishing tendency, a need to be taken care of, to punish others, to avoid facing unwelcome facts, and so forth.

Deviant illness behavior not only interferes with recovery and rehabilitation of the patient, but it also readily brings him into conflict with the health team, resulting in mutual hostility and recriminations. A psychiatric consultant is usually asked either to change the patient's behavior or to remove him from the scene. This is one of the most trying tasks facing the consultant. He is usually called in when the conflict is open. He encounters a hostile, angry, and suspicious patient and exasperated doctors and nurses. His first task is to gather information and appraise rapidly the dynamics of the interaction. He must mediate between the patient and the staff and explain in acceptable terms their respective behavior to the contending parties. An excellent autobiographical account of a dramatic conflict on a neurological ward has been written, with the author's encouragement, by an intelligent patient who had sustained severe head injury followed by post-traumatic epileptic seizures and mild delirium.[23] The patient expressed her fear and anger by making excessive demands on the staff and by developing multiple hysterical fits in addition to cerebral seizures. One extended psychiatric consultation resulted in the subsidence of the mounting despair of the patient and disruption of the ward routine.

Psychiatric Disorders

At times psychiatric disorders may mimic neurological disease. This is particularly true of conversion hysteria and of depression manifested primarily by somatic symptoms, such as headache, paresthesiae, fatigue and weakness, and so forth.[6] Many neurological disorders have a marked psychological component that can play a part in precipitating, aggravating, and maintaining the symptoms. Migraine, narcolepsy, backache, atypical facial neuralgia are just a few examples of syndromes and symptoms whose management calls for collaboration between neurologists, neurosurgeons, and psychiatrists.

TEACHING AND RESEARCH

Liaison psychiatry implies more than provision of consultations on request. Its mediating role has already been stressed. In addition, liaison psychiatrists are involved in teaching medical students and health professionals working in the given specialty. Much of this teaching consists of informal discussions with the staff and of providing a role model for a comprehensive approach to diagnosis and treatment. A more formal, patient-centered conference is a valuable teaching method. The author has reported on such a joint clinical conference that he used to conduct at the Montreal Neurological Institute.[5] It could be argued cogently that a liaison psychiatrist should be attached to every neurological department. He would certainly not remain idle!

A liaison psychiatrist is also strategically placed to engage in collaborative research on the borderlands between neurology and psychiatry. Only a few worthwhile research projects can be mentioned—the relationship of life stress to the precipitation of strokes[24] and the psychological rehabilitation of the stroke patient,[25] psychological aspects of the postconcussional syndrome[26] and patterns of recovery from head injury,[27] psychological sequelae of subarachnoid hemorrhage,[28] psychological factors in multiple sclerosis,[29] the study of pain,[30] the causes and management of depression common in Parkinsonism,[31] psychological aspects of migraine,[32] psychosocial aspects of epilepsy,[33] sexual functioning in paraplegics[34] and in patients with temporallobe epilepsy,[35] the relationship of schizophrenia to disorders of the limbic system,[36] application of behavior modification in the management of the brain-damaged,[19] and countless other joint research ventures that could contribute to a better understanding of the brain-behavior relationships as well as to improved patient care. Both neurology and psychiatry can only gain from their still tentative attempts at a rapprochement.

REFERENCES

1. Woodger JH: Biology and Language. Cambridge, Eng., Cambridge University Press, 1952, p 286
2. Toulmin S: The mentality of man's brain, in Karczmar AG, Eccles JC (eds): Brain and Human Behavior. New York, Springer, 1972, p 409
3. Rose AS: The integration of neurology into psychiatric education. Am J Psychiatry 123:592–594, 1966
4. Wilson WP, Wells CE, Irigaray PJ: Should psychiatry and neurology integrate? Am J Psychiatry 128:617–622, 1971
5. Lipowski ZJ: Psychiatric liaison with neurology and neurosurgery. Am J Psychiatry 129:136–140, 1972
6. Lipowski ZJ, Kiriakos RZ: Borderlands between neurology and psychiatry: Observations in a neurological hospital. Psychiatry Med 3:131–147, 1972
7. Lipowski ZJ: Organic brain syndromes: An overview and classification, in Benson DF, Blumer D (eds): Psychiatric Aspects of Neurologic Disease. New York, Grune & Stratton (in press)
8. Liske E, Forster FM: Pseudoseizures: A problem in the diagnosis and management of epileptic patients. Neurology (Minneap) 14:41–49, 1964
9. Engel GL: Conversion symptoms, in MacBryde CM, Blacklow RS (eds): Signs and Symptoms (ed 5). Philadelphia, Lippincott, 1970, pp 650–68
10. Aring CD: Observations on multiple sclerosis and conversion hysteria. Brain 88:663–674, 1965

11. Fullerton DT, Munsat TL: Pseudo-myasthenia gravis: A conversion reaction. J Nerv Ment Dis 142:78–86, 1966

12. Kirshner LA, Kaplan N: Conversion as a manifestation of crisis in life situation: A report of seven cases of ataxia and paralysis of the lower extremeties. Compr Psychiat 11:260–266, 1970

13. Lipowski ZJ: Psychiatry of somatic diseases: Epidemiology, pathogenesis, classification. Compr Psychiat 16:105–124, 1975

14. Lipowski ZJ: Delirium, clouding of consciousness and confusion. J Nerv Ment Dis 145:227–255, 1967

15. Marsden CD, Harrison MJG: Outcome of investigation of patients with presenile dementia. Br Med J 2:249–252, 1972

16. Hachinski VC, Lassen NA, Marshall J: Multi-infarct dementia. Lancet 2:207–209, 1974

17. Wells CE (ed): Dementia. Philadelphia, Davis, 1971

18. Bennett R: Social isolation and isolation-reducing programs. Bull NY Acad Med 49:1143–1163, 1973

19. Fowler RS, Fordyce WE: Adapting care for the brain-damaged patient. Am J Nurs 72:1832–1835, 1972

20. Plutzky, M.: Principles of psychiatric management of chronic brain syndrome. Geriatrics 29:120–127, 1974

21. Shontz FC: Physical disability and personality: Theory and recent research. Psychol Aspects Disability 17:51–63, 1970

22. Lipowski ZJ: Physical illness, the patient and his environment: Psychosocial foundations of medicine, in Arieti S (ed): American Handbook of Psychiatry (ed 2), vol 4, ch 1. New York, Basic Books (in press)

23. Lipowski ZJ, Stewart AM: Illness as subjective experience. Psychiatry Med 4:155–171, 1973

24. Gianturco DT, Breslin MS, Heyman A, et al: Personality patterns and life stress in ischemic cerebrovascular disease. I. Psychiatric findings. Stroke 5:453–460, 1974

25. Zankel HT: Stroke Rehabilitation. Springfield, Ill., Thomas, 1971

26. Lidvall HF, Linderoth B, Norlin B: Causes of the post-concussional syndrome. Acta Neurol Scand 50 (suppl 56):1–144, 1974

27. Najenson T, Mendelson L, Schechter I, et al: Rehabilitation after severe head injury. Scand J Rehabil Med 6:5–14, 1974

28. Storey PB: Psychiatric sequelae of subarachnoid haemorrhage. Br Med J 3:261–266, 1967

29. Surridge D: An investigation into some psychiatric aspects of multiple sclerosis. Br J Psychiatry 115:749–764, 1969

30. Sternbach RA: Psychophysiology of pain. Psychiatry Med (in press)

31. Brown LG, Wilson WP: Parkinsonism and depression. South Med J 65:540–545, 1972.

32. Mitchell KR, Mitchell DM: Migraine: An exploratory treatment application of programmed behaviour therapy techniques. J Psychosom Res 15:137–157, 1971

33. Horowitz MJ: Psychosocial Function in Epilepsy. Springfield, Ill., Thomas, 1970

34. Fitzpatrick WF: Sexual function in the paraplegic patient. Arch Phys Med Rehabil 55:221–227, 1974

35. Blumer D: Sexual function in temporal-lobe epilepsy, in Benson DF, Blumer D
     (eds): Psychiatric Aspects of Neurologic Disease. New York, Grune & Stratton,
     1975
36. Torrey FE, Peterson MR: Schizophrenia and the limbic system. Lancet 3:942–
     946, 1974

PART III

Psychiatric Consultation: The Perennial Problems in the Hospital

John J. Schwab

Introduction

The next seven chapters deal directly with the problems constituting the bulk of the psychiatric consultant's work in the general hospital. Viewing these problems brings into focus the major aspects of the consultant's role. In handling psychiatric emergencies, assessing the meaning of patients' physical symptoms, recommending management programs for those with chronic pain or delirium, gauging suicide risk, and working with dying patients and the bereaved, the consultant functions as a physician who uses his knowledge of medicine and his skills as a specialist in human behavior. His role as a practitioner of comprehensive medicine, therefore, is basic to other major aspects of his role as an interpreter of data to staff and family and as a model for others in his approach to patients.

The hospital situation tends to isolate patients artificially. In the hospital the patient is removed from the social setting in which all illness arises, and often his meaningful interpersonal contacts are drastically curtailed. Thus, the hospitalized patient must be regarded as a "displaced person." When the consultant does not have an in-depth understanding of significant events that precipitate emergencies or heighten the risk of suicide, he sees the patients only as "cases," and, consequently, his therapeutic endeavors may be more evanescent than lasting. In the first chapter of the section, "The Psychiatric Emergency," Straker points out that as the consultant gains experience with the perennial problems in psychiatric consultation in the hospital, he acquires a growing realization of the importance of the lack of social support systems as causes of emergencies, delirious reactions, suicide attempts, and sustained physical symptomatology. The influence of the social setting on illness, the cultural relativity of symptoms, and the human being's age-old need for support systems comprise a theme fundamental to the discussions of consultation work in the hospital.

As a consultant in the general hospital, the psychiatrist learns quickly that it is necessary to dismiss the dichotomous conceptions of illness—either functional or organic—that have led too often to an incomplete comprehension of patients' difficulties and fragmented treatment programs. Patients who present as psychiatric emergencies and those with physical symptoms, including pain and/or delirium, frequently are suffering from concurrent physical and emotional illnesses. In 1965 Palerea stated, "The presence of concurrent significant medical and psychiatric illnesses appears to be the rule rather than the exception."[1] Supporting evidence for this statement comes from numerous sources, including the controlled study by Matarazzo and his associates, which showed that in both medical and psychiatric inpatients and outpatients the increased number of medical symptoms correlated positively with an increased number of psychiatric symptoms.[2] Those authors asserted, "The number of medical symptoms is a good predictor of psychiatric symptomatology, and vice versa." In 1957 Hinkle and Wolff concluded from their comprehensive evaluation of illness in relatively healthy populations that "those people who had the greater number of bodily illnesses, regardless of their nature, and regardless of their etiology, were the ones who experienced the greater number of disturbances of mood, thought, and behavior."[3] These findings bear directly on the subject matter in this volume presented by Wahl in his chapter, "The Patient Whose Physical Symptoms Mask a Psychiatric Disorder," and by McCreary and Jamison in their chapter, "The Chronic-Pain Patient." Wahl's discussion of physical symptoms masking a psychiatric disorder reflects the breadth and depth of his clinical experience, his knowledge of the diversity of the psychophysiologic expression of disease, and his humility in approaching the variations and vicissitudes of human experience as it is manifested by hospitalized patients in distress.

In working with patients in the general hospital, the consultant should be wary of a propensity for making a case for psychogenic etiology and should be alert to the presence of concurrent physical and mental illness. Psychiatric symptomatology can mask medical illness, mild or serious, acute or chronic. Endocrine dysfunctions that tend to make their appearance gradually and are difficult to diagnose in their early stages because the symptoms may be numerous, ill defined, and often bizarre, may be incorrectly labeled "neuroses." Furthermore, since these disorders often occur in midlife, about the time of the climacteric when life's disappointments are readily apparent and when the body no longer functions as smoothly and agilely as before, the symptoms may be perceived as indicators of mental illness and the underlying endocrine disease neither fully investigated nor adequately treated. In reviewing 30 years' experience with psychiatric endocrinology, Bleuler emphasized the intimate relationships between hormones and emotions.[4] He asserted flatly that all patients with endocrine disorders, regardless of the adequacy of substitutive therapy, showed at least minor psychic and behavioral changes.

Patients with endocrine diseases such as hypothyroidism are too often diagnosed "depressed." The hypoparathyroid patient's muscle spasms and bizarre sensations caused by tetany may mislead the physician to make a diagnosis of conversion reaction. The electrolyte disturbances accompanying hyperparathyroidism, particularly when there are renal complications, may produce an acute brain syndrome with the typical features of delirium.

Working with the patient who complains of chronic pain can be discouraging for the psychiatric consultant when he is relatively unaware of the meaning of the pain to the patient and when he does not consider the associations between pain and helplessness, guilt, and the need for expiation. Moreover, complaints of chronic pain have numerous social and cultural variations, as shown by Zborowoski in 1952; his research in New England revealed that patients who came from Jewish and Italian backgrounds tended to display more emotional responses to pain than did the typical "Old Americans."[5] In evaluating patients whose main complaints are chronic pain, the consultant should heed the bruised Don Quixote's words to the commiserating Sancho Panza: "Other men's wounds are easily borne."[6]

Delirious reactions not only constitute emergencies but also indicate that such medical patients' prognoses are poorer than those of other general medical patients. Guze and Cantwell reported that in Barnes Hospital the mortality rate of patients with organic brain syndromes was 17 percent compared with the general mortality rate of 3.7 percent.[7] Age was not the major factor accounting for the increased mortality in the patients with delirium; 13 percent of those under the age of 50 who had organic brain syndromes died. Psychiatric consultants in general hospitals soon learn that the medical staff is not always alert to the onset of delirium. In many instances the medical and nursing staff dismiss the predelirious phase—characterized mainly by increased apprehension, some overt nervousness, and difficulty sleeping—as a not unusual stage of convalescence. Opportunities for early diagnosis and prompt treatment are missed. Furthermore, when the patient is presenting as a management problem, he is likely to be diagnosed as "possibly schizophrenic" by the staff and treatment to prevent the development of full-blown delirium is not initiated. Instead, as Jones points out in his chapter, "Delirium," many of these patients are given moderate doses of sedatives or tranquilizers, doses that tend to obtund their already diminished faculties and potentiate the onset of delirium.

Litman's chapter, "The Assessment of Suicidality," furnishes the psychiatric consultant with valuable guidelines for gauging suicide risk. The consultant needs to maintain a high level of awareness of the significance of deprivation and the lack of social support systems as factors that produce despair. Also, he should be alert to familial interactions, which, on occasion, may drive the patient to suicide. Another important consideration is the increase in the suicide rate among young adults and groups whose suicide rates previously were very low. Currently, the suicide rate for blacks is rising, and for nonwhite females it is at the highest point in American history.[8] Attempted suicide and/or suicide is an index of psychosocial malaise and, as Litman points out, is the result of sociocultural and familial as well as individual and medical factors.

The care of the dying patient is becoming a serious problem. The devaluation of our belief systems strikes at the root of one of man's Ur needs (described by Masserman[9] as the basic need to find a philosophy, belief or faith that gives meaning and coherence to life and death). This has resulted in a shifting of the responsibility of the care of the dying patient away from the family and the clergy to hospital and professional caretakers. Furthermore, advances in modern technologic medicine have removed many of nature's defenses that palliated the experience of dying. For example, life support systems and vigorous therapy prevent coma and pneumonia. Traditionally, pneumonia was known as the friend of the aged and the infirm. The family's deathwatch has been supplanted by "medical and nursing care"; as a consequence, closeness is being replaced by the more professional ministrations of hospital employees.

In view of these considerations we are compelled to ask about the psychiatric consultant's goals with the dying patient. Should he attempt to help him achieve some degree of equanimity if possible? In order to develop equanimity, to what extent should the dying patient use the mechanism of denial? We should ponder Spinoza's assertion that it is necessary for human beings to preserve certain illusions in order to live as well as to die.[10]

Many writings on the dying patient seem to be aimed at benefiting the hospital staff and the family rather than the patient. They enable others, not the dying patient, to assuage guilt and at times help them bolster their own counterphobic defenses against death. But instead of propounding lofty abstractions, Weisman, in his chapter, "The Dying Patient," emphasizes that the consultant needs to refine the art of interviewing and let the interview material guide him in his work with the patient. Weisman's other suggestions, illustrated by common sense questions and answers, will assist the consultant in his work with the dying patient.

As we consider the growing need to work with dying patients, we should recall LeShan's statement, "The therapist who works with patients in a catastrophic situation may find to his surprise that there are real rewards in the work that he did not expect. . . . Working with people who are under the hammer of fate greatly increases one's respect for them and makes one proud of being a human being."[11]

The final chapter in this section, "Postvention: The Care of the Bereaved," by Shneidman, should be mandatory reading for all physicians, not only psychiatric consultants. The model that he presents—prevention, intervention, and postvention—can be generalized to the care of countless medical patients and their families, not only the bereaved.

The authors of this section do not shy away from the seriousness of the problems that they are describing. Instead, they acknowledge the complexity of their work and offer the benefits of their experiences to the consultant to enable him to function effectively in his roles as a practitioner of comprehensive medicine, a specialist in human behavior, an interpreter to family and staff, and a model for students and other professionals.

REFERENCES

1. Palerea EP: Medical evaluation of the psychiatric patient. J Am Geriatr Soc 13:14, 1965

2. Matarazzo RG, Matarazzo JD, Saslow G: The relationship between medical and psychiatric symptoms. J Am Soc Psychol 62(1):55, 1961

3. Hinkle LE, Wolff HG: Health and the social environment: Experimental investigations, in Leighton A, Clausen J, Wilson R (eds): Explorations in Social Psychiatry. New York, Basic Books, 1957, 105–137

4. Bleuler M: Principal findings based on 30 years' experience in endocrine psychiatry, in Usdin G (ed): The Psychiatric Forum. New York, Bruner/Mazel, 1972, pp 39–43

5. Zborowoski M: Cultural components in responses to pain. J Soc Issues 13:16, 1952

6. Cervantes Mde: Don Quixote of La Mancha, trans by Walter Starkie. New York, Signet, 1964

7. Guze SB, Cantwell BP: The prognosis in organic brain syndromes. Am J Psychiatry 120:878, 1974

8. Schwab JJ, Warheit GJ, Holzer CE: Suicidal ideation and behavior in a general population. Dis Nerv Sys 33:745–748, 1972

9. Masserman JH: The Practice of Dynamic Psychiatry (ed 2). Philadelphia, Saunders, 1961

10. Spinoza B: The Ethics. New York, Tudor, 1936

11. LeShan LL: Some observations on the problem of mobilizing the patient's will to live, in Kissen DM, LeShan LL (eds): Psychosomatic Aspects of Neoplastic Disease. Philadelphia, Lippincott, 1964, pp 109–120

Manuel Straker

13
The Psychiatric Emergency

The psychiatric emergency has many faces. It is shaped by the crisis characteristics, by the personality style, and by the specific features of the setting in which it finds expression. The emergency may erupt at home, at work, in the streets, or in a social setting, reflecting the past experience, the immediate life situation, and the responses of the environment. One major arena for consultation-liaison activities exists within the hospital, where emergencies of all kinds occur as everyday experience. The psychiatrist works in the emergency room and in areas at the boundaries between the organic disorders and the less well understood emotional and behavioral disturbances. His interest may focus on a patient in turmoil, or on staff agitation about patient behavior or the discouragement experienced as a treatment failure looms or death claims another victim. Interpersonal conflicts can emerge between patient and staff (contaminating the therapeutic environment) or between staff and staff, or it may involve the family, the ward milieu, or the hospital community. Under such conditions, and no matter what the origin, the patient is still the ultimate victim. Consultant-liaison functions at times may appear to move far afield, but the basic commitment remains to support and assist patient care.

The larger population served by existing diagnostic and treatment resources has changed the old narrow concept of the psychiatric emergency. The emergency of the past was restricted to the determined suicide attempt, to outbreaks of homicidal aggression, or to outbreaks of bizarre behavior beyond the tolerance of the environment. A crisis mobilized the limited community resources then available. The patient was confined in the city or county jail or committed for treatment to a psychiatric hospital or a state institution.

Many developments have taken place since World War II. There is alteration of psychiatric boundaries through an increased public acceptance of the need for psychiatric care and expanded treatment techniques. "The psychotic and severely neurotic are not the only ones now seen as patients; there are also the unhappy, the poor, the deviant, the socially deprived, the unsuccessful, and the unfulfilled."[1] Psychiatric patients now present new clinical syndromes.[2] The increased range of patients has also been reflected in a rapid expansion of treatment resources, which are established in the mainstream of community life. The formerly isolated state institution is now supported by a network of other resources, including the psychiatrist in private practice, the general hospital psychiatry unit, the community mental health center, storefront clinics, and the psychiatric hospital or institute. A promising new outreach technique extends psychiatric services into the heart of the ghetto by utilizing bidirectional cable television as the medium for patient-physician contact.[3] Specialized groups have developed influential roles in the delivery of mental health services. These organizations include the alcoholics anonymous groups, suicide prevention centers, drug dependency treatment centers, and others that are less well established.

DEFINITIONS

Frazier broadly defines the *emergency* as "any urgent psychiatric condition, functional or organic, for which immediate treatment would increase the likelihood of recovery, or provide urgently needed protection."[4] The emergency state is so designated by the patient, the perturbed family, the referring agency, the escorting police, or the therapist examiner. Most emergencies involve an acute condition "with people who are frightened, desperate, hopeless, driven by self-destructive impulses, or paralyzed by conflict and anxiety."[5] Any combination of factors that threatens to overwhelm the available coping resources of the individual can precipitate the "emergency state." After assessment the situation may be reconceptualized as a suicidal act or serious risk, a loss of control with bizarre or assaultive behavior, a panic state, a turmoil marking an incipient psychotic break, a confusion or delirium resulting from drug overdosage, alcohol, or a postictal state, or any other sudden disorder of homeostasis, no matter what the precipitants may be.

"The psychiatric emergency refers to (1) socially disruptive or deviant behavior or (2) personally overwhelming feelings of catastrophe, rather than to a particular diagnostic category of mental illness."[6] There is either an intrapsychic crisis, an interpersonal conflict, or a series of social problems and environmental stressors that strain the coping resources. However, when the therapeutic response is shaped only by the major precipitants, it will usually turn out to be inadequate therapy. Appropriate action includes a number of steps. The first requirement is to provide immediate support and relief of symptoms. The basic elements of the crisis need to be clarified and sorted out. One needs to identify the major conflicts as well as the nature of the patient's

Table 13–1

Presenting Symptoms by Frequency

Symptoms	Ranked First	Ranked Second
Depression	67	14
Suicide attempt	6	5
Anxiety	20	27
Intoxication	8	16
Assaultive	7	13

responses. In addition to the task of making the diagnosis, the assessment includes consideration of the patient's ego strengths, consideration of the environment supports and resources, and consideration of those realistic options available for practical problem-solving action. All of the supportive elements need to be combined in a multifactorial helping approach. A successful outcome is marked by the disappearance of the crisis reaction and a return of reorganized and effective coping mechanisms, while an untreated crisis can result in suicide, psychosis, or severe disability.

COMMON PRESENTING SYMPTOMS

The presenting behavior of emergent patients is described in a study by Glasscote and his associates.[7] Their data, collected from 114 completed questionnaires, have a wide base and seem to provide a fair representation of general experiences. In Table 13–1 only the five major presenting symptoms revealed in the study are reproduced. In the discussion that follows these common syndromes will be briefly described—depression, suicide, anxiety, intoxication, and assaultiveness.

Depression

The variety of depressive reactions is extensive. Depression is the most frequently occurring emotional disturbance. Common to all types is the marked loss of self-esteem, a loss of hope about the future, and a pervasive sadness from which the patient cannot be easily distracted. Self-blame, guilt feelings, and some anguish and agitation are present, along with changes in the usual psychomotor activities. This is a high-risk group for suicide. In spite of the recognized high frequency of depression, many cases remain undiagnosed and untreated, particularly when the depressive affect is masked, expressed mainly through somatic disturbances or other variants.

Treatment requires supportive and frequent contact. Environmental support systems need to be assessed and used effectively. Uncovering psychotherapeutic explorations are best delayed until ego functions are more adequate. Antidepressant medication offers symptom relief in approximately 70 percent to 80 percent of patients within four to six weeks of therapy onset. Alertness to suicide risk is important. In doubtful situations, it is recommended that the patient be hospitalized. Only there is 24-hour observation, support, and external control possible. Where the suicidal risk is overwhelming and unrelieved, electroshock therapy is indicated as a lifesaving measure.

Suicide

Wayne studied the admissions to a private psychiatric hospital.[6] He designated 20 percent of admissions as emergencies; of this group, 40 percent were depressed and suicidal. Suicide can occur without warning and unpredictably, but this is rare. Usually, clues are provided by patient behavior, thought content, direct threats, or covert help seeking. The special-risk group includes patients who are severely depressed or schizophrenic. The time of greatest danger occurs during the period when the patient is entering a depressed state or is emerging from it. Many suicides are completed when the therapist's vigilance relaxes in the face of an improving patient.

In the emergency room the first task is to distinguish the serious suicidal risk from the manipulative gesture, whose goal is not death-related. In the absence of objective tests, careful clinical assessment is necessary. Family suicidal attempts and past suicidal acts in the personal history are significant. The recent crisis needs evaluation, and suicidal thoughts and threats are to be noted. The role of the significant other is often central to the patient's fate.[8] The patient's support systems—family, social, cultural, and religious—must be considered. Diagnosis will lead to a clear plan of treatment whose aim is to provide lifesaving protection and to reverse the existing crisis.

Anxiety

Typically, the anxiety attack is already subsiding by the time that the emergency room is reached. The patient always has lingering fears and misinterpretations about the unusual sensations just experienced. A careful history and physical examination can deal with the issue of significant organic disease. A psychotherapeutic approach calms the patient. Anxiolytic medication may be useful as an early intervention and assist further exploration. It is evidence of therapeutic failure when the patient drifts into a recurring or chronic state or learns to rely on barbiturates, alcohol, or other self-medications to maintain the existing defences against anxiety.

Intoxications

A state of intoxication depends upon dosages, acquired tolerance, potentiation by other drugs, personality traits, racial background, and physical condition. Usually psychotomimetic drugs produce symptoms only while the intoxicant is in the system. In some instances symptoms may last for days, weeks, or months after the ''trip'' is over, either in flashbacks (especially for LSD and sometimes marijuana) or by initiating a profound psychological disorder.

Drug withdrawal symptoms may be characteristic. Such symptoms may follow the abrupt cessation of physically addicting drugs taken in large doses over a prolonged period. This holds for alcohol, barbiturates, amphetamines, opiates, and others. A drug psychosis usually presents with confusion, disorientation, perceptual distortions, vivid hallucinations, bizarre behavior, panic, chaotic turmoil, delusions, and CNS depression or excitement, depending on the drug used. The triad of coma, pinpoint pupils, and respiratory depression indicates opiate overdosage. Coma, respiratory depression, and nystagmus point to barbiturate poisoning, while fixed and dilated pupils are indicative of poisoning from anticholinergics. Furthermore, the ingestion of drug combinations produces confusing clinical states.

The withdrawal from opiates is marked by lacrimation, rhinorrhea, back pain, GI distress, piloerection, and mydriasis. Ambulatory detoxification with methadone over a 10-day period is now a firmly established practice. Withdrawal from barbiturates or alcohol can produce an acute brain syndrome, including confusion, disorientation, delirium, agitation, anxiety, insomnia, motor restlessness and tremors, and convulsive seizures. Seizures can also follow withdrawal from diazepam, glutethimide, meprobamate, and a number of minor tranquilizers. Convulsions may also follow the use of strychinine, high doses of amphetamines, and LSD.

Table 13–2 summarizes the effects of drugs that are commonly abused. All personnel who serve in an emergency psychiatric service should be thoroughly familiar with these drugs, the type of presentation that are commonly associated with them, and the withdrawal symptoms.

TREATMENT

A 1973 general hospital emergency room survey indicates that overdosage constitutes 6.2 percent of all emergency medical admissions, that 44 percent of these patients had current or recent psychiatric treatment, and that the most frequent intoxicant was diazepam (Valium) and/or nonbarbiturate hypnotics.[10]

Psychiatric emergency room tasks concern identifying life-threatening poisonings, treating those that may not survive transfer, and managing the milder intoxications. Psychotherapeutic support is necessary to reduce anxiety.

Table 13–2

Comparison Summary, Selected Effects of Commonly Abused Drugs*

Drugs	Dependence	Intoxication	Withdrawal	Flashbacks
Alcohol	Marked	Depression of sensorium and respiration Pupils normal	Gastritis Convulsive seizures	None
Barbiturates	Marked	Depressed CNS and respiration Nystagmus	Convulsive seizures	None
Opiates	Marked	Pinpoint Pupils Analgesia Depressed sensorium and respiration	GI upset Lacrimation Rhinorrhea Gooseflesh	None
Glutethimide	Marked	Coma Respiratory depression Dilated pupils Laryngeal spasm	Convulsive seizures Hyperpyrexia Delirium	None
Amphetamines	Mild	Hypertension Dilated pupils Convulsive seizures Tachycardia Paranoid psychosis Hypomanic behavior	Depression Organic brain syndrome	Occasional

Minor tranquilizers	Marked	Sensorium depression Pupils not unusual	Similar to barbiturates	None
Marijuana	Absent	Conjunctivae injected Giddiness Drowsy Perceptual changes May lead to hallucinations, psychosis	None specific	Occasional
Anticholinergics	Absent	Acute psychosis Dilated fixed pupils Tachycardia Hallucinations	Mydriasis	None
Phenothiazines	Absent	Rigidity Akasthisia Drowsy Dystonia Increased psychosis	Possible tardive dyskinesia	None

*Modified reproduction from Dimijian and Radelat.[9]

Watchful support and talking down a "bad trip" may be all that is needed. In the latter instance Valium 10 mg I/M or I/V may be helpful. When respiratory depression is not present, one can use small doses of barbiturates, Valium 10 mg I/M, or modest doses of oral chlorpromazine 25–50 mg (except for cases of anticholinergic poisoning). Close monitoring of vital systems is essential. Intravenous fluids and anticonvulsant medication are to be given when appropriate.

The methods of treatment of substance ingestion at the Brentwood VA Hospital include

(1) *Removal of stomach contents* by emesis or gastric lavage. An empty stomach stops further absorption and reduces risk of aspiration.

(2) *Careful monitoring* of vital functions requires intensive care instrumentation, with interventions as required to support cardiac or respiratory failure.

(3) *Excretion assistance* by intravenous fluids, forced diuresis, or lifesaving hemodialysis.

Identification of the drug is made by history, clinical findings and biochemical laboratory screening. The situation is often complicated by the ingestion of a number of different drugs at the same time.

If opiate overdosage is suspected, immediate and repeated administration of nalorphine hydrochloride is lifesaving. Other routine measures include establishing an adequate airway, checking blood pressure, treating status epilepticus by diphenyl hydantoin 200 mg I/M, and diazepam 10 mg I/V. The phenothiazine induced extrapyramidal reaction or dystonic crisis is quickly relieved by Cogentin 1–2 ml I/M (benztropine mesylate) and followed by oral medication.

Assaultive Behavior

Public myths frequently confuse mental illness with assaultive behavior. Actually this is a rarity. Assaultive behavior may emerge during the confusion state of a profound intoxication with alcohol or drugs, during psychomotor seizures, in a postictal furor, or as an expression of an "episodic dyscontrol syndrome." It can also occur during a manic excitement or in response to persecutory delusions in a paranoid panic. Alcohol plays an important role in precipitating assaultive attacks.

Supportive interest, a clear explanation of intentions, and firm persuasion are helpful in calming the patient. Confrontation is a last resort. If absolutely necessary, it is best to present a sufficient show of force and authority so that the patient will choose not to fight. Physical restraints may be needed until the patient has regained self-control. Sedation and tranquilization are invaluable, repeated as needed, to provide a few hours of rest, which is helpful in terminating the attack. The therapist needs to consider that other drugs may have been imbibed or prescribed, and must anticipate synergistic effects or overreactions to the drug selected. One may choose sodium amytal 500 mg I/V, Valium 10–20 mg I/M or I/V, Thorazine 25–50 mg I/M, repeated as required, while nursing supervision is arranged. Prophylactic anticonvulsants are given if seizures are anticipated. The present drug of choice for an impending alcoholic delirium is either Librium 100 mg I/M repeated as necessary or Haldol 2–5 mg I/M, together with 5 percent dextrose in water I/V and vitamin-B complex I/V. This brief review clearly indicates that effective psychiatric emergency room treatment includes a combination of psychological, biological, pharmacotherapeutic, and environmental modalities.

Admission Area Survey

A computer-assisted survey* of admission applicants to the Brentwood Veteran's Administration Hospital in Los Angeles, a psychiatric hospital of 470 beds, confirms the findings of Glasscote and his associates about the presenting behavior of emergent patients. During a two-week period in September 1974 there were 171 applicants who made 182 visits to the evaluation/ admission area, which is open 24 hours daily. The area is manned by an assessment team consisting of a nurse clinician, social worker, and psychiatrist. A multidiciplinary team approach is the rule for the examination of every applicant prior to disposition. Patients can be held overnight for crisis treatment or for observation. The data gathered by the team for the 1974 survey follows:

Data

Age Of the applicants, 38 percent were under age 30, 23 percent were age 50 and older, while 39 percent were between ages 30 and 49.

Marital. 25 percent of the total were married, 43 percent were unmarried, and 28 percent were divorced or separated. Data not completed for 4 percent.

Admission. For 51 percent it was a first application to this hospital.

Duration. One out of 5 (20 percent) described the onset of symptoms as acute, recent, a matter of days or weeks. An illness duration of months was given by 14 percent, years for 51 percent, unknown 14 percent.

Referral Source. Although several provided multiple referral sources, most gave a simple source of referral. The figures that follow include both types of sources: 62 percent were primarily self-referred, 30 percent by a social agency, 24 percent by family, and 7 percent by police.

Precipitants. A number of applicants described multiple precipitants. By fre-

*Assisted by the Data Analysis Unit of Program Evaluation and Health Services computing facility of the University of California at Los Angeles. Sponsored by the National Institute of Health Special Research Resources Grant RR-3.

quency, health complaints topped the list with 44 percent, bizarre behavior followed with 42 percent, social crises with 38 percent, and a need for protection with 24 percent.

Diagnosis. Psychoses were diagnosed in 43 percent of the applicants. This included schizophrenia in 36 percent (undifferentiated 25 percent, paranoid 11 percent), psychosis unspecified 2 percent, manic-depressive 3 percent, organic brain syndrome 2 percent. Alcoholism, chronic and acute, was the main diagnosis for 29 percent of the applicants. Depressive reactions were diagnosed for 7 percent, drug dependent state 4 percent, neurosis 4 percent, personality disorder 4 percent. The major skew toward schizophrenia at younger ages and alcoholism in middle age is not unusual in veteran populations applying for treatment. The remainder included psycho-physiological reaction, no diagnosis, and other diagnoses.

Disposition. The team admitted 60 percent as inpatients, 14 percent were referred to other community agencies for assistance, and 9 percent were assessed, counseled, or otherwise treated to resolve the immediate problem and received no further referral. The remaining 17 percent were referred for ambulatory care.

Selected Variables

Comparison of Acute Onset and Chronic Illness. Computer assistance with collected data compared age, precipitants, source of referral, diagnosis, and disposition. No major differences emerged. Of the acute onset cases, 78 percent were treated by Brentwood programs, compared with 72 percent of the more chronic patients. Among the patients under 30 years of age in Brentwood treatment, 45 percent presented acute problems compared with 35 percent for the more chronic type.

Comparison of Marrieds with Divorced/Separated. The spouse provided referral incentive and support to obtain help for 42 percent of the marrieds who applied for treatment; otherwise the differences in diagnoses were insignificant between these groups.

Police Referral and 72-hour Holds. This involved 20 patients. The incidence of psychoses was 60 percent, of which 55 percent total were schizophrenics. For these 20 patients, bizarre behavior was given as the main precipitant for 70 percent, Social problems were major factors for 40 percent, need for protection for 35 percent. Multiple precipitants were described in several cases. Within the total of 171 patients, 3 percent came to hospital on 72-hour holds. Almost all of these were brought by police.

Need for Protection. For 44 patients the need for protection was the primary precipitant. The diagnoses showed 45 percent of this group were schizophrenics, 18 percent were depressed, 16 percent were diagnosed alcoholic. The remaining 21 percent carried a variety of other diagnosis. The staff response was to admit 75 percent (compared to 60 percent overall), while an additional 9 percent were referred for outpatient care. Additional surveys were directed to the post–Vietnam era veteran, those diagnosed alcoholic, and those referred back for agency care.

The data do not identify the psychiatric emergency per se. It is possible that greater urgency attended illness of recent onset, although decompensations in a chronic process may, as readily, trigger crisis reactions in the patient or the environment. Another possibility is that the data collection could include inaccuracies. It is surprising to find that the acute group and the chronic group were so similar in many details. This suggests that the Brentwood VA Hospital essentially treats a chronic illness population, no matter how the admission status may present to the examining staff.

The data underscore the difficulty in evaluation and definition of subjective perceptual differences, such as those reflected by the terms emergency, urgent, acute, subacute or chronic. Like beauty, the psychiatric emergency lies chiefly in the eye of the beholder.

It is when one looks beyond the statistical demographic data to the individual case study that the real meaning of "emergency" comes into focus. This reflects a state of acute turmoil and imbalance. It arises when problems and conflicts facilitate the discharge of acute emotions which exceed the coping capacities of the individual and the tolerance or limits and controls of the environment.

PSEUDOEMERGENCY

A comment must be made about the pseudoemergency. In such a situation there is "scapegoating" of the patient by "surrounding others." These individuals can be spouse, family, or others who may accompany the patient to the emergency room and, in confidence, provide a highly distorted version of the crisis. The description may simply express projective behavior or serve other motives that have little to do with the patient's actual behavior.

Within the hospital ward environment the consulting psychiatrist may be called to the "emergency." It may turn out that his visit is invested with the hope that he will become the savior for a difficult situation. The consultant may find that the staff relations are in turmoil, or that disproportionate anger or empathy is evoked within the staff toward the patient.

Obviously in all of these situations it is important to realize that the consultation request includes an unstated conflict, and it is necessary to explore the charged situation with tact and sensitivity. Confrontation (as an interpretative technique) has limited indications or success. Addition of data permits a reformulation of the original statement to a more appropriate problem definition.

TREATMENTS FOR THE PSYCHIATRIC EMERGENCY

Any unit that aims to respond to psychiatric emergencies should have the capability to deal effectively with the full range of psychiatric disturbances 24 hours a day. Needed is a team of professionals and paraprofessionals who possess the skills and the resources to carry out necessary interventions. It is required wisdom to understand patient behavior before definitive action is taken.

"Flying blind is difficult in an aircraft, and dangerous in psychotherapy."[11]

The initial tasks of the team include a rapid assessment and immediate attention to relief of acute symptoms. Further evaluation is needed to complete a diagnostic appraisal of the crisis. Further intervention is determined by a growing understanding of the patient's pathology and resources and the contributing role of family, social, and environmental factors. The optimal decision for immediate treatment is one that encourages maximal patient participation in selecting among the available options. Once the emergency subsides, further thought is given whether to limit the intervention to the present crisis or to plan continuing treatment. Beyond the relief of immediate symptoms, the major objective is to utilize alternatives to hospitalization when possible and to avoid progress toward chronicity. The responses to the emergency, therefore, involve immediate supportive intervention, diagnosis, and crisis intervention or brief therapy. Brief hospitalization can be very useful. This may be possible in an emergency room bed or on a 72-hour unit. Other alternatives include admission to a backup psychiatric unit bed or referral for continuing aftercare to a suitable community agency or to an outpatient treatment service.

The capabilities of a particular unit will reflect its staff, its goals, and its organization. A psychiatrist who is willing to make house calls practices both primary and secondary prevention. Treating the patient in his own environment allows for more accurate observations, involves the family from the first, and generally is more effective in calming the crisis. As part of the treatment of the lower-class patients, Behrens reports benefit even from brief house visits by the clinic therapist.[12] Torrey[13] describes the Russian system, where an on-call ambulance team responds to emergencies by making home visits. A similar home-visiting crisis team is rare in the United States.

In many hospitals a limited emergency consultation service is provided by an on-call resident, with a backup senior resident or staff member. The patient is examined in the outpatient area or in the general emergency room.[14, 15] In a university health center the sole service provider generally is the faculty psychiatrist.[5] Alcoholics Anonymous volunteers respond to the alcoholic in crisis, while other volunteers monitor the "cry-for-help" telephone call in the suicide prevention center.[16] In more complex units the emergency team consists of several professionals; in the most sophisticated units the team involves a psychiatric nurse, a social worker, possibly a psychologist, and a psychiatric resident, with one or more senior staff as consultants. Such an organization can best fulfill the multiple tasks of a comprehensive emergency service and provide in-depth patient care, as well as opportunities for teaching and research.[17]

Blane and his associates reviewed the national scene for existing acute psychiatric services in the general hospital. Their report refers to the Bronx (New York) Municipal Hospital Services,[19] the Elmhurst (New York) City Hospital Clinic,[20] and the Massachusetts General Hospital (Boston)

Emergency Ward.[21] In their opinion, the "typical consumer of general hospital emergency services is the unreflective lower-class patient. They use the emergency service in place of the neighborhood doctor, who is no longer available."[18] The San Mateo (California) County General Hospital Emergency Clinic reports that 3 percent of its applicants are true emergencies, 27 percent are urgent, and the remainder elective. Of those admitted to the hospital, 50 percent are suicidal risks or recent attempters.[22]

Autonomy of the emergency unit is recommended for optimal function.[23] Emergency services, whether partial or more complete, have evolved in many areas and are designated under various labels, such as walk-in clinics, trouble-shooting clinics, crisis centers, brief therapy clinics, and so on.

The prevailing philosophy also shapes the emergency unit's development and determines staff roles. Morrice[24] offers the hypothesis that much mental illness is the result of an unresolved social crisis situation and that social factors are the major precipitants of hospital admission. He concludes that "the non-professional holds the key in community and emergency psychiatry. The role of the doctor becomes that of support and consultation rather than direct service to the patient. The answer lies in the fuller and more enthusiastic use of nonprofessionals and of professionals who are at present untrained in mental health." Similar ideas are reflected in the organization of community health centers in various cities in the United States. These centers have as their staffs such personnel. Unfortunately, the initial high hopes for success have not been fulfilled. The scope of paraprofessional activities and responsibilities is increasing, but a final balance for effective team function has not yet evolved. There is no doubt that sophisticated service is best provided when a variety of team member skills is harmoniously harnessed towards the common goal of helping the patient.

CRISIS INTERVENTION

The review of published reports clearly indicates that there are wide differences in presenting populations and problems. While variations in psychiatric labeling may play some role in these differences, other idiosyncratic features are decided by the location of the clinic, by the characteristics of the cachement population, and by a host of social and cultural factors. The incidence of psychosis varies in the presenting population at emergency units. One report gives the figures as 32 percent,[17] another 44 percent,[25] two others 50 percent,[15, 26] and still another 60 percent.[4] It is the general consensus that availability of hospital backup beds is essential to permit the effective operation of an emergency service. This view is supported by a Canadian hospital study,[27] by a United Kingdom community study,[28] and by United States reports.[14, 15, 22] The substantial incidence of psychoses in the applicant population indicates that this group evidences major deficits of function. In addition to gross disturbances of behavior, thought, affect, or perception, there is usually a reduced tolerance to stressful life events. Under circumstances of an acute conflict or crisis, whether external or internal, hospitalization provides the supportive and structured environment where appropriate understanding and treatment is delivered to the patient in turmoil.

The emergency state signals the presence of acute distress. This arises from a crisis accompanied by the failure of the normal coping responses to resolve the conflict or meet the overwhelming threat. The attempts at adaptation become more primitive as regression occurs. With continued unremitting anxiety and an unrelieved crisis, there is increasing disorganization, the abandonment of the usual reality boundaries, and a strong possibility of chaotic purposeless behavior. The abuse of alcohol or drugs facilitates dysinhibition and dyscontrol.

The immediate interventions should provide support, rest, a protective and sheltered environment, and external redefinition of reality boundaries. Therapeutic responses that accomplish these objectives are those that demonstrate interest, firmness, kindness, and professional competence. Such a response encourages the beginning recovery from the chaotic state and supports the attempts at ego reorganization (''pulling oneself together''). The therapist involvement offers renewed hope to the patient and counters exaggerated fears and suspicions. It permits some relaxation. The primitive ego mechanisms operational within the patient tend to assist the rapid development of sustaining transference affects, partly because of the heightened state of suggestibility present under these conditions. Sedation can also be very helpful; if appropriately given, it can reduce panic but still leave the patient accessible to interview contact and available for early explorations of the crisis.

Aided by support from the therapist, the necessary examinations can take place. Family, friends, or others may add invaluable data. An interview with these individuals aims to clarify the immediate problems, to provide clues about usual personality and coping styles, and to develop information about the patient's strengths and family resources. The collection of these data, together with observed patient behavior, transference responses, and physical findings, provide the basis for the initial diagnostic impression and treatment formulation. In addition, the therapist is scanning various action plans during this initial contact. The most obvious needs may lie in providing social or legal assistance, or intervening in marital or family counseling relationships.

Such interventions cannot be standardized. The therapeutic focus is on the present, and the aim is to achieve adaptive resolution. The decision may be for brief crisis intervention, which aims at treatment termination after six to ten interviews. Home visits may be appropriate. As a recovery progresses, the patient can and should increasingly participate in decisions about continuing treatment.

Reaching a treatment goal shared by patient and therapist is a necessary development. In uncomplicated situations many therapeutic objectives may be telescoped and condensed into one or two contacts. In other situations the clinical state dictates the wisdom of observing the patient over some hours, overnight, or longer.

Brief therapy can have beneficial long-lasting effects beyond the immediate crisis.[20, 29]

> Emphasis is placed on the patient's ego strength and demands are made upon the patient to maintain his or her part of the therapeutic contract. The therapist must maintain the balance between supportive closeness and the proper separateness. He maintains a firmly based reality position and does not yield to the patient's pathological demands. Via identifications with the therapist and a growing insight into the origins of the crisis, a strengthening of the patient's adaptive capacities may ensue.[6]

The effective application of brief therapy tests all of the resources of the skilled therapist. He must be capable of risk taking, within acceptable limits. Menninger states, "The art of medicine consists in knowing how to make shortcuts, and when it is wise and permissible to do so."[30] Direct interpretations should be made only when it can lead to constructive change. Unwise confrontation can lead to panic, acting out, increased denial, or suicide.[20] In contrast, clarification to the patient in meaningful terms helps to reach the goal of crisis resolution.[29] However, for some patients the crisis resolution is only the first step into a period of continuing therapy.

PREVENTION OF EMERGENCIES

The prevention of all psychiatric emergencies is not an attainable goal. Overwhelming anxiety or depression or the presence of denial or projection as major pathological defences can prevent help-seeking behavior until others are forced to intervene. The emergency room patient population also has its own characteristics that inhibit the prevention of emergencies. The visit is often impulsive, and recommended investigations or follow-up appointments are not kept.

In ghetto and culturally alien communities in particular, the psychiatrist is perceived as a judgmental figure whose major function is to decide who goes to the state hospital.[5] Therefore, those in need of treatment do not seek aid except under extreme pressure. On the other hand, there are times that a patient does seek help, and the psychiatrist may fail to meet the clinical situation effectively, misreading the patient's needs, expectations, or psychopathology. Ruedy reports that 44 percent of overdoses are patients in current or recent psychiatric treatment.[10]

The whole issue of early intervention ultimately depends upon educational efforts in the field of mental health. Constant efforts need be exerted to convey to the public at large what the possibilities are and what the limitations are. It is equally disastrous to "undersell" or "oversell." Educational training of the "gatekeepers" to treatment is essential. These basic helpers in human affairs include teachers, the clergy, family physicians, the police, social and welfare workers, public health nurses, interested volunteers, and others who come into frequent contact with human problems and suffering. It is a great challenge to focus educational efforts so as to stimulate interest and learning and to encourage a deeper commitment to one's neighbors and community. The importance of education of the patient himself cannot be overestimated. It is the crucial factor in maintaining contact and following instructions for prescribed medication.

The application of epidemiological methods to psychiatry is in its infancy. High-risk populations need to be defined and preventive programs developed. For those who seek help, an early response is essential, and it is also essential to provide follow-up care for those who are mentally ill. Treatment dropouts need an active outreach follow-up. A well-organized consultation-liaison psychiatry service in a hospital can perform major preventive work—not only in providing needed attention to individual patients, but also by assisting staff to understand behavioral dynamics and group interactions and to alert them to the presence of the emotional overtures in medical or surgical patients. The usefulness of liaison work in hemodialysis units, in intensive care units, and other high-anxiety-level environments is obvious.

In addition, prevention of emergencies rests with the adequacy of our resources for treatment. There are major gaps and deficiencies in the network of resources required to respond to existing mental health problems. In order to mobilize such support, psychiatry must also learn the skills of political process, to lobby when it is important to do so, and to stand and act clearly as the "agent for the consumer." Every community gets the kind of care that its people are willing to pay for. When needs and resources are in better balance, the psychiatric emergency will be less frequent than it is at present.

REFERENCES

1. Straker M: Schizophrenia and psychiatric diagnosis: An editorial. Am J Psychiatry 131:693–694, 1974
2. Schimel JL, Salzman L, Chodoff P, et al: Changing styles in psychiatric syndromes: A symposium. Am J Psychiatry 130:146–155, 1973
3. Straker N: Bi-directional cable TV: A new technique for mental health services delivery. Paper presented at Veteran's Administration Hospital Brentwood, Los Angeles, August 23, 1974
4. Frazier S: Comprehensive management of psychiatric emergencies. Psychosomatics 9:7–11, 1968
5. Farnsworth D: Psychiatric emergencies. Int Psychiatry Clin 7:227–235, 1970
6. Wayne G: The psychiatric emergency: An overview, in Wayne G, Koegler R (eds): Emergency psychiatry and brief therapy. Int Psychiatry Clin 3:3–8, 1966
7. Glasscote R, Cumming E, Hammersley D, et al: The Psychiatric Emergency: A Study of Patterns of Service. Washington, DC, American Psychiatric Association and National Association for Mental Health, 1966
8. Straker M: Clinical observations of suicide. Can Med Assoc J 79:473–479, 1958
9. Dimijian G, Radelat F: Evaluation and treatment of the suspected drug user in the emergency room. Arch Intern Med 125:162–170, 1970.
10. Ruedy, J: Acute drug poisoning in the adult. Can Med Assoc J 109:603–605, 1973
11. Ewalt JR, Zaslow S, Stevenson P: How non-psychiatric physicians can deal with psychiatric emergencies. Mental Hospitals 15:194–196, 1964
12. Behrens M: Brief home visits by the clinic therapist in the treatment of lower-class patients. Am J Psychiatry 124:371–375, 1967
13. Torrey E: Emergency psychiatric ambulance services in the USSR. Am J Psychiatry 128:153–157, 1971
14. Ungerleider J: The psychiatric emergency. Arch Gen Psychiatry 3:593–601, 1960
15. Bernstein M, Straker N: A study of Mt Sinai emergency room patients seen by psychiatric residents. Mt Sinai J Med 38:480–488, 1971
16. Kaplan M, Litman R: Telephone appraisal of 100 suicidal emergencies. Am J Psychother 16:591–599, 1962
17. Straker M, Yung C, Weiss L: A comprehensive emergency psychiatric service in a general hospital. Can Psychiatr Assoc J 16:137–139, 1971
18. Blane H, Muller J, Chafetz M: Acute psychiatric services in the general hospital II. Current status of emergency psychiatric services. Am J Psychiatry 124:37–45, 1967
19. Coleman M, Rosenbaum M: The psychiatric walk-in clinic. Israel Ann Psychiatry 1:99–106, 1963
20. Bellak L: Comprehensive community psychiatry programs at city hospital, in Bellak L (ed): Handbook of Community Psychiatry and Community Mental Health. New York, Grune & Stratton, 1964
21. Chafetz M: Acute psychiatric services in the emergency ward. Mass Gen Hosp News 222:1–3, 1963
22. Trier T, Levy R: Emergent, urgent, and elective admissions. Arch Gen Psychiatry 21:423–430, 1969

23. Jacobson G: Emergency services in community mental health. Am J Public Health 64:124–128, 1974
24. Morrice J: Emergency psychiatry. Br J Psychiatry 114:485–491, 1968
25. Guido J, Payne D: 72-hour psychiatric detention. Arch Gen Psychiatry 16:233–238, 1967
26. Hankoff L: Emergency psychiatric treatment. Springfield, Ill., Thomas, 1969
27. Blais A, Georges J: Psychiatric emergencies in a general hospital outpatient department. Can Psychiatr Assoc J 14:123–133, 1969
28. Johnson J: Psychiatric emergencies in the community. Compr Psychiatry 10:275–284, 1969
29. Jacobson G: Some psychoanalytic considerations regarding crisis therapy. Psychoanal Rev 54:649–654, 1967
30. Menninger K: The Vital Balance. New York, Viking, 1963

Charles William Wahl

14

The Patient whose Physical Symptoms Mask a Psychiatric Disorder

There is a whole category of psychiatric disorders that do not, at least on first view, seem to be psychological in character. The presenting symptoms are usually physical rather than ''mental,'' and the patient's psychiatric difficulties are occult rather than overt. Not only are the symptoms those of physical illness, but the patient himself is usually convinced that he is physically ill. In such cases the physician, too, impelled by the whole course of his training to first consider the organic causes that may produce the symptoms, may not at once recognize the basically psychiatric character of the patient's complaints. Such symptoms may closely simulate those of an organic illness that may already be present. These are among the clinician's most taxing and challenging problems.

WHY THE SUBTERFUGE OF PHYSICAL SYMPTOMS

There are a variety of reasons why symptoms may be employed as a cover-up for psychiatric difficulties. The first and most obvious is that it is still, to many persons, debasing and humiliating to have emotional problems but quite acceptable to have a physical illness. Often this cultural bias is reinforced by the attitude of the physician who may share that prejudice. Second, physical illness evokes a wide variety of helping responses. If a degree of incapacity warrants admittance to hospital, this may be equated by the patient with the receipt of loving care, the fulfillment of dependency longings, or an honorable retreat from life's problems and responsibilities that pride might not otherwise afford.

The contrast of these conditions with those of a primarily psychiatric illness is most striking. Not only does the psychiatric patient usually feel ashamed of being ill, but he often finds that he is an object of dread and aversion to others. If treatment in a psychiatric hospital is necessitated, this is equated with being "put away"—a far cry from the situation of a comfortable bed in a medical hospital where he can be solaced by visitors, surrounded by gifts of candy and flowers, and deluged with get-well cards.

In addition to these situational and cultural disadvantages, there are also unconscious intrapsychic reasons that impel the patient to focus upon the physical aspects of his symptoms. The words *hurt, ache, pain,* and *sore* do double duty in our language. They may refer to strictly physical or strictly psychic states. Since the pains of the body are easier to endure than those of the mind, an unconscious substitution can take place. If the mechanisms of repression, denial, displacement, and reaction formation are used excessively as a way of avoiding psychical conflict and emotion, "body language" is employed instead. The mind always chooses what it regards as the lesser of two evils. Physical suffering may be unconsciously viewed as preferable to psychic suffering and may also act as a guilty expiation of the latter. However, the relationships between mind and body are subtle and complicated. A patient cannot be expected to be aware of the physiological and biochemical disturbances that accompany or presage mental turmoil. The bent of his entire education, as indeed is also the physician's, reinforces the concept that physical pain or alteration of function is produced only by structural abnormality and is wholly physical in character. All of these factors combine to facilitate a focusing of attention and concern on physical rather than psychic distress. Hence, the most frequent initial manifestation of a psychiatric problem will usually be a complaint of physical symptoms—particularly in an admission to a general hospital. It is here, consequently, rather than in a psychiatric facility, that such patients are first seen and their disease most easily diagnosed and treated.

CLASSIFICATION OF PATIENTS WITH PROBABLE PSYCHIC STRESS

Illnesses in these patients occur is several categories. There are patients who have unquestioned organic disease but who have concomitant psychic stresses that alter or complicate its management. An example is the patient with an overmastering fear of death or disability in relation to the primary disease. Other examples are instances in which the symptoms or complaint are manifestly disproportionate to the exciting organic cause.

The largest group is made up of patients who have physiologic or biochemical changes produced by acute or chronic psychic stress.[2] Examples are the usual psychosomatic illnesses and specifically those states of alteration of function that closely mimic organic diseases—for example, psychogenic muscular dystonia, hyperventilation syndrome, cardiospasm, pylorospasm, aerophagia, psychogenic hypoglycemia, splenic flexure syndrome, tension cephalalgia and status medicamentosus. In a third group are patients with concomitant organic or psychophysiological illnesses in multiple combination. Another category is made up of patients with intense convictions of disease or those who have psychogenic interference with motor function without biochemical or physiological alteration, as in the conversion hysterias.

A fifth category includes patients with psychiatric condtions such as depression, anxiety, or apathy produced in consequence of the experience or anticipation of an illness or a therapeutic procedure. Examples are panic antecedent or subsequent to a surgical or obstetrical procedure or an intensified fear of disability or death.

These common categories by no means exhaust the possibilities. All of these patients have, however, certain characteristics in common that are helpful in diagnosis:

1. Usually there is disproportionate concern regarding the symptoms (with the exception of the bland indifference of the conversion hysteric).
2. The symptoms range widely in character and are not consistent with the usual pattern of organic disease syndromes.
3. The onset of symptoms is concurrent and often co-temporal with states of conflict and stress that the patient is unable to acknowledge or handle.
4. The symptoms are static and, unlike organically induced symptomatology, neither advance nor diminish.
5. There is usually a personal and family history of psychic and psychosomatic disorders.
6. Other concomitant psychiatric disorders are usually encountered.
7. There may be evidence of secondary gain or advantage accruing to the patient as a result of his illness.

ADVANTAGE OF GENERAL HOSPITAL ADMISSION FOR PSYCHIATRIC CONSULTATION

It is generally considered that the treatment of patients whose psychiatric difficulties are expressed though the means of physical symptoms is one of singular difficulty. Somatic expression of psychic difficulties is presumed to be indicative of massive repression, which prevents honest consideration by the patient of his underlying problems.[3, 4, 5]

In my experience the converse is the case. These patients are particularly accessible to psychiatric help and intervention, and one of the major reasons for this accessibility is the direct consequence of the hospital admission.[6, 7, 8, 9]

As physicians, we are habituated to hospitals. They are places in which we learn, treat, and work. They have, therefore, a variety of pleasant and reassuring connotations to us. To the patient who does not share this background, however, the hospital is often an alien world, and to be put into a hospital is an anxiety-producing experience. Except for imprisonment, no other circumstance in our society requires one to surrender more of his personal liberty, prerogatives, and identification.

Consider the state of the patient in the hospital. He is restricted by convention and necessity to a white rectangle, three feet by six feet, and is often required to maintain a special set of postures for long periods. For most of the time he is isolated from persons of his own choosing or is exposed to other sick patients who have problems, suffering, and idiosyncrasies of their own. Whatever his extramural fame or worth, he often cannot show his individuality or status by dress but, like everyone else, must wear a hospital gown and take a bed number. The hours, methods, and character of his awakening, eating, and sleeping are specifically regulated. The privacy of the body and the bowel habits which are among the most personal of functions, have to be greatly modified from his usual patterns. The patient also finds himself with a huge amount of time on his hands with very limited means of filling it. Access to his doctor and nurse is usually much less than he would wish. In addition to the natural worries about himself attendant upon any illness and the financial and other concerns resultant from it, he is often exposed to the sights of suffering and death that may have been quite foreign to his usual experience.

In short, the hospital experience can be—and usually is to some degree—frightening, and the fear is compounded if the physical symptoms for which the patient is admitted are, in fact, emotionally based. It is well for us to remember that the ''sick role'' is often no bowl of cherries, magnifying, as it does, the loss of major identity of oneself as a working, healthy, self-sufficient, and self-directed person.

Paradoxical as it sounds, however, these implicit conditions serve to operate as decided advantages in the psychiatric consultation, and it is not difficult to see why this would be. The patient in a hospital often feels helpless in an alien and frightening environment. His full and individual self may be depersonalized to an identification as ''that case of gall bladder in room 227.'' The regression and the heightened dependency upon others that inevitably accompany illness are intensified in a patient of this kind, yet he finds that the physician and the nurses cannot satisfy his increased need for time, explanations, and reassurance. Hence, the psychiatrist, who is not only specifically trained in the techniques of communication but is also prepared to spend the time required to get to know him fully and well, is usually extremely welcome.

In a fraction of the time that would otherwise be required, there usually develops with such patients a state of strongly positive transference. This occurs since states of physical illness, acting in concert with the previously mentioned special conditions that characterize a stay in hospital, induce and intensify the kind and quality of regression that is achieved by the organically well patient only after many hours of outpatient psychotherapy. It is an axiom of psychoanalytic theory that access to the deepest repressions and to the conflictful material that patients defend against can only be effected in the posture of a strongly positive transference and with the development of that state of regression that will recapitulate and make more easily accessible early childhood repressed memories. The experience of being put in hospital and the organic illness can intensify and reinforce the physician-patient relationship; as a result, deeply repressed and highly relevant material becomes quickly accessible and utilizable by the patient.

The fortunate consequence is that with such patients it is often possible to achieve striking psychotherapeutic results, not only toward alleviation of the presenting symptoms, but in the modification of the underlying character structure as well. With no other group of patients is this so fully possible.

In fact, this occurs so regularly that it is with just such categories of patients that the techniques of short-term, intensive, insight psychotherapy were developed by Deutsch, Jelliffe, and others, and it is with such patients that these techniques are primarily taught and demonstrated to residents in psychiatric training.[10]

PSYCHIATRIC CONSULTATION IN A GENERAL HOSPITAL SETTING

The method of psychiatric consultation, and the psychotherapeutic work that follows it, should proceed somewhat as follows:

At the outset, provision is made for privacy. The patient cannot be expected to speak candidly and openly of things that trouble him if he can be overheard. If necessary, the patient's bed should be moved to an unoccupied room. Then, after the therapist has introduced himself to the patient and has explained the purposes of the interview, the patient is encouraged to describe in detail the nature, course, and progression of the symptoms.

Listen to the patient. This helps him in three ways. First, it permits the patient to ventilate or abreact his emotions. It gets things off his chest; this in itself affords considerable relief. Second, the stimulus of calm attention fosters a focusing of the patient's attention upon the causes, primary and contributory, of his disquietude. It helps him to organize his addled thoughts, and this is vastly reassuring. Third, it gives the physician an opportunity to obtain a broader cross section of the patient's personality and ways of relationship and enables the patient to better delineate his life situation.

This listening by the physician need not be prolonged. It seems to me that the usual reason that we fail to listen to patients is that we feel that it is not likely to be effective unless it is in the usual psychiatric 50-minute session. Nothing could be further from the case. A few minutes may suffice to permit the patient to gain relief. The patient is more interested in the doctor's willingness to listen and in the doctor's interest in his welfare rather than in the quantity of time spent.

"Key" Signs in an Interview

Careful attention is paid not only to the order or lack of it with which the history is related, but also specific note is made of the "key words," these being the reiterated or idiosyncratic expressions or words that appear with unusual frequency in the stream of the patient's discourse. These are interrogatively repeated to the patient in a subtle manner by the examiner in order to evoke further associational material. Since they indicate emotionally laden conflicts, they produce in association material concerned with memories, events, and personages that often have a significant relationship to the genesis and progression of the symptoms.

Careful note is also made during the interview of occult signs of anxiety and the coincident appearance of these with the events and personages being discussed. The most reliable of these signs prove generally to be the subtle twitchings of the muscles of the face, particularly the periorbicular and infraocular muscle groups and the twitching of the toes. Particular note is also taken of the disparity between the consciously evinced anxiety and the signs of unconscious anxiety as shown by an elevated pulse rate, heightened skin temperature, hyperhidrosis, and increased muscle tension.

Often the psychosomatically ill patient has all of the physiological signs of anxiety without being aware of the conscious emotion or effect that usually accompanies them. A helpful test is to note the response to anxiety-induced questions when interspersed with questions that are more benign. In highly anxious patients the contrast in reaction between the two is greater than in other patients. The patient should also be asked to describe the personalities of the significant figures of his past and present life. Careful attention must be paid to the content and the affect of his responses as well as to the scope and character of these descriptions. The covertly anxious patient will be, usually, unable to

describe or accept mixed, conflictful, or ambivalent feelings regarding significant persons of the present or past.

The Meaning and Significance of Symptoms Uncovered

As the interview progresses, several characteristic things are discovered.
The symptoms of the illness in a psychiatric disorder may be found to have
appeared coincident with some conflictful event or circumstance in the patient's
life. In addition, the symptoms usually manifest what has been called the
autoplastic effect, which is to say that the patient's individual conception of his
illness bears little relationship to medical fact but rather shows evidence of a
highly personal distortion relevant from his own life history. Even educated
persons will often display a number of bizarre and magical ideas concerning the
funtioning of the body parts that are related to the painful symptoms. In
addition, there is also usually evidence that the illness or symptoms subserve
some unconscious paleological, unwitting purpose to the patient. For example,
the illness may operate as an assuagement of guilt, a suffering to guarantee
immortality, a fulfillment of premonitory feelings of nemesis; or the illness may
demonstrate anniversary reactions that are the development of a set of
symptoms similar or identical to those experienced by some ambivalently
regarded person in the past at the same chronological period. And last, there is
usually evidence of a concomitant secondary gain, that is, the symptoms often
enable the patient to achieve some gratification that would not otherwise be
available to him or enable him to ''fail with honor.'' From all of these data, the
history and the communication of the patient as well as his relationship to the
physician, the meaning and significance of the symptoms can be investigated
and understood.

PSYCHIATRIST'S ROLE DURING A CONSULTATION

Explain to the patient. Being outside the patient's skin, the physician can
delineate often more clearly than can the patient some of the immediate
determinants and concomitants of his anxiety and assist the patient in seeing
these. He can also by dint of his special knowledge of people—how they work
and function and the kind of things that plague and trouble mankind—
illuminate areas not clearly seen by the patient. Moreover, the physician's
knowledge of how states of tension and emotion affect physiological and
biochemical function permit him to explain and to account for the patient's
production of the symptoms, which are usually terrifying or at least disconcert-
ing to the patient.

Explore with the patient his life and feelings. Help him to see the relationship in time between emotional stress and the conflicts that he may be repressing and the emergence of his frightening or painful symptoms. When the patient can identify with your dispassionate attitude and view himself more objectively, there is a great diminuation in anxiety.

Comfort and reassure. It is the custom today, particularly for psychiatrists, to sneer at these two words. To do so is shortsighted and stupid. They represent valuable adjutants in any physician's professional skills.

Use drugs sparingly. Each new tranquilizer has its vogue largely because so great a need exists in medical practice for such an agent and because so many prove disappointing in their effect and disadvantageous or harmful in their application. It is known that a condition of sustained anxious stress affects many of the homeostatic body mechanisms. To design a drug that will restore all of these without insalubrious side effects is well nigh impossible. It is the sad fact that we do not have a good pharmacological agent that is fully satisfactory in the treatment of these conditions.

Do not overstudy the patient. This procedure alarms far more than it reassures.

It is good to remember also that these simple measures are so effective when practiced by a competent and warm physician because of the special magical role with which our society invests him. He stands dealing as he does with matters of life, death, succor, and aid, *in loco parentis*. This lends a paleological efficacy to small efforts that, when practiced by others would not be so effective as when practiced by the physician. As a mythic figure, the physician has a degree and quality of influence for good that, embroiled in his own vicissitudes, he is often prone to overlook or forget.

REFERENCES

1. Kubie L: The ontogeny of anxiety. Psychoanal Rev 8:78–85, 1941
2. Saul L: Physiological effects of emotional tension. in Hund J (ed): Personality and Behavior Disorders. New York, Ronald, 1944
3. Stekel W: Conditions of Nervous Anxiety and Their Treatment. London, Kegal Paul, Trench, Trubner, 1923
4. Sullivan H: The theory of anxiety and the nature of psychotherapy. Psychiatry 12:3–13, 1949
5. May R: The Meaning of Anxiety. New York, Ronald, 1950
6. Wahl CW: Unconscious factors in the psychodynamics of the hypochondriacal patient. Psychosomatics 4:9–14, 1963
7. Wahl CW: Iatrogenic neuroses, their production and prevention. Dis Nerv Supts 28:318–322, 1967
8. Wahl CW: Psychodynamics of the allergic patient. Ann Allergy 18:1138–1143, 1960

9.   Wahl CW: The psychosomatic emergency. Calif. Med 105:276–280, 1966
10.   Wahl CW: The technique of brief psychotherapy with hospitalized psychosomatic patients. Int J Psychoanal Psychother 1:69–82, 1972
11.   Wahl CW: The differential diagnosis of normal and neurotic grief following bereavement. Psychosomatics 11:104–106, 1970

Charles McCreary and
Kay Jamison

15

The Chronic-Pain Patient

CHRONIC PAIN

One wonders why pain is such a mystery. Although pain is a common phenomenon experienced by almost everyone, the universality of the experience seems to overshadow its complexity. Acute pain from some specific injury or illness has lifesaving importance as a warning sign of bodily damage. However, chronic pain does not have such lifesaving utility; in fact, often it is very debilitating, demoralizing, and life-threatening.

Chronic pain is defined here as persistent pain that is usually a daily experience for a period of at least six months, is often incapacitating, and frequently interferes with a person's daily functioning. Such chronic pain may have physical findings related to it, but usually there are no specific underlying disease processes that can be alleviated by known medical treatments. The experience of chronic pain involves a complex interaction of perceptual, motivational, and cognitive components. Melzack maintains that chronic pain has multiple determinants and that there are no specific pain pathways for this phenomenon.[1]

Sternbach, Wolf, Murphy, and their associates point out that the most common form of chronic pain is low-back pain.[2] There are other medical syndromes involving chronic pain, such as anesthesia dolorosa, postherpetic neuralgia, causaliga, migraine, phantom limb pain, arthritis, and so forth. These syndromes all show persistent pain that represent diseases of central areas, the spinal cord, or nerve pathways, or they may reflect wounds or other injuries to peripheral nerves. In addition, chronic pain may exist in the absence of any injury or disease process. Engel has suggested an analogy between chronic pain and phenomena such as visual and auditory hallucinations that do not involve sensory stimulation.[3]

Two major psychiatric disorders are often found in chronic-pain patients. Hysteria is typically used to explain chronic pain of psychogenic origin. Yet, it may also be part of a psychophysiological reaction. Unfortunately, clinicians and researchers too often confuse these disorders and do not adequately define the kind of chronic pain that they are discussing. Such confusion leads to fruitless arguments about whether chronic pain does or does not involve physical findings.

The treatment of chronic pain is often a frustrating and difficult task for medical specialists. We believe that consultation from the behavioral sciences is especially crucial for the proper understanding and treatment of patients with this problem. Melzack points out some of the reasons for the difficulties in understanding and treating this disorder.[4] He notes that traditional medicine teaches a specificity theory of pain; this theory proposes that the intensity of the pain experience is directly proportional to the extent of tissue damage and that there are specific pain receptors, neural pathways, and central mechanisms underlying the pain experience. Melzack gives evidence that pain is not a simple function of tissue damage, but rather it involves complex psychological processes, such as attention, anxiety, suggestion, prior learning experience, and a wide variety of other cognitive variables.

Because of this specificity theory, and due to certain factors in our Western culture (for example, the assumption of total relief from pain), physicians often feel that they must completely cure their patient's pain by isolating and removing a specific and single source. Patients present themselves with the same set of expectations and typically react with disappointment if physicians disagree with this simplistic model of pain. Rather than confront patients directly in regard to their expectations, physicians often encourage the expectation of a specific push-button way of alleviating pain. They may prescribe a variety of pain-relieving medications; if these do not work, they may continue to suggest more drastic—and yet still disease-specific—diagnostic and medical procedures.

In order to examine some of the complexities of chronic pain, this chapter will review current theory and research relevant to the issue. It will discuss ways to measure pain, examine theoretical approaches to explain and treat pain, consider empirical research on the personalities of chronic-pain patients, and review various studies that have tried to identify patients who are at high risk for not responding to traditional medical-surgical treatment of chronic pain. Finally, certain recently developed treatment approaches for chronic pain will be briefly described.

MEASUREMENT OF PAIN

A variety of procedures has evolved for the measurement of clinical pain. Physicians rely on these techniques to assess both acute as well as chronic pain. These procedures will be contrasted with methods that have been developed to measure experimentally induced pain.

The objective assessment of pain has remained, in many ways, intriguingly illusive. The difficulties in the communication of the pain experience are well known to patients, physicians, psychologists, and philosophers. Keele described a few of the problems intrinsic in the description of pain: (1) the difficulty in finding words to describe such an unusual if not unique experience (and here Keele quotes Virginia Woolf: "Let a sufferer try to describe a pain in his head to a doctor, and language runs at once dry"); (2) the confusion about what features of this experience are relevant to the observer; and (3) difficulties in remembering the experience.[5] Approaching the problem of pain from a linguistic point of view, Melzack and Torgerson have discussed the varieties of pain in the following manner: "Pain refers not to a specific sensation which can vary only in intensity, but to an endless variety of qualities that are categorized under a single linguistic label."[6] Likewise, Petrovich wrote about the multiplicity of factors involved in the perception of pain, for example, age, sex, race, cultural background, interpersonal variables involved in the origin and locus of pain, the agent and person responsible for it, and the situation and context in which the pain experience takes place.[7] He, as many authors have done, emphasizes the importance of differentiating the perception of pain from the reaction to pain.

What then are some of the methods of assessing pain that have evolved? Perhaps it is useful to start with clinical medicine's approach to pain evaluation as it is there that many of the relevant questions are necessarily, and most importantly, raised. Serjeant[8] has noted that not only is pain the most common chief complaint of patients and that pain is the most common and valuable symptom available to an examining physician, but that there are over 400 items listed under "pain" in French's *Index of Differential Diagnoses*. Clinical medicine, which traditionally has had to rely on verbal reports and visible-audible indications of pain, typically inquires into the history of the pain experience (including the severity, frequency, duration and course, type, location), the response to an elicited pain, and the clinical significance of the absence of pain. Additionally, Fordyce has outlined the major bases for the formation of inferences about both clinical and experimentally induced pain: (1) afferent stimuli, (2) autonomic arousal signs, (3) visible-audible signs of pain, (4) verbal report, and (5) interference with activities, such as being unable to work or drive, having to remain confined to bed, and so on.[9]

Since there is such a high degree of subjectivity in such an important area, it is only natural that many investigators would attempt to make order from veritable chaos and would try to begin an objectifying and quantifying process. Melzack and Torgerson were interested in further understanding the language and description of pain.[6] By taking the words that had been used to describe pain, they found that the words, or adjectives, could be classified into three major groups: (1) sensory—temporal, spatial, brightness, dullness, and so forth; (2) affective—tension, autonomic, fear, punishment; and (3) evaluative. They stressed the distinction between the sensory-discriminative and the motivational-affective dimensions obtained and felt, as many other authors have, that both dimensions are clearly affected by such intra- and interpersonal variables as attention, past experience, and the meaning of the situation. Pain is thus defined by them as being in "multidimensional space and comprising several sensory and affective dimensions."[6]

Yet another series of approaches to the measurement of pain fall within the field of psychophysiology. Many techniques have been used in the experimental production and evaluation of pain, including the application of such stimuli as electrical currents, hot test tubes and radiant heat to the skin, with pain measures consisting of either subjective report of the pain experience, physiological responses from the subject, or the length of time that the subject can experience the stimulation. Another commonly used method of inducing pain experimentally is the tourniquet technique used by Smith, Lowenstein, Hubbard, and their colleagues.[10] With this procedure the subject squeezes a hand exerciser approximately 20 times after a tourniquet is inflated around his upper arm; the measurement in this instance is the amount of time between the end of the squeezing and report of different levels of pain (slight, moderately distressing, very distressing, and unbearable).

Two major criticisms have been leveled against such psychophysiological studies. First, it is impossible to replicate the psychological factors involved in ongoing or chronic pain (such as fear, hopelessness, interference with lifestyle, and so on) under such time-limited experimental situations. Second, the reliability of threshold changes when analgesics are given to the subject during these procedures makes pain evaluation somewhat suspect. Sternbach and his coworkers have attempted to integrate clinical and psychophysiological techniques into their evaluation of pain.[11] Thus, a patient is asked to rate his clinical pain on a scale of 0 to 100, which is a clinical, subjective evaluation, and he is then asked to compare this pain with the pain experience through experimentally induced pain (using a variation of the tourniquet technique); the ratio of the clinical pain level to the maximum "untolerable" tolerance time (multiplied by 100) is then a measure of the patient's tendency to minimize or maximize his pain experience.

Other techniques being used in the assessment of pain include the measurement of different physiological responses to painful stimuli (for example, blood pressure changes, withdrawal reflexes, pulse rate, and pupillary dilations) as well as sensory detection analysis. The multiplicity of measures available is an index of the complexity of the problem of pain evaluation. Katz and Bresler, in a grant application, made the following point:

> "The perception of pain perfuses all levels of CNS functioning since it reflects an integration of *sensory* (i.e., noxious) stimulation, *affective* and *motor* reactions to the pain sensation, *motivational* and *emotional* reactions to the primary threat of continued pain, and *cognitive* interpretation

of the entire event . . . as a result there is no single index which can unequivocally indicate the presence or absence of pain.[12]

MODELS TO EXPLAIN AND TREAT CHRONIC PAIN

There appear to be two major psychological models for the understanding and treatment of chronic pain. The *psychodynamic model* views chronic pain as a symptom reflecting deep-seated, largely unconsciousness, psychopathological processes. This approach focuses on complex interpersonal aspects of the pain experience and stresses early childhood experiences as fundamental etiological factors. Early in life, according to this view, pain becomes associated with the anticipation of comfort and reunion with a significant love object. Continuing into childhood, pain and punishment become closely associated. Typically, pain becomes a signal for the child that he has been ''bad''; therefore, pain often evolves into an important way for the child to handle guilt feelings and earn reacceptance from parent figures. Furthermore, this approach stresses how pain may often become associated with aggressive and sexual feelings in childhood. Engel describes this fundamental process:

> Beginning from a primitive protective system, pain evolves into a complex psychic mechanism, part of the system whereby a man maintains himself in his environment. Both as a warning system and as a mechanism of defense, pain helps to avoid or ward off even more unpleasant feeling states or experiences and achieved, albeit at a price.[3]

The psychodynamic view regards pain as a symptom that involves self-inflicted punishment that serves to ease feelings of guilt. Unconsciously, patients with pain complaints do not believe that they deserve success or happiness and feel that they must pay a price for whatever happiness they have. Typically, these patients are chronically depressed; however, they do not experience their depression in terms of internal psychological processes, but rather they explain their pessimistic outlooks toward life largely as a consequence of either their pain or another form of externalized misfortune. Such persons often present themselves to others in a stoical fashion and typically portray themselves as a martyr tolerating pain, thereby, earning overt comfort and covert expiation of guilt.[3]

The suggested treatment of pain for this approach involves the exploration and uncovering of the unconscious conflicts that prompt its expression. The psychodynamic model assumes that when these conflicts are made conscious, the patient will see that they are no longer appropriate to his current life situation.

The second major psychological approach, the *behavioral model,* questions the general applicability of the disease model as an explanation of chronic pain. This approach suggests that pain behavior (symptoms) may not be under the exclusive control of some underlying pathology, such as unconscious conflicts or actual physical disease. Rather, this model maintains that pain is a learned behavior that is governed largely by consequences in the patient's environment. The proper way to understand pain is to observe pain behaviors and the systematic consequences of these behaviors in the patient's life. Fordyce, a major spokesman for the behavioral approach in treating chronic pain, maintains that pain complaints can be changed by modifying such consequences.[9] He suggests two basic procedures: (1) decrease pain behaviors by withdrawing the positive reinforcements, such as attention, rest, medications, compensation, and such, that have typically followed these complaints or (2) increase the rate of incompatible behaviors by reinforcing them with appropriate positive reinforcers. Fordyce maintains that many alleged pain behaviors have been learned as a way of avoiding pain and do not require the presence of pain stimuli in order to continue to occur.

There are approaches to the understanding and treatment of chronic pain that combine the psychodynamic and behavioral perspectives. Szasz[13] and Sternbach[14] have emphasized viewing pain as a form of communication and interpersonal manipulation that often involves games between the patient and the doctor. Sternbach describes the game of "painmanship" as the doctor's effort to confirm his professional identity by diagnosing pain and relieving suffering and the patient's goal of establishing his identity as a suffering person with undiagnosable problems. He maintains that because of disease, injury, or emotional conflict, a person experiences continued pain and comes to think of himself as a chronic invalid. This becomes the person's identity, and all his interpersonal interactions take the form of "games" designed to maintain this identity. The patient is unwilling to give up his pain, and when the doctor fails to relieve his suffering, as he usually does, the doctor assigns the patient to another diagnostic category such as hysteric or "crock." Sternbach suggests a variety of psychodynamic and behavioral approaches to deal directly with these pain games.[14]

PERSONALITY CHARACTERISTICS OF
CHRONIC-PAIN PATIENTS

In the United States the psychometric instrument most frequently used to assess the personality characteristics of patients with chronic pain is the Minnesota Multiphasic Personality Inventory (MMPI). There appears to be an amazing consistency of findings using this instrument. Hanvik, over two decades ago, reported that patients with acute and chronic low-back pain that had no physical findings were distinctly different from low-back pain patients with clearcut organic problems.[15] Patients without physical findings showed the "conversion V" configuration—elevations on MMPI scales Hs (hypochondriasis) and Hy (hysteria) with scale D (depression) relatively lower. However, patients without physical findings still had significantly higher D scores than patients with organic evidence. Patients with organic pathology had generally normal personality profiles, while patients with the "functional" profile showed signs of emotional disturbance. These "functional" patients have been described as having a strong need to interpret their circumstances in a logical and socially acceptable manner and as displacing emotional conflicts onto somatic concerns. Typically, they are very defensive and repressed, and they resist suggestions of any weakness or unconventionality in their character. In general, they are described as egocentric, immature, and dependent. Their complaints of pain appear to allow them to avoid the awareness of anxiety and conflict, though at some considerable cost in emotional control and repression.[17]

Some researchers have not found clearcut differences between "functional" and "organic" chronic-pain patients. Sternbach found higher scores on Hs and Hy in patients with chronic versus acute pain and also in patients who had some litigation involved in their pain complaints; however, he did not find this difference in patients with and without physical findings.[18] Sternbach feels that many chronic-pain patients have a real disease or injury that becomes associated with severe feelings of depression, helplessness, and hopelessness. Most patients seem to be able to recover from the immediate effects of their illness. However, certain persons, who may have core emotional conflicts that involve deep-seated feelings of depression and hopelessness, if injured, are likely to dwell on and utilize pain complaints to avoid dealing with these basic emotional problems. Sternbach labels these patients as depressed with psychophysiological reactions. They need their pain to survive, but at a cost of repression and the acceptance of a life-style of chronic invalidism.

It is important to ask why some have reported scales Hs and Hy from the MMPI do differentiate functional from organic pain while others have not found this result. Two basic reasons emerge. Swartz and Krupp have found that older medical patients tend to have elevations on Hs and Hy and these scales are not as useful in making the functional versus organic dichotomy.[19] Sternbach reported that his patients were in their early forties while Hanvik did not report the ages of his patients.[16] One might suspect that Sternbach's patients were older. The second reason for the contradictory evidence may involve the criterion for evidence of physical findings. Hanvik's criterion seemed to be more stringent than Sternbach's. Sternbach may have included many more "borderline" cases in his organic category.

A review of these research findings leads to the following conclusions. Two basic personality types with chronic pain stand out. First, there are those patients with *la belle indifference* who do not readily admit depression and who fit the description usually labeled conversion hysteria. These patients have elevations on scales Hs and Hy with relatively lower D scores. A second type of patient looks more depressed than the former type and appears to be more likely to have definite physical findings associated with pain complaints. Such patients may be more appropriately regarded as depressed with a psychophysiological reaction.

The impression should not be left that the MMPI is the only instrument used to assess personality characteristics of chronic-pain patients. In Great Britain the Eysenck Personality Inventory (EPI) has been used on such patients, and patients with chronic pain have shown consistently higher neurotic scores (anxiety and obsessions) than a normal comparison group.[20] Further research is needed to see whether other personality instruments identify characteristics of chronic-pain patients.

USE OF PSYCHOLOGICAL DATA
IN THE PREDICTION OF OUTCOME
TO MEDICAL OR SURGICAL INTERVENTION

Several investigations have been done in order to examine the value of different psychological variables in predicting outcome of medical and/or surgical intervention with chronic-pain patients. All of these studies evidenced significant methodological difficulties in terms of sampling procedures, the nature of the statistical analyses, and the criteria used for outcome; however, despite these limitations, there are certain consistencies in the results across studies. Wiltse and Rocchio were interested in determining which patients would respond well to surgery and would thus be "good surgical risks."[21] Their study sample comprised 130 patients with low-back pain who had no previous history of back surgery and no significant organic complications; the surgical intervention consisted of a chymopapain injection to one to three interspaces of the lower spine. Psychometric and demographic data were obtained from the patients and included the Cornell Medical Index, the Quick Test (as a measure of intelligence), and the MMPI. The outcome criterion was the surgeon's rating, one year after surgery, of objective improvement (physical examination findings, muscle weakness, reflex changes, and so forth) and his rating of functional or symptomatic improvement. The hypochodriasis and hysteria scales from the MMPI were found to be the best predictors of functional improvement from surgery; Wiltse and Rocchio concluded that "patients with very low scores (54 and below), for example, were 90 percent certain of showing good or excellent functional improvement while only 10 percent of patients whose scores were extremely high (85 and above) showed this degree of improvement.''[21]

Phillips compared 58 patients with low-back syndrome (patients without any demonstrable or significant organic components to their presenting symptoms) to 72 fracture patients.[22] In addition to finding that the patients with the low-back syndrome had significantly higher scores on the MMPI's ''neurotic triad'' scales (hypochondriasis, depression, and hysteria), he also found that the amount of neuroticism, as reflected by the MMPI, was negatively correlated with the prompt completion of a rehabilitation program and was also negatively correlated with the prompt and effective abatement of symptoms. On the other hand, Sternbach, in his prediction work on successful outcome from either psychological or surgical intervention, found that the relationship between the classic conversion V on the MMPI (that is, patients with elevations on Hs and Hy and with D relatively low) and successful outcome was unclear.[2] He also concluded that when the dominant MMPI profile was neurotic depression, the prognosis was good and that when the hypochondriasis was markedly elevated, the prognosis was poor.

Wiffling, Klonoff, and Kokan studied 26 male patients with spinal fusions, comparing those patients with successful surgery with those with non-successful surgery; they also compared the patients on the basis of whether they had had one or more than one surgical procedure.[23] Psychometric instruments used included the Wechsler Adult Intelligence Scale (WAIS), Cornell Medical Index, Mooney Problem Check List, and MMPI; the outcome criterion was a three-point rating scale filled out by the surgeon ascertaining whether he felt the surgical results were good, fair, or poor. The results indicated that there were no differences among groups on either the WAIS or the Mooney Problem Check List but that there were differences on the MMPI. Those patients with good surgical outcome scored significantly lower on the following MMPI scales: hypochondriasis, hysteria, depression, and the low-back pain scale. Those patients with a history of a single operation scored significantly lower than those with a history of multiple surgeries on three of the same four scales (Hy, D, Hs).

In an analysis of the relationship between demographic, medical, and psychological factors and successful outcome in a rehabilitation program for patients with low-back disorders, Nagi, Burk, and Potter studied the case records of 125 admissions to the Ohio Rehabilitation Center.[24] The outcome criteria consisted of improvement in various performance areas, such as driving, eating, dressing, ambulation, and work activities, as well as the degree to which the patient fulfilled the expectations of the clinical team; the psychological factors were defined as the ''degree to which psychological disorders contributed to the patient's disability'' and were measured by psychiatric ratings and psychological testing (unspecified). These researchers concluded that the amount of psychological contribution was negatively correlated with success on the program, that the nonachievement group suffered more from emotional and other personal problems than did the high-achievement group.

Pheasant and Holt and their colleagues at Orthopedic Hospital in Los Angeles tested a series of predictive hypotheses on two samples (an initial sample of 95 and a second, cross-validation sample, of 94) of low-back pain patients.[25] Both groups of patients were interviewed and completed a battery of psychological tests; additionally, they were each rated daily in an attempt to assess their level of functioning. The general outcome criterion (established as a difference score between pre- and posttreatment measures) was one of disability or, as Pheasant and Holt defined it, the amount of interference that the patient was having in daily living. On the basis of their data the authors concluded,

> The group having the poorest rated response to treatment had a correspondingly larger incidence of maladjustment indications . . . the patient's response to treatment was inversely related to the extent of neurotic symptomatology as clinically interpreted from the MMPI . . . in conclusion, minimal support (from the MMPI) did exist for the hypothesis that anxiety, tension, and worry are negatively correlated with response to treatment, but that other data (IPAT and CMI) were essentially nonconfirmatory and more study is required before a firm conclusion is possible.[25]

Beals and Hickman investigated certain environmental and psychological characteristics that predicted return to work for patients injured on their job and treated in a special physical rehabilitation center.[26] Their sample consisted of 180 acute and chronic patients who had injuries to their extremities or back. They used MMPI scores and clinical impressions of physicians and psychologists as the basis for predicting recovery. They found greater psychopathology in back-injured patients than in extremity-injured patients and in chronic, polysurgical, versus acute patients. In addition, patients with greater psychopathology (shown by elevations on the Hs and Hy scales) demonstrated a decrease in likelihood of returning to work. The authors suggest that in certain patients psychological distress involving hypochondriacal and hysterical symptoms leads to a chronic condition of vocational maladjustment and poor response to medical-surgical intervention.

It can be seen that across all of these studies there is a general and fairly consistent tendency for indices of psychological well-being, or ''adjustment,'' to be positively correlated with a good response to medical and/or surgical intervention in chronic-pain patients. High scores on MMPI scales Hs and Hy seem to be consistently related to poor response to medical treatment for chronic pain, especially low-back pain.

NEW DIRECTIONS AND OVERVIEW

There are a number of promising treatment approaches for chronic-pain patients that often involve combinations of psychological and noninvasive medical procedures. Drawing on research citing raised pain thresholds of yogis in a meditative state, reports of the high alpha content during meditation and studies of operant conditioning of alpha waves, Gannon and Sternbach attempted alpha conditioning on a patient with severe and chronic headache.[27] They found that the patient was able to prevent pain by going into a high alpha state before the headache began; however, he was not able to rid himself of pain by achieving a high alpha state once the pain began.

Shealy, reporting the results of six years' experience with electrical stimulation for pain control on over 1500 chronic pain patients, concluded that external electrical stimulation is of great benefit, especially in screening patients, and that dorsal column stimulation (involving the implantation of electrodes at the level of the dorsal columns of the spinal cord) was of great value for selected patients, but only as a last resort.[28] He maintained that drugs, the most frequent treatment for chronic pain, are "almost totally useless except in very specialized situations" and that traditional destructive procedures— cordotomy, cingulumotomy, rhizotomy—are "not only useless (except in cancer) but they cause far more harm than good, and they interfere with the success of other procedures." He stressed the importance of recognizing personality factors as of prime importance in dealing with chronic-pain patients and recommended psychological treatments, such as behavior modification, as well as the establishment of multidisciplinary, regional pain centers for patients with chronic pain.

Acupuncture has been suggested as a promising method for healing chronic pain. Katz and his associates reported relief using this method in patients with a variety of pain syndromes, and they noted a relationship between response to acupuncture and hypnotizability in their patients.[29]

The techniques mentioned do not exhaust the list of developing treatment approaches. Furthermore, it appears that chronic pain is being treated with a wide range of "home remedies" such as over-the-counter medications and physical therapies (heat, cold, and so on.) Clearly, more research is needed to evaluate the efficacy of all such treatments. Most likely, the effectiveness of particular procedures is interrelated in a complex manner with personality characteristics of patients. There is increasing evidence that certain personality traits aid in the identification of patients who will show poor response to the traditional medical-surgical procedures.

Perhaps the phenomenon of chronic pain is too diffuse and complex to allow the development of a relatively homogeneous set of effective therapeutic interventions. However, certain factors appear to emerge from the commonalities of many of the procedures reported to be beneficial. Those techniques involving combinations of medical and psychological methods, recognizing the multidimensionality of the pain experience, seem particularly effective.[30] Likewise, those methods that give the patient a feeling of hopefulness and a sense of control over his pain appear promising.[4]

It is clear that chronic pain presents a great challenge for the fields of medicine and the allied helping professions. Traditional understanding and current treatment approaches are being severely criticized.[1, 28] For example, pharmacological approaches are regarded with increasing alarm because of the problems of unwanted side effects and the potential for fostering addiction; ablation techniques are being questioned not only because of their relatively high morbidity rate, but also because of the too frequent return of pain following significant neurosurgical destruction.

Certain refreshing and innovative views and findings appear to be giving direction to a way to meet the challenge of chronic pain. It seems especially important that behavioral science consultants, who work with the medical specialists in the treatment of these patients, adopt a multidimensional model of pain and attempt to dispel the traditional unidimensional approach of most medical practitioners.

REFERENCES

1. Melzack R: The Puzzle of Pain. New York, Basic Books, 1973, p 71
2. Sternbach R, Wolf S, Murphy R, et al: Aspects of chronic low back pain. Psychosomatics 14:52–56, 1973
3. Engel G: Psychogenic pain and the pain-prone patient. Am J Med 26:899–918, 1959
4. Melzack R: Psychological concepts and methods for the control of pain, in Bonica JJ (ed): Advances in Neurology, vol 4. International Symposium on Pain. New York, Raven, 1974
5. Keele KD: The pain chart. Lancet 255:6–8, 1948
6. Melzack R, Torgerson WS: On the language of pain. Anesthesiology 34:50–59, 1971
7. Petrovich DV: The pain apperception test. J Psychol 44:339–346, 1957
8. Serjeant R: The Spectrum of Pain. London, Rupert Hart-Davis, 1969
9. Fordyce W: Pain viewed as learned behavior, in Bonica JJ (ed): Advances in Neurology, vol 4. International Symposium on Pain. New York, Raven, 1974
10. Smith GM, Lowenstein E, Hubbard JH, et al: Experimental pain produced by the submaximum effort tourniquet technique. J Pharmacol Exp Ther 163:468–474, 1968
11. Sternbach R, Murphy R, Timmermans G, et al: Measuring the severity of clinical pain, in Bonica JJ (ed): Advances in Neurology, vol 4. International Symposium on Pain. New York, Raven, 1974
12. Katz RL, Bresler DE: Chronic pain: Acupuncture, hypnosis, and control of pain. USPHS grant application, 1974

13. Szasz T: Language and pain, in Arieti S (ed): American Handbook of Psychiatry Vol 1. New York, Basic Books, 1959, p 982

14. Sternbach R: Varieties in pain games, in Bonica JJ (ed): Advances in Neurology, vol 4. International Symposium on Pain. New York, Raven, 1974, 423–430

15. Sternbach R: Pain Patients: Traits and Treatment. New York, Academic Press, 1974

16. Hanvik L: MMPI profiles in patients with low back pain. J Consult Psychol 15:350–353, 1951

17. Lachar D: The MMPI: Clinical Assessment and Automated Interpretation. Los Angeles, Western Psychological Services, 1974, p 46

18. Sternbach R, Wolf S, Murphy R, et al: Traits of pain patients: The low back ''loser.'' Psychosomatics 14:226–229, 1973

19. Schwartz MS, Krupp NE: The MMPI ''conversion V'' among medical patients: A study of incidence, criteria, and profile elevation. J Clin Psychol 27:89–95, 1971

20. Woodforde J, Merskey H: Personality traits of patients with chronic pain. J Psychosom Res 16:167–172, 1972

21. Wiltse LL, Rocchio PD: Predicting success of low back surgery using psychological tests. Paper presented at the American Orthopaedic Association, Hot Springs, Virginia, 1973

22. Phillips EL: Some psychological characteristics associated with orthopaedic complaints. Current Practice of Orthopaedic Surgery 2:165–176, 1964

23. Wiffling FJ, Klonoff H, Kokan P: Psychological, demographic, and orthopaedic factors associated with prediction of outcome of spinal fusion. Clin Ortho P 90:153–160, 1973

24. Nagi SZ, Burk RD, Potter HR: Back disorders and rehabilitation achievement. Chronic Dis 18:181–197, 1965

25. Pheasant HC, Holt JM: Low-back disorders: Psychological, demographic, and organic correlates of response to treatment. Orthopedic Hospital Report. Los Angeles, 1973

26. Beals R, Hickman N: Industrial injuries of the back and extremities. J Bone Joint Sur 54–A:1593–1610, 1972

27. Gannon L, Sternbach R: Alpha enhancement as a treatment for pain: A case study. J Beh Ther Exper 2:209–213, 1971

28. Shealy C: Six year's experience with electrical stimulation for control of pain, in Bonica JJ (ed): Advances in Neurology, vol 4. International Symposium on Pain. New York, Raven, 1974

29. Katz R, Kao C, Spiegel H, et al: Pain, acupuncture, hypnosis, in Bonica JJ (ed): Advances in Neurology, vol 4. International Symposium on Pain. New York, Raven, 1974

30. Greenhot J, Sternbach R: Conjoint treatment of chronic pain, in Bonica JJ (ed): Advances in Neurology, vol 4. International Symposium on Pain. New York, Raven, 1974

Robert O. Jones

16
Delirium

DEFINITION

A delirium (acute brain syndrome) is a psychotic disorder characterized by a lowering of the level of cognitive functioning with accompanying changes of affect (generally one of suspicion and fear) and perceptual changes (illusions, hallucinations, and delusions). These changes result from a global impairment of cerebral metabolism occurring from a variety of causes. There is the potentiality for recovery if the cause is removed; if not, there may be progress to irreversible brain change (a chronic brain syndrome). This possibility of permanent damage and the possibility of harm during the period of confusion makes the diagnosis and treatment of delirium a matter of great importance.

To the above criteria, Engel and Romano would add as a requirement the presence of a marked slowing of the electroencephalogram, which closely parallels changes in the level of consciousness.[1]

OCCURRENCE

Delirium represents the most commonly occurring psychosis in general medical and surgical practice. It makes mockery of any hospital and doctor who claim that they do not see psychiatric patients. Delirious patients are on the medical wards as complications of a wide variety of medical illnesses, on the surgical wards as a frequent postoperative complication, on the opthamology wards following cataract surgery, on the obstetric service in the postpartum period—in fact delirious patients are anywhere where there are sick people. One could equally say that any place where drugs are prescribed for people, there will be deliriums too.

Many consultants with a great deal of experience in general hospital work estimate that about 15 to 20 percent of all psychiatric consultations in a general hospital are for delirium. Lipowski and Titchner and his associates in their survey of 200 surgical patients at the Cincinnati General Hospital found that 22 percent of these randomly selected patients were psychotic at some time during their hospital stay, and of this group over a third had deliriums.[2, 3] Our experience at the Victoria General Hospital in Halifax is that about 20 percent of the consultations from nonpsychiatric services are acute brain syndromes. These, of course, represent the more serious problems; there are no figures that would indicate the number of mild to moderate that are treated successfully by these services themselves.

Many patients with delirum are disturbed troubled people. They try to get out of bed, are noisy, and are considered a nuisance by the medical and nursing attendants. Causing trouble quickly results in consultation.

There is evidence that there are at least an equal number of quiet delirious patients, who lie in bed puzzled and perplexed, frequently making polite and normal responses to superficial social remarks, who are not recognized as delirious, and who may even be considered good patients. Engel and Romano[1] and Lipowski[2] have made this point forcibly.

The first thing that the general hospital consultant must develop is a knowledge that many delirious patients will not be referred to him until their condition has been in existence long enough to become irreversible or when the patient's puzzlement and perplexity has caused a tragedy, such as falling head first down the fire stairs when the patient is looking for the bathroom. *A high degree of suspicion and constant vigilance of patients are necessary attitudes for the consultant to instill in his medical and nursing colleagues.*

Finally, we can expect an increase in the number of referrals of delirious patients. Unfortunately, our ability to produce delirium is increasing far more rapidly than our ability to recognize and deal with it. As we get bigger and better ways of producing brain damage, as we get more potent drugs that are frequently toxic to cerebral tissue, as we get more prolonged and serious surgical procedures, with frequent periods of anoxia, as the population ages, deliriums are certain to increase in frequency.

ETIOLOGY

The necessary factor in the etiology of the delirious reaction is the production of a global disturbance of brain metabolism, which may occur from a wide variety of causes—a wide variety that increases every day. Before we discuss those causes, it is of the greatest importance to realize that there is an identifiable population at risk. The recognition of this group and the appropriate management of this population may prevent the development of delirium. The general hospital consultant should strive to have his medical and nursing colleagues appreciate this. There are certain features of the population at risk that they should look for when treating patients.

First, those who already have some degree of brain damage. The best example is the aging person with early arteriosclerotic or senile brain change. A few doses of barbiturate given to such a patient are extremely effective in producing a delirium. *The greatest caution should be exercised in prescribing drugs, particularly sedatives, for aging people.*

The frightened and lonely person is a candidate for delirium. The person who comes into the hospital not knowing what is going to be done to him, who has no supportive relationship with a doctor or anybody else on the staff, and who is cut off from his own family is particularly prone to delirium. Titchner and his colleagues showed many years ago that the elderly surgical patient's chances of developing a delirium varied inversely with the number of visitors that he had.[3]

Those suffering from sensory deprivation also are high-risk delirium patients. The person who is cut off from sensory input that relieves fear, helps with orientation, and resolves confusion should be watched closely. Ophthamologists have known this for a long while. They have experienced delirium with their cataract patients, who developed a so-called "black-patch" delirium. Sensory deprivation as a factor in delirium is becoming increasingly apparent to cardiologists. The experiences of patients in two intensive care units in the same hospital, without selection, looked after by the same staff and with the same methods, showed that deliriums developed much more frequently in a unit without windows than the unit with windows.

Sleep deprivation is still another prevalent factor in arousal of delirium. The person who, for one reason or another, has lost a good deal of sleep very often is at increased risk.

The typical high-risk patient, then, is the aging man or woman with some arteriosclerosis in an intensive care unit, sleeping poorly, having few visitors, and given a barbiturate. Here is one place where the consultant can do some preventive psychiatry.

The direct etiological factors of delirium include exogenous intoxication—that is, intoxications from outside the body—and endogenous intoxications—that is intoxications produced from within the body. Drugs generally administered by doctors lead all of the rest in causing exogenous intoxications that have caused delirium. Indeed, the history of medical therapeutics can be traced in the etiological factors in delirium through the ages. In my lifetime, for example, I have seen things "progress" from the time when I saw many deliriums as the result of bromides, then large numbers from barbiturates, and now from the newer tranquilizers such as Valium. All of the old drugs (Digitalis, Atropine, and so on) and most of the new given to susceptible people in the right dosage will result in delirium. In the drug field alcohol deserves special mention—either during its increasing intake or with its sudden withdrawal—as a primary precipitant of delirium. The street drugs, of course, will frequently cause delirium as well. Endogenous intoxications that frequently bring the onset of delirium are:

1. Infections such as in the postoperative period, in pneumonia, in hepatic or kidney failure, and many more
2. Disturbances of cerebral nutrition (such as severe anemias), cardiovascular disorders, or vitamin deficiencies (such as pellagra)
3. A wide variety of metabolic disorders (such as electrolyte imbalance) and many endocrine dysfunctions (such as hyperthyroidism)
4. Trauma
5. Epilepsy and its several manifestations
6. Infections generalized with a high fever or infections of the nervous system (such as encephalitis)

CLINICAL FEATURES

The psychiatric liaison-consultant is usually called to the other services of the hospital when a patient becomes restless and disturbed. The history of the delirious patient generally includes some medical or surgical problem of the nature already mentioned. The behavior disturbance may have rapid or gradual onset. In the early or prodromal stages symptoms may be mild and transient, with difficulty in concentration, in thinking coherently, and with accompanying anxiety, mild depression, or apathy. Sleep may be disturbed by vivid dreams or nightmares. The severity of the condition will vary and is apt to be worse at night. It is very likely the night nurse who first makes the diagnosis. A particularly alert ward staff will find a number of other patients with cognitive difficulties of the quiet perplexed kind mentioned as will the consultant who makes regular rounds in the wards of the hospital in addition to the psychiatric ward.

From a careful examination of a patient in the onset of delirium, it will be possible to demonstrate a disorder of ''grasp,'' which designates an inability to comprehend relationships among elements of one's environment and relate them meaningfully to oneself and one's past experience and knowledge. At the beginning, and indeed throughout the course of the illness, the severity of the delirium will vary from moment to moment and nearly always retain its original pattern of being worse at night. Further examination will show disturbances in orientation, with time usually being first affected and then place and persons. Characteristically, the delirious patient mistakes unfamiliar places and persons for familiar ones; for example, he regards the hospital as his home.

A third characteristic disturbance is that of attention; the patient has difficulty fixing his attention and maintaining it on any particular subject or concern. Memory defect is generally present too. Recent memory tends to be more severely impaired than remote, but as the delirium progresses, retention and recall will also be affected. Occasionally the patient will confabulate.

These cognitive changes are the sine qua non of delirium, but there will also be affective changes evident. Fear and suspicion is frequently the most common change, but some patients are apathetic, some depressed, some angry and excited.

The final member of the triad that is usually present in delirium is disturbances of perception. The delirious patient soon experiences illusions, hallucinations, and delusions, the latter frequently of the fearful types. Statistically, delusions and visual hallucinations are most common, and the presence of visual hallucinations should always make one suspect an organic brain syndrome. The patient's behavior will be appropriate to these cognitive difficulties. The patient may be restless and frightened, trying to get out of bed to get away from his fancied dangers or lying in a puzzled, perplexed state. Accidents may occur because of this confusion. There may be a progressive reduction in the level of consciousness so that the patient lies in bed increasingly unresponsive to environmental stimuli but manufacturing his own stimuli through his visual hallucinations and illusions. The muttering delirium or picking bugs off the bedclothes or out of the air is the stereotype of this further development.

There are three possible results of delirium:

1. Through treatment or spontaneous elimination of the cause, recovery with little or no impairment of cerebral functioning
2. A progressive impairment of cerebral functioning leading to a chronic brain syndrome
3. Coma and death

DIFFERENTIAL DIAGNOSIS

Only rarely is it difficult to make a differential diagnosis of delirium. The crucial point is to find evidence of some degree of cognitive impairment tending to fluctuate in severity. Careful history taking and mental status examination will usually make the diagnosis. Tests usually given in the sensorial part of the mental status examination—for example, serial subtraction, digit span, simple calculation, orientation questions, and simple psychomotor tests—will usually provide evidence of the cognitive slipping. From the laboratory the electroencephalogram can be a most important aid. There is a characteristic slowing of the basic frequencies. The electroencephalogram mirrors closely improvement or deterioration.

MANAGEMENT

Having made a diagnosis of delirium, what must a consultant do? The following seem to me to be the steps, in the order of importance, to take:

1. Protect the patient.
2. Provide continuous good nursing care.
3. Attend to the general medical condition.
4. Investigate the cause of the condition so that it may be treated or eliminated.
5. Provide sedation. *Caution*, only the minimal amount.
6. Prescribe an adequate convalescence period.

The first and necessary step is to protect the patient. Delirious patients are not generally suicidal, but they get into serious trouble, which may involve mistaking a window for a door and going through it in their fear. Thus, they need protection, which is best provided by a nurse who is comfortable with the patient and takes her responsibility for care seriously.

There will be the need for continued good nursing care, preferably given, as much as possible, by the same nurse. One person spending a significant period of time with the patient may quiet his fears, give reassurance, help to keep him oriented, and attend to his physical and psychological needs. He should be reassured by explanation, telling him that the confusion that he is experiencing is not unusual or abnormal in the kind of situation that he is in and informing him as to the way in which he perceives things may be altered by drugs, diseases, toxins, and so on. A patient should be told that this state of affairs is not rare or without precedent, that it will improve, that it is not serious or permanent, and that it can be treated. The psychological explanation should embrace the facts that all illnesses and changes in sensorium produce fear and panic and that these emotions when repressed and unacknowledged arouse conflicts, worries, and anxieties from earlier life. The patient should have an opportunity to consider these fears, to examine them, and to communicate them to his physician or some other staff member. Obviously, the patient will be completely dependent on regular medical and family visitation.

Good nursing care is of the utmost importance. If this cannot be provided on a regular basis by the hospital, then bring in friends and relatives who can protect the patient and at the same time provide some frame of reference in the real world to which he is accustomed. Some familiar person should be in the room, which should be well lighted, thus cutting down on the possibilities of misperceptions. Frequent orientation statements by whoever is present are helpful: "You are in Ward 9-B at the Victoria General Hospital." "This is Sunday, June 16th." Careful explanation of all diagnostic or surgical procedures repeated and repeated may well prevent or contain the delirium.

Having attended to all that, one pays attention to the general medical condition—the electrolyte balance, adequate hydration, nutrition, vitamin supplies, and the like.

When general measures have been instituted, one then looks for the cause with the hope that this may be treated or eliminated. Not uncommonly, it is not found. One of the most important things to do is to scrutinize carefully the patient's drug regime. Almost any drug in a susceptible person, even in minute doses, may precipitate a delirium. (In one week I have seen three atropine deliriums. One, a distinguished colleague, became wildly psychotic following the preoperative injection of 0.6 mg of atropine. Another absorbed enough atropine from an ointment containing belladonna for bleeding piles to produce this effect.) Almost every day several new drugs appear that will produce delirium; for example, drugs such as Xylocaine, used in an intensive care unit, may be one of the precipitators of delirium in that situation. Frequently there is nothing to do but promote elimination of the drug by all channels; sometimes specific remedies are available. We used to see bromide deliriums and sodium chloride was said to be useful in replacing the bromide ion. The anticholinergic drugs such as scopolamine and atropine, as already mentioned, may produce a serious delirium. Green has reported prompt relief of this kind of delirium by physotigmine given intravenously, the dose being twice that of the anticholinergic drug previously administered.[4] Sometimes treatment of the cause will demand antibiotics, surgical procedures, and so forth. Again, the occurrence of a delirium may precede the evidence of developing physical pathology by several days and should always lead to immediate careful physical survey.

Sedation should be used as little as possible, but in most deliria of any degree it will be necessary either for the patient or for his wardmates. It should be remembered that delirious patients are always worse at night; therefore, the sedation should be saved for that period if possible. It should be given early in the evening before the patient becomes psychotic and should be given in adequate dosage.

The greatest mistake that I have seen in a general hospital in the management of delirious reactions is using sedation in inadequate dosage. In the days when paraldehyde was used, such was the case. Now with the use of phenothiazines, the same criticism is valid. Generally the medication of choice is a phenothiazine given in adequate dosage. What phenothiazine is used should mostly depend on the physician rather than the condition that he is treating. In delirium the drug will often have to be given intramuscularly or intravenously; so one needs a nonirritant drug, potent in small doses, with a very considerable margin of safety in its use. At the Victoria General Hospital, perphenazine B.P. (Trilafon) 5 mg intramuscularly repeated in an hour, if necessary, but generally every four hours, has given good results. Whatever drug is chosen should be continued until things are under control and then gradually reduced. What the physician should do is to learn two or three phenothiazines and be comfortable in their use. The exhibition of any phenothiazine with which the physician is comfortable in adequate dosage is good treatment, and the physician's knowledge is more important than the individual drug. There are certain exceptions to this, the one of most importance being the treatment of the delirium of alcoholism, either in the predelirious state or when delirium tremens has developed. Here the phenothiazines are inappropriate because they reduce the convulsive threshold. There is much evidence in the literature that chlordiazepoxide (Librium) is very much a superior drug, both in terms of efficacy and in terms of safety. Again, our method in the delirium associated with alcoholism is to give 100 mg of chlordiazepoxide intravenously (this is safe and to be preferred to the intramuscular route, which is much less predictable), every four hours for 24 to 40 hours. With improvement in the delirium gradually introduce the drug orally, with slow reduction over the next week. Support in favor of chlordiazepoxide is found in the report of Favazza and Martin.[5]

On a few occasions it is exceedingly difficult to control the overactivity of delirium with drugs, and we have followed the practice of giving a small number of ECTs, which, strangely enough, has been effective in controlling the severity of the delirium.

Finally, it is important that the patient with delirium have an adequate convalescence period. Relapse is common when treatment is discontinued and responsibility returned to the patient too soon.

IN CONCLUSION

It is fitting to conclude this discussion by reiterating the original statement that delirium is an extremely common illness that every physician is going to recognize and treat many times during his practice. It is also a condition that provides a fascinating opportunity to learn much about body and mind interaction. Awareness of its frequency and skill in its treatment are a necessary part of armament for the practitioner of medicine in whatever field.

REFERENCES

1. Engel G, Romano J: Delirium, a syndrome of cerebral insufficiency. J Chronic Dis 9: 260–277, 1959
2. Lipowski ZJ: Delirium, clouding of consciousness and confusion. J Nerv Ment Dis 145:227–255, 1967
3. Titchner J, Zwerling I, Gottschalk L, et al: Psychosis in surgical patients. Surg Gyn Obs 102:59–65, 1956
4. Green L: Anesth Analg 50:2, 1971
5. Favazza A, Martin P: Chemotherapy of delirium tremens: A survey of physician's preferences. Am J Psychiatry 131:1031–1033, 1974

Robert E. Litman

17
The Assessment of Suicidality

Psychiatrists are asked to assess the suicidality of patients in different settings and under a variety of circumstances. This assessment is essential for two purposes: (1) the immediate survival of the patient and (2) the patient's long-term therapy goals. It is first necessary to make certain immediate decisions, such as whether the patient should be admitted to a psychiatric unit and to what degree special precautions against suicide should be taken; second, the evaluation of suicide risk is an important element among others in the evolution of ongoing treatment plans for every patient.

The two objectives are not necessarily contradictory, but neither are they congruent. Treatment goals for most patients including achieving greater freedom, self-direction, and personal responsibility. Yet, short-range survival goals put the emphasis on the safety and security of the patient at the expense of independence, autonomy, and responsibility. Suicidal patients who are legally committed to a psychiatric hospital dramatize the therapeutic dilemma. Which are more important, the patient's survival, safety, and security or the patient's autonomy, freedom, and dignity? Posed as philosophical issues, these eternal dilemmas have no conclusive answers. Luckily, in practice, aided by common sense, knowledge, and experience, the patient can usually be assisted toward both survival and dignity.

The most important element in the psychiatric assessment of suicidality is the time dimension. Does the patient's suicidal behavior represent an acute, time-limited crisis reaction, or does it represent a chronic, long-lasting lifestyle? The prognosis, and therefore the rational treatment approach, depends upon this diagnostic distinction. Current models of crisis intervention appear to be effective suicide prevention for those patients who are actually in a crisis. A crisis model implies that persons were in reasonable harmony with their environment until a life stress event occurred such as a separation or death, which threw them into emotional perturbation that represents the crisis.

227

If suicidal patients are in crisis, there should be great emphasis on insuring their temporary safety and security since the patients may be expected to recover completely, and an impulsive suicide would be most regrettable.

By contrast, crisis interventions are relatively ineffective with persons who have a long history of chronic or repetitive suicidal behaviors as part of a self-destructive style of life. They are chronically depressed, or make repeated suicide attempts, have masochistic personal relationships, and abuse drugs and alcohol. Their suicidal behaviors do not represent crises so much as repetitive behavior patterns. For these persons the treatment plan should emphasize the gradual amelioration of self-destructive life-styles, with rather less emphasis on active intervention to insure the safety of the patients. It must be admitted that psychiatrists have not developed, to date, highly effective treatment techniques to alter rapidly the self-destructive life-styles of many of these persons who are at high suicide risk.

WHY DO PEOPLE COMMIT SUICIDE?

Several years ago I tried to answer for myself the question of why people commit suicide by obtaining and personally reading all of the suicide notes discovered in Los Angeles over a period of two consecutive years. During that time there were almost 3000 committed suicides and almost 1000 suicide notes. My task turned out to be a peculiarly distressing and disappointing one—distressing because there was so much human misery recorded in the coroner's files and in the suicide notes, disappointing because the notes failed to provide an explanation for the question, why suicide. Suicide notes tend to be stereotyped and uncreative. The most typical note says, ''I am sorry. I love you. Please forgive me. I have to do this.'' The next most common items in notes are instructions: ''My car is parked across the street.'' ''Please pay Stan back the $20 I borrowed.'' ''Police, this is a suicide.''

Some persons give reasons for the act of suicide. They express regret over a lost lover, apprehension about sickness, unwillingness to be a burden. Often, the communications describe fatigue, exhaustion, and a need to escape. ''I just can't stand it any more, I am too tired to go on.'' The notes seldom (less than 10 percent) express anger or reproach. Humor is absent. The general mood of those notes that express feelings is one of hopelessness. However, there are those exceptional messages that convey a confident religious faith in a happy afterlife.

Behavioral scientists have studied retrospectively the lives and circumstances surrounding individual suicides by interviews with surviving relatives and friends, a method sometimes called ''psychological autopsies.'' After collecting these materials, psychiatrists have no great difficulty in making retrospective psychiatric diagnoses on 90 percent of those committed suicides. Typically, about 40 percent of the committed suicides are given the diagnosis of "affective disorder"; 20 to 25 percent of the committed suicides suffered from chronic alcholism; 10 to 15 percent were schizophrenic; 20 to 25 percent could be diagnosed as chronic behavior disorder or personality maladjustment. Psychiatrists feel that these individuals should have consulted psychiatrists. The general public recognizes a moderate degree of association or relationship between suicide and madness, although, of course, most psychotic persons do not commit suicide and most persons who committed suicide were not psychotic.

There are other reasons why many persons who are in danger of making a suicide attempt or of actually committing suicide are seen by psychiatrists on the patients' own volition or because they were referred by others. Suicidal people are ambivalent in their intentions; wishes to die or to escape coexist with wishes to continue living. People approaching suicide are often perturbed and confused, and they have difficulties in communicating. Suicidal persons often express feelings of depression and anxiety, and other people around them also become anxious and distressed. Ambivalence, perturbation, confusion, communication problems, depression, and anxiety—these are conditions that are generally accepted as suitable for psychiatric intervention. Finally, there is a tradition that suicide is usually an expression of mental illness, and, therefore, prevention should be in the hands of psychiatrists, backed up when necessary with legal sanctions. Thus, society has assigned to psychiatry the role of safeguarding and rehabilitating suicidal persons, a task that is complex, difficult, hazardous, and sometimes impossible.

The difficulties are not only practical but theoretical. Although we know a lot of the circumstances and the reasons given for individual suicides, we do not have a satisfactory theoretical explanation for suicide. Sociological theorists tend to view suicide as an expression of deviance. Low suicide rates are associated with societies that tend to be more structured, with more explicit social roles, in which most people tend to be very much like all of the other people. High suicide rates are associated with societies in turmoil, where social roles are unclear. Some social theorists assert that the more deviant the individual, that is, the fewer social roles that person shares with other people, the higher the risk of suicide for that individual. In general, suicide rates for large social units, such as countries, tend to remain relatively stable over long periods of time and change only in response to rather obvious, large-scale events, such as wars, depressions, or rapid changes in population characteristics. Many of the younger sociologists feel that theories derived from statistical collections have not been very helpful; they look toward psychological data from individuals who have committed suicides or near suicides to provide more useful information.

It must be admitted, however, that there is no universally accepted psychological theory of suicide. In large part, this is because psychology and psychiatry do not provide, at present, a satisfactory theory of human behavior, normal or abnormal. Psychoanalysis probably owes its longevity to the fact that it offers the only comprehensive theoretical approach to understanding how human beings feel, think, and act. Psychoanalysis offers quite elegant formulations for understanding dreams, slips of speech, and symbolic behaviors, but psychoanalysts have a harder time understanding or predicting actions in the real world. A review of the writings of Sigmund Freud, the founder of psychoanalysis, indicates that he tried to explain the "enigma" of suicide as he encountered it in his clinical material and in his personal relationships. It was necessary for him to revise his basic theoretical constructions several times in order to deal specifically with problems of masochism and self-destructiveness.

My theoretical model for suicide follows closely Menninger's adaptation from Freud.[1] The key concept is fragmenting of the personality. According to this theoretical orientation, there is a suicide potential in all of us, a degree of self-destructiveness that ordinarily is tamed, controlled, and overcome through our healthy identifications, ego defenses, and constructive habits of living and loving. When the ordinary defenses, controls, and ways of living and loving are ineffective or break down under stress, people may then feel forced into suicidal behaviors. At such times they feel helpless, hopeless, and abandoned, and they may or may not be aware of a great deal of unexpressable aggressive tension. Thinking becomes stereotyped and constricted; alternatives cannot be imagined. It is because of these characteristics of suicidal states of mind that suicide notes are psychodynamically unrevealing.

QUANTIFYING SUICIDE RISK

The most effective approaches at the present time to assessing suicidality are pragmatic (atheoretic) and holistic, in that they sample a wide variety of traits, characteristics, and behaviors.[2, 3, 4] Follow-up studies of patients who were seen originally in emergency medical settings after suicide attempts, or who were treated in psychiatric hospitals, or who had called emergency telephone counseling services compared committed suicide victims with persons who did not commit suicide within one or two years. Certain items, or combination of items, are more closely associated with suicidal outcome, thus predicting a higher suicide risk.

What is the quantitative translation of the concept "high suicide risk"? Customarily, suicide rates are reported as suicide deaths per 100,000 population per year. The suicide rate for the entire United States population is approximately 11. In the so-called suicide capital of the nation, San Francisco,

Table 17–1
Risk Defined as Suicide Probability

Suicide Probability	"Risk"
0–5/100,000	Nonrisk
5–50/100,000	Normal (minimal) risk
50–500/100,000	Suicidal with low risk
500–5,000/100,000	Suicidal with moderate risk
Over 5,000/100,000	Suicidal with high risk

the suicide rate is approximately 30. Suicide rates obviously fluctuate according to such variables as age, sex, and geographic location. For persons who have been in touch with the Suicide Prevention Center in Los Angeles, the suicide rate has been approximately 1000 (1 percent a year) in the two years following contact with the center. Studies of persons who attempted suicide indicated a suicide rate of 1000 to 2000 (1 to 2 percent) in the two years following the suicide attempt. In an effort to quantify what is meant by "low" or "high" suicide risk, there is a suggested classification of suicide probability presented in Table 17–1.

According to this classification scheme, unselected suicide-attempt cases are "moderate" suicide risks. Certain subcategories of suicide attempters are "high risks." A "highest-risk" sample was described by Moss and Hamilton.[5] They selected patients who were in a psychiatric hospital because of "high-lethality" suicide attempt and had, in addition, obvious mental illness. The suicide mortality of this group was 22 percent over several years, with a majority of the deaths occurring in the first year of follow-up. The authors felt that it is possible to identify potential high-risk suicide cases. The big problem is how to reach these patients with effective treatment, which requires maintaining long-term therapeutic contacts.

Patients in psychiatric treatment have, in general, a "low" suicide risk amounting to an expectation of a mortality of 100 over 100,000, which is about 10 times that of the unselected population, according to reports from Pokorny[6] and Babigian and Odoroff.[7] There are at least two types of moderate-risk psychiatric patients—those who have a diagnosis of depression or manic-depressive illness[6] and veterans who have had psychiatric hospitalization with special attention drawn to their suicidal status.[8] [9] A history of chronic alcoholism carries with it a suicide risk comparable to being a psychiatric patient, namely, low.[10, 11]

Certain social indicators provide a special clue to suicidal lethality in suicide attempters. An outstanding example is the living arrangement "alone" for suicide attempters as reported by Tuckman and Youngman.[12] The combination of these two features, namely, suicide attempt and living alone, predict a suicide rate of 7140.

Table 17–2

Examples of Predicted Suicide Risk

Type of Case or Group	0–5/ 100,000 Nonrisk	5–50/ 100,000 Minimal	50–500/ 100,000 Low	500–5,000/ 100,000 Moderate	Over 5,000/ 100,000 High
SPC* cases (unselected)				X	
Selected high-risk SPC cases					X
Suicide attempters seen in hospitals				X	
Psychiatric patients			X		
Suicidal psychiatric patients				X	
Manic-depressive psychiatric patients				X	
Young men		X			
College students		X			
Age under 12	X				
Young female with no obvious turmoil	X				
Old females		X			
Young female suicide attempters			X		
Female, repeated suicide attempts				X	
Old man, lives alone			X		
Heroin addicts			X		
Chronic alcoholics			X		
Depressed alcoholic middle-aged male, SPC					X
Suicide attempter, lives alone					X
Serious suicide attempter in a mental hospital					X

From reference 3.

*SPC = Suicide Prevention Center, Los Angeles

Examples of predicted suicide risk are presented in Table 17–2. This table illustrates that it is possible to place many individuals into the low to moderate clinical risk groups on the basis of brief history and demographic data. It is even possible to diagnose high risk in a few persons on demographic data alone. However, for diagnosing high lethality usually a clinical examination of the current mental status of the individual is needed.

To some extent, the weighting of information that may predict suicide depends upon the setting. For persons in contact with the Los Angeles Suicide Prevention Center, the significant items are listed in Table 17–3.

Note that absence of current stress (items 9, 11) and unwillingness to accept help (items 6, 8) are suicide predictors in this setting. For comparison, a study of suicide attempters from the Payne Whitney Psychiatric Clinic failed to

Table 17-3
Los Angeles Suicide Prevention Center Prediction Items

Variable in Rank Order	Content of Item	Direction For Suicide
1	Age	Older
2	Alcoholism	Yes
3	Irritation-rage-violence	No
4	Lethal prior behavior	Higher
5	Sex	Male
6	Accept help now	No
7	Duration of current episode	Longer
8	Prior inpatient psychiatric treatment	No
9	Recent loss-separation	No
10	Depression-somatic	Yes
11	Loss of physical health	Less
12	Occupational level	Higher

From reference 3.

designate factors predicting suicide except the following: the patients (7 of 300) who died within a year from another suicide attempt were predominately former inpatients with long-standing psychiatric disturbances who were making no progress in treatment.[13]

PSYCHIATRIC INTERVIEW

The contribution of the psychiatric consultation to the overall assessment of suicidality is dependent completely upon the ability of the consultant to develop a relationship of confidence, trust, and intimacy with the patient. The decision as to whether the patient must have immediate protection and anti-suicide precautions depends in large part on certain highly personal feelings. These feelings are painful to discuss in many cases and often make the patient feel vulnerable and exposed.

The psychiatrist in the interview inquires as to how the patient feels "now." Are there feelings of anxiety, guilt, sadness, or remorse? Has the patient made preparations for suicide by securing a weapon, practicing a method, planning a funeral, making a new will, writing a farewell note? Has the patient set a deadline for suicide? Are there certain conditions without which life is not worth living? Is all this in relationship to a recent specific stress, especially a loss? Positive answers to any of the above questions raise possibilities of immediate danger of suicide.

The most important source of information, as well as potential assistance, is the family and close friends of the patient. Frequently the most significant information revealing suicidal trends comes from a spouse. One important aspect of suicidal behaviors and suicidal attempts is the communication effort. What message is the patient trying to get across? Can the psychiatric consultant act as an intermediary or a negotiator in a tense interpersonal situation? The psychiatric consultant assessing suicidality plays a double role as diagnostician and therapist. Whether or not a successful referral can be made depends upon the relationship that has been established.

Suicide attempts and suicide rarely occur within hospital walls. At times an alcoholic may impulsively steal a bottle of rubbing alcohol or a box of pills from the nurses' station and ingest them. Psychiatric consultants should be aware that postoperative confusion can be dangerous, especially with older persons, and such confused persons may jump from a window or open balcony. Probably the only type of patient who will deceive the psychiatric consultant by masking continuing suicidal intentions is the schizophrenic who has had some previous experience with psychiatrists. One clue that the patient is indeed schizophrenic is provided by a history of suicide attempts that included unusual or bizarre features. Occasionally a patient who has been seen by a psychiatric consultant to the medical service after an overdose reports honestly to the psychiatrist a resolution of suicidal feelings, which are then reactivated during a visit from a spouse or other intimate enemy. If there is a possibility of such a visit, it would be well to alert the nursing staff to monitor the interaction.

If the consultant assesses the suicidality as high risk, hospitalization in a psychiatric unit is probably the best disposition, both for the patient's safety and also as a place to reevaluate personal relationships and personal resources and to plan for future activities. Even the best hospital units, however, are only relatively secure, and the treatment is only relatively effective. In my opinion the most important aspect of the therapy of the acutely suicidal person is the *transition* in the therapeutic process from preoccupation with safety, security, and survival to concern over life-style, interpersonal relationships, and self-direction. The main problem with hospitalization is that this transition can be delayed or confused. There is a question as to how useful legal commitment is for the purpose of preventing suicide. As indications for commitment have been tightened and reduced in California, there has not been an epidemic of suicide in patients prematurely released from enforced psychiatric hospitalization, which I view as an expedient that should be used sparingly with high selectivity and thoughtful deliberation. The argument for commitment is that the suicidal urge is time-limited and that the future of the patient should be protected against transient turmoil of his personality. Two weeks of persuasion and discussion should be sufficient, however, to enable a patient to repair fragmented ego controls, and this should put an upper time limit on commitment.

From the standpoint of the patients' safety the best precaution against suicide, in or outside of a hospital, is the presence of other people. This may mean a more or less continuous monitoring of a patient by family, by other patients, and by the staff. Suicidal persons should not have a single room, and they should never be placed in isolation. Common sense dictates that windows and doors should be secure and that poisonous materials should not readily be available. It is a good idea to have regular patient meetings that include, from time to time, a review by the patients of possible danger areas and dangerous objects in the ward environment. Although ease of communication from patients to staff to physicians and back aids greatly in forestalling suicidal actions in hospitals, it should be stated explicitly that there is no certain way to prevent anyone from committing suicide anywhere if the individual is wholly dedicated to self-death, since many people have committed suicide in maximum security areas of hospitals and prisons.

CONCLUSION

The assessment of suicidality is a complicated, difficult, and hazardous task. Important items to be considered include age, sex, history of prior suicidal behavior, duration of the current episode, alcoholism, recent outburst of irritation, rage or violence, willingness to accept help now, current stress situations, and the presence of psychiatric disorders, especially depression but also including schizophrenia. Chronic psychiatric patients who have made previous suicide attempts and who are making no progress in their psychiatric treatment are extremely high suicide risks. There is no certain method to prevent suicide. Continuous monitoring on a person-to-person basis in a psychiatric unit offers the best security available. The essential aspect of treatment, however, is the transition from antisuicide precautions to concern over life-style, interpersonal relations, and self-direction.

REFERENCES

1. Menninger K: The Vital Balance: The Life Process in Mental Health and Illness. New York, Viking, 1963
2. Neuringer C (ed): Psychological Assessment of Suicidal Risk. Springfield, Ill., Thomas, 1974
3. Litman R: Prediction models of suicidal behaviors, in Beck A, Resnik H, Lettieri D (eds): The Prediction of Suicide. Bowie, Md., Charles, 1974
4. Brown T, Sheran T: Suicide prediction: A review. Life Threatening Behav 2:67–98, 1972
5. Moss L, Hamilton D: The psychotherapy of the suicidal patient. Am J Psychiatry 112:814–820, 1956

6. Porkorny A: Suicide rates in various psychiatric disorders. J Nerv Ment Dis 139:499–506, 1964
7. Babigian H, Odoroff C: The mortality experience of a population with psychiatric illness. Am J Psychiatry126:470–480, 1969
8. Porkorny A: A follow-up study of 618 suicidal patients. Am J Psychiatry 122:1109–1116, 1966
9. Eisenthal S, Farberow N, Shneidman ES: Follow-up of neuropsychiatric hospital patients. Public Health Reports 81:977–990, 1966
10. Kessel H, Grossman G: Suicide in alcoholics. Br Med J 2:1671, 1961
11. Rushing W: Individual behavior and suicide, in Gibbs J (ed): Suicide. New York, Harper & Row, 1967
12. Tuckman J, Youngman W: Identifying suicide risk groups among attempted suicides. Public Health Reports 78:763–766, 1963
13. Kiev A: Prognostic factors in attempted suicide. Am J Psychiatry 131:987–990, 1974

Avery D. Weisman

18
The Dying Patient

Death is such a commonplace event in a hospital that a psychiatric consultant is seldom called upon simply because a patient is dying. It is wholly possible for a psychiatrist to become rather expert in offering consultation and brief therapy to medical and surgical colleagues (the ambiguity is deliberate) without ever being asked for an opinion about better ways to manage a patient with a fatal illness.

Nevertheless, because death is part of human life, and sickness is a significant event that is likely to have psychosocial ramifications, fatal illness falls within the scope of psychiatric participation. Conversely, psychiatrists who venture into this field usually find the encounter with dying patients most rewarding and instructive, both for patients and for themselves. It can also be a very taxing effort. Even the consultant needs help, and he should not hesitate to share and discuss his concerns and doubts with others. He will discover countertransference, including denial, devaluation, resentment, and identification, in about as naked a form as possible. If a psychiatrist is afraid of working in vain or finds a dying patient particularly obnoxious in the sense of being odious, then he is working with a sense of vanity or specious delicacy. In either case he would be wise to turn the patient over to someone else and go no further. Actually, this often happens unwittingly. A consultant may briefly talk with a terminal patient, just as he consults about an incurable psychopath, then he writes a short note, advising long-term social service support, and leaves.

WHEN IS A PSYCHIATRIST CALLED UPON?

As a rule, psychiatric consultation in a general hospital is requested only when other experts find that a patient's *behavior* is too baffling or too agitating to manage by ordinary means. A dying patient by definition is one who has not responded to curative measures and now can be offered only symptomatic or

237

palliative treatment. When "nothing further can be done," and a patient or family confronts the professional staff with anxiety, depression, hostility, or other threats, then the help of a psychiatrist may be requested. Recently, with the rise of consumerism, patients' rights, and the demands of social workers and nurses, psychiatrists are not permitted to escape easily from consultations and conferences about dying patients.

A dying patient is not merely someone with a fatal illness, but a person who has already passed through a series of procedures, has been disappointed, frustrated, and disillusioned and is facing still another uncertainty, the sickness unto death.

If a psychiatrist waits to be asked for help, he will not only wait in vain, but he will not be equipped to deal with the manifold problems presented in the terminal phase. Incurable disease, irreversible injury, incipient bereavement, and the secondary sufferings imposed by partial griefs and psychosocial predicaments make it imperative for a psychiatrist to *seek out* dying patients, without waiting for his colleagues to solicit help in prescribing psychotropic medicines or cooling off an agitated, distraught patient. Although hospital psychiatrists like to identify themselves with medical and surgical colleagues, their task is different. Belatedly psychiatrists are discovering death as an obligatory phase of human experience. Not only does life take place in the midst of death, but the social unit, of which a patient is a part, may also suffer and become ill as a result of loss and bereavement. Consequently, death for the psychiatric consultant is more than palliation: it is a summons to alleviate suffering and to ensure significant survival for a patient, who is a person within a social unit.

WHAT IS A DYING PATIENT MOST CONCERNED ABOUT?

Most people tend to see a dying patient either as someone who, for practical purposes, is already dead or as a living person minus almost everything else that signifies being alive in the first place. Any person who expects little of themselves, of the world, and of the future is in despair, whether he is in fact suffering from a fatal illness or not.

The predominant concerns of dying patients are those of living people plus inherent anxiety about annihilation, alienation, endangerment, and the encroachment of physical and social disability. Naturally, these may not be self-evident, especially during an initial interview. Predominant concerns may be disguised by defensive maneuvers, medications, and the disinclination of professionals to investigate. However, in general terms, we can commonly recognize the following: *health, existential concerns, work and finances, family, friends (significant others), religion,* and *self-appraisal.*

Few dying patients are utterly unaware that death is almost at the threshold. But it is reasonable to expect patients to seek relief of symptoms (health), to wonder about their progress or its lack ("What is happening? Must I die now?") as an expression of existential concerns. They may ruefully reproach themselves for being unable to work and support the family because this, after all, identifies a significant role. When a patient voices concern about significant others, it often hides a question that implies loneliness, abandonment, or repudiation by, and sometimes of, other people. Religious concerns are usually assigned or abrogated by very sick patients. The chaplain is certainly more experienced and much more acceptable to patients with religious concerns than is the psychiatrist. Finally, like most people, sick or not, dying patients continue to judge themselves on the basis of one value system or another. The difference at this time is that self-appraisal (the simplest version asks, "Am I a good person? Could things have turned out differently?") is retrospective as well as prospective. Vulnerable patients talk about past regrets, current problems, discrepancies between aspiration and achievement, and, to the keen or compassionate listener, they may even wonder audibly what life would have been, if only. . . .

The balance and weight of significant concerns vary from person to person. Some patients are less articulate and are guided more by bodily functions. They are not accustomed to expressing themselves, and in many instances the mist of medication and misery obscures the psychiatrist's clear view. Nevertheless, very human and natural fears about being engulfed are often overlooked by those too eager to help. They seek to reassure but do not pause to look into the predicament of being alive and afraid to die.

WHAT CAN A PSYCHIATRIST REALLY DO?

Surprisingly enough, sincere and sophisticated professionals ask whether talking with patients is really worth the time and trouble. The psychiatrist is usually very busy, and there are other people who can support a dying patient and give specific assistance as well. The chaplain, social worker, and nurse are trained and already have established social roles within the hospital that make psychosocial interventions more acceptable. Leaving aside special knowledge of medicine and psychiatry, including the ability to recommend psychotropic drugs, a psychiatrist still does not have to justify talking with people in trouble. He simply goes beyond the impersonal facts of sickness into the interpersonal domain of relationships and then to the privacy of very intrapersonal concerns, which are very difficult to get at without a considerable background of experience, interest, and supervision. The simplest aim of psychiatric intervention is to promote a better death. Since every person has only one death to die, a psychiatrist may help in discovering how a dying patient's regular life-style and personality, coping strategies, values, and vulnerability can be brought to a focus. Awareness that life and death are not necessarily enemies should help in understanding the context in which death occurs.

Broadly considered, what a psychiatrist does for the dying patient can be divided into two categories: (1) evaluation and (2) safe conduct.

Evaluation

Psychiatric evaluation of a dying patient underscores the importance of communication as an element of care and of the psychiatrist as an instrument of that care.

The psychiatrist asks himself several questions in the course of evaluation. What kind of reality does this patient have? What has he been living for, and what is he now dying to? What are the salient forces in this patient's social and emotional field, now and in the past? These questions supplement the medical problem of what a patient is dying from.

It is part of the psychiatric approach to recognize that dying and death may not invariably be a tragic outcome of incurable illness. Rather, because death always occurs within a psychosocial context, it can be both timely and even an occasion for maturational development. Another question, therefore, is, How can we make this death acceptable, even appropriate, under the circumstances?

Medical and surgical interventions are intended to relieve the primary sufferings brought on by the disease. Psychosocial management tries to alleviate the secondary sufferings related to social and emotional complications. These secondary sufferings are called *vulnerability*. In addition to identifying areas of concern, the psychiatrist differentiates between several kinds of vulnerability: denial, annihilation anxiety, alienation, endangerment, encroachment, and destructive dysphoria.

Denial may be very useful under certain circumstances, but militantly preserved, denial tends to be regressive and magical when it is the only coping strategy available. *Annihilation anxiety* is characterized by hopelessness, helplessness, dread about imminent extinction, and fears about having no future whatsoever. *Alienation* includes feelings of abandonment, diminished self-esteem, lack of mutuality in relationships with significant others, and repudiation of those who would be helpful. *Endangerment* expresses fears and despairs, coupled with anger and lack of appreciation for whatever has been done. It is being a passive victim who cannot protest or expect a reasonable response. *Encroachment* is a sense of drastic constriction in time, space, autonomy, and effective operations. Dying patients suffering from encroachment become scornful of their own weakness in not being able to walk, talk, feed themselves, and so forth. Finally, *destructive dysphoria* is a conviction that all is over. The dying patient feels exhausted and apathetic. In some cases the patient who is unable to find relief may talk about suicide and wanting to die and in a few situations, may even attempt suicide, directly or indirectly.

Safe Conduct

The purpose of safe conduct is to guarantee and restore to the powerless the rights and safety of which they have been deprived. Too often death is regarded as a failure of treatment. The dying patient becomes tangible evidence of failure, and, as a result, people looking after the dying move away, lose interest, substitute drugs for personal presence, or simply put the patient into one category or another, disregarding the individuality of the person.

Safe conduct does *not* mean that a psychiatrist, say, comports himself safely, in the manner best fitted for office practice. In other words, he is prepared for a give-and-take encounter, sharing what seems appropriate without feeling guilt. Kübler-Ross has described a series of stages: denial, anger, bargaining, depression, and acceptance. While some dying patients do, in fact, follow such a sequence, it is by no means invariable. Nor should the psychiatrist expect these stages to turn up with preordained regularity. In fact, the interests of safe conduct may not be most effectively served if the psychiatrist simply looks for salient features of "stages."

Throughout the dying process denial and acceptance intermingle; sometimes one is stronger than another, but usually they are present together. The psychiatrist is not immune from each of these stages himself. The chief value of the Kübler-Ross staging concept is not merely to call attention to changes in a patient's attitude, but also to monitor how the psychiatrist accepts or rejects the reality of certain death. Safe conduct means that we help keep someone alive as a significant person through informed communication, compassionate concern, and intelligent use of support systems.

Support systems are social and psychological strategies designed to recognize problems and do something about them, to revise and reorder priorities, and to fortify coping strategies most likely to alleviate vulnerabilities (secondary suffering). What is a dying patient able to do? Whom does he want to see (if anyone)? How can we restore a measure of self-esteem? What can we do to influence this patient and to change his surroundings so that a more appropriate death is feasible? Can we indicate that the patient matters, without becoming maudlin, or starting to mourn ourselves? Ideally, a dying patient should be helped to acknowledge and accept the plight, without undue vulnerability. Confrontation should be followed by efforts to redefine and relieve the obstacles to the realization of death. All the while, the psychiatrist remains accessible by dealing with his own anxieties, which, curiously enough, frequently parallel those found in the patient.

STRATEGIES FOR INTERVENTION

The general principles outlined need to be fleshed out with precepts and precautionary suggestions. Nothing is too obvious to mention. For example, *sit down and establish eye contact*. There is no set speech or sequence of questions. The dying patient usually has something to say on his own behalf. It may be a question, but more often it is a complaint.

Learn to listen. Listening involves not only signs of vulnerability in the patient, but also indications that the psychiatrist himself is uneasy. Some patients are more inclined to talk than are others. It is not true that every patient, given a chance, will immediately unburden himself about death and dying. *Telling or not telling* the so-called truth (''Why don't I feel better?'') about the prognosis (''Will I live or die?'') is not the primary question. Comparatively few patients ask about their prognosis. Learning to listen enables a psychiatrist to revise any question so that with tact, forebearance, and candor a more relevant question can be appropriately answered. *Modulate the truth* with the needs of the patient, not with your own needs. *Do not support regressive symptoms*; allow for the exhaustion and disability that most dying patients contend with.

Ask yourself what the patient would be like without the disease or what he was like during healthier times. Having done this, you will find it easier to accept the patient on as high a level of competence as possible, consistent with the present circumstances. *Talk about how the illness has changed the patient*, emphasizing expectations and disappointments. Support systems are encouraged by acceptance of the patient in the here-and-now with an appraisal of vulnerability and available coping strategies. If, for example, a patient seeks to deny, a psychiatrist should wonder what he might do to alter this strategy and replace it with reasonable awareness. ''What bothers you most about being so sick,'' one might ask. ''Whom have you talked to about what's happening to you?'' Anticipate bereavement of significant others, and talk, if possible, about *how the patient anticipates bereavement*. The central idea behind interventions with dying patients is not so much to verbalize about death as it is to accept the reality of death as a precondition of talking and being together.

Marshal every possible bit of support if you decide that support is inadequate or misdirected. The function of a psychiatrist is to be a *productive counterforce* against sickness and vulnerability, but the psychiatrist need not become an adversary of the professional staff. Therefore, *collaboration* is indicated, whenever feasible, to improve communication and trust.

The art of interviewing has fallen into quiet disregard within the past decade, perhaps coincidentally with the devaluation of psychodynamic psychiatry. Nevertheless, skillful interviewing is a necessity in consulting and following dying patients. A prepared interviewer does not need to be told what to say. His interventions are the result of discovery and improvisation, based upon the leading problems *right now* for that individual patient. Cliches, overly prompt reassurances, displacement of primary concern to peripheral and impersonal issues, and philosophical aphorisms are contraindicated. If a dying patient is adamantly disinclined to talk about anything, the psychiatrist need not be alarmed about the lack of verbal material for formulation. As a rule, a dying patient asks very little beyond essentials, and when a few leading questions bring forth even fewer responses, it may be because time itself matters even less. Nevertheless, many things, silent or spoken, can be crowded into the moment.

Common questions are "Why are you coming to see me? What's wrong with me that my doctor has asked a psychiatrist to visit?" Common answers might be "I go to see many patients in the hospital. Because I am a psychiatrist, I think about the many things that bother people, especially patients who have been sick as you have been. If I can, I'd like to know you better. How would you say you're feeling, right now?"

A most instructive principle in following patients who are dying is that of resisting *iatrogenic distortions*. These are usually shown by doctors who offer false or misleading hopes, undue pessimism, overly academic comments, antipathy to the patient, the staff, or the situation as a whole. Psychiatrists should expect that a dying patient will repeat himself, asking the same questions over and over, but not heeding the answers. Repetition is a way of dealing with reality, particularly one that baffles and intimidates. There is a temptation to combat anxiety by subtly avoiding the source of threat. It is well to remember that hope is not an expression of blind confidence in unlimited survival. Most dying patients do not expect this. But it is fair to do everything possible to enhance self-esteem by reinterpreting events in such a way that death will come almost as a matter of timely choice, not brute necessity.

Fear of death is practically universal. Psychiatrists should realize, however, that many smaller fears are covered by the enormity of this ultimate dread. *Basically, the death we fear dying is of losing the life we never lived.* If this paradox is understood, then death is more tolerable. For the psychiatrist, even in the absence of a scenario, the scenery can be moved around. The stage is set, accommodating itself to the best way of yielding up what is no longer ours.

REFERENCES

Feifel H (ed): New Meanings of Death. New York, McGraw-Hill, 1975
Kübler-Ross E: On Death and Dying. New York, Macmillan, 1969

Shneidman ES: Deaths of Man. Quadrangle/New York Times Book Co, New York, 1973

Weisman AD: On Dying and Denying. New York, Behavioral Publications, 1972

Weisman AD: The Realization of Death: A Guide for the Psychological Autopsy. New York, Aronson, 1974

Edwin S. Shneidman

19

Postvention:
The Care of the Bereaved

Grief and mourning are not diseases, but their deleterious and inimical effects can often be as serious as though they were. The recently bereaved person is typically bereft and disorganized. Long-standing habit patterns of intimate interpersonal response are irreversibly severed. There is a concomitant gale of strong feelings, usually including abandonment and despair, sometimes touching upon guilt and anger, and almost always involving a sense of crushing emptiness and loss. In light of these psychological realities it comes as no surprise that individuals who are acutely bereaved constitute a population "at risk."[1-9]

Excluding Freud's indispensible paper, "Mourning and melancholia," published in 1917,[10] much of the important work on this topic has been done only since 1944.[11-17] In general, these studies point out that grief and mourning may have serious physical and psychological concomitants (in the way of heightened morbidity and even a greater risk of death), and they explicate some of the dimensions of bereavement as well as ways of helping the bereaved.

This chapter will not be an attempt to replow the ground so fertilely turned by others, especially Parkes in his chapter "Helping the bereaved" in his book *Bereavement* in which he discusses the role of the funeral director, the church, the family doctor, and self-help organizations, among others.[9] Instead, the discussion will be limited to what I know best, namely, my own work with bereaved persons.

A specific example will be useful at the outset. Here are some excepts from a taped session with a young adult widower whom I had seen for several months after his wife died. She was a university student (whom I came to know in a course on death and suicide that I taught). She died of scleroderma. This session is three years after her death.

DR. S: Now to start with, your relationship with Edith was unusual in that you knew she was ill from the beginning.

MR. H: That's correct, I first met her ten years ago, she was 18. It was just after her illness had been diagnosed and her parents, if I remember correctly, told me about it when they saw that we were becoming serious, after we had been courting for some time. And I really didn't know exactly what the disease was, I mean as far as life span was concerned. I wonder why I didn't try to find out more. Maybe I was afraid; I don't know. I knew her life would be shortened, but I don't think I really allowed myself to think about it or to find out exactly what it was. It was terminal about eight years after. I have thought about it, because it seems to me strange of my not pursuing it. She was the first girl I guess I really had a good meaningful relationship with, and I think I might have been very frightened to find out the truth. But I didn't want to know . . . The more I think of it the more I really realize I think I blocked a tremendous amount out.

DR. S: Her death was not totally unexpected to you. When she came into the hospital, she was struggling and you knew she was failing. How were you told that she was dead, and then what happened?

MR. H: The doctor that had been attending her told me when I came in that morning to see her, and he brought me aside. He took me somewhere. I think he gave me a tranquilizer. I was extremely impressed with him. I was probably in shock, but I remember the clear thing I did feel was some sense of relief that I don't have to wait any longer. That incredible waiting that I realized I had been going through was suddenly over. But then there was this, I don't know . . . I went home alone from the hospital, alone, really alone. I really don't recall what happened the rest of the day. I think that a good friend of ours stayed with me that night. I was feeling very freaked out. I must have gone around for maybe a week or so before I really began to feel the loneliness and her loss. I finally stopped running around taking care of everybody, and really felt the mourning, really felt her loss. It was a feeling inside of having an incredible emptiness. I felt sort of at a loss, kind of wondering how my life was going to continue. How it possibly could go on. Everything sort of like disintegrated. Sort of like a piece of me just was kind of lost.

DR. S: What helped you the most?

MR. H: I don't know that there's anyone thing that helped me the most. Perhaps Susan probably has helped a lot. Even though it was after a year, she forced me to the issue of dealing with Edith, really moving her out of the apartment and started showing me things. About six months after Edith died, I went around and grabbed everything that had anything to do with her and put them in boxes and shoved them in the closets; but still Edith was in the closet. She was still there. We moved things around the apartment to make it different. I started doing some of those things, but she just kept saying that she really felt it wasn't her place, that it was still Edith's. She wanted it to be hers. So she did force me a great deal.

DR. S: Did you get rid of all her things?

MR. H: Oh, no. As a matter of fact we have some pottery that Edith had made that we use, that I had never thought of using before.

DR. S: Do you sleep in the same bed that you had before?

MR. H: Yes, but I've moved the bed in the room and I sleep on the other side of the

bed. I've told Susan that the bed used to be in a different location and I never made anything of it. I did this about six months after Edith died, before I met Susan. I did a few
things, painted one of the walls, and a few things like this, rearranged the furniture. But
there was still the other thing. It was very hard for me to commit myself to Susan. This
was a big problem. This is over two years now. We've been married for several months
and had been going together for two years. I took all that time to make a commitment.

Dr. S: Why was that?

Mr. H: I don't know. I searched in myself a lot for what it was. And I wasn't really
able to grab it. I'm sure that part was really there. A part of it was the holding on. I'm sure
that was also a large part of it. I don't think it was until Susan and I were married that we
went through all the boxes in the closets, took all the stuff and decided either to throw it
away or use it, to get it out of the closet, literally and figuratively.

Dr. S: Did you make any inquiries as to Susan's state of health?

Mr. H: Susan is very healthy. I don't recall. I might have asked her, but I'm conscious of the fact that I certainly noticed her health. She's also younger than I am by a few
years and I thought of that. You know what that means. I think part of that means that I
don't want to live longer. I don't want her to die before I do. I'm sure that's there. I'd be
surprised if it weren't. . . .

Dr. S: I knew Edith and then I knew you. How did that work out?

Mr. H: Well, I think I came to you; I'm not sure if it was because you knew her. I
think that was part of it, because you did know her and you knew me through her. But I
think it was because of you yourself. I felt you were the type of person who could help
me.

Dr. S: In what way?

Mr. H: I can't recall, whatever, but I think that some of the things that you said at
the time helped me, helped to alleviate my desperation that I felt. A few times I did come
in I was feeling pretty desperate. Completely kind of lost and floundering. But that
worked out . . .

PURPOSE OF POSTVENTION

I prefer to think of the work with the bereaved person as a process that I
have called *postvention:* those appropriate and helpful acts that come *after* the
dire event itself.[17, 18, 19] The reader will recognize prevention, intervention,
and postvention as roughly synonymous with the traditional health concepts of
primary, secondary, and tertiary prevention, or with the concepts of immuniza-
tion, treatment, and rehabilitation. Lindemann has referred to "preventive
intervention." It would be simpler to speak of postvention.

As I have described in *Deaths of Man*, postvention consists of those
activities that serve to reduce the aftereffects of a traumatic event in the lives of
the survivors.[17] Its purpose is to help survivors live longer, more productively,
and less stressfully than they are likely to do otherwise. I will attempt to
summarize my observations in the following paragraphs.

Reactions of Survivor Victims

It is obvious that some deaths are more stigmatizing or traumatic than others: death by murder, by the negligence of oneself or some other person, or by suicide. Survivor victims of such deaths are invaded by an unhealthy complex of disturbing emotions: shame, guilt, hatred, perplexity. They are obsessed with thoughts about the death, seeking reasons, casting blame, and often punishing themselves.

The investigations of widows by Parkes are most illuminating.[9] The principal finding of his studies is that independent of her age, a woman who has lost a husband recently is more likely to die (from alcoholism, malnutrition, or a variety of disorders related to neglect of self, disregard of a prescribed medical regimen or common-sense precautions, or even a seemingly unconscious boredom with life), or to be physically ill, or emotionally disturbed than nonwidowed women. The findings seem to imply that grief is itself a dire process, almost akin to a disease, and that there are subtle factors at work that can take a heavy toll unless they are treated and controlled.

These striking results had been intuitively known long before they were empirically demonstrated. The efforts of Lindemann, Caplan, and Silverman to aid survivors of "heavy deaths" were postventions based on the premise of heightened risk in bereaved persons.[11, 13, 15] Lindemann's work, which led to his formulations of acute grief and crisis intervention, began with his treatment of the survivors of the tragic Coconut Grove nightclub fire in Boston in 1942 in which 499 people died.[11] Silverman's projects, under the direction of Caplan, have centered around a widow-to-widow program.[13, 15] These efforts bear obvious similarities with the programs of "befriending" practiced by the Samaritans, an organization founded by the Reverend Chad Varah (1966) and most active in Great Britain.[22]

Death a "Disaster"

A case can be made for viewing the sudden death of a loved one as a *disaster* and, using the verbal bridge provided by that concept, learning from the professional literature on conventionally recognized disasters—those sudden, unexpected events, such as earthquakes and large-scale explosions, that cause a large number of deaths and have widespread effects. Wolfenstein has described a "disaster syndrome": a "combination of emotional dullness, unresponsiveness to outer stimulation and inhibition of activity. The individual who has just undergone disaster is apt to suffer from at least a transitory sense of worthlessness; his usual capacity for self-love becomes impaired."[23]

A similar psychological contraction is seen in the initial shock reaction to catastrophic news—death, failure, disclosure, disgrace, the keenest personal loss. Studies of a disastrous ship sinking by Friedman and Lum and of the effects of a tornado by Wallace both describe an initial psychic shock followed by motor retardation, flattening of affect, somnolence, amnesia, and suggestibility.[24, 25] There is marked increase in dependency needs with regressive behavior and traumatic loss of feelings of identity and, overall, a kind of "affective anesthesia." There is an unhealthy docility, a cowed and subdued reaction. One is reminded of Lifton's description of "psychic closing off" and "psychic numbing" among the Hibakusha, the survivors of the atomic bomb dropped on Hiroshima:

> Very quickly—sometimes within minutes or even seconds—Hibakusha began to undergo a process of "psychic closing off"; that is, they simply ceased to feel. They had a clear sense of what was happening around them, but their emotional reactions were unconsciously turned off. Others' immersion in larger responsibilities was accompanied by a greater form of closing off which might be termed "psychic numbing."[14]

POSTVENTION: AN ONGOING THERAPY

Postventive efforts are not limited to this initial stage of shock; they are more often directed to the longer haul, the day-to-day living with grief over a year or more following the first shock of loss. Typically postvention extends over months during that critical first year, and it shares many of the characteristics of psychotherapy: talk, abreaction, interpretation, reassurance, direction, and even gentle confrontation. It provides an arena for the expression of guarded emotions, especially such negative affective states as anger, shame, and guilt. It puts a measure of stability into the grieving person's life and provides an interpersonal relationship with the therapist that can be genuine, in that honest feelings need not be suppressed or dissembled.

Parkes distinguishes four phases in the bereavement process: numbness, yearning/protest, disorganization, and reorganization—but in general we ought to view "stages" of recovery from death (and especially we need to view the so-called stages of the dying process) with a liberal and flexible mind.[7]

Characteristics of the Postventive Session

In order to appreciate the nature of postvention, it is necessary to touch upon some important characteristics of the interaction between the bereaved victim and the therapist,* specifically the difference between a *conversation* (or "ordinary talk") and a *professional exchange*— recognizing that postventive

---

*The person who systematically attempts to help the bereaved individual is either a therapist or is acting in the role of a therapist. He cannot escape this role. This is not to say that many others—relatives, dear friends, organization (e.g., church) members, neighbors—do not play important, perhaps the most important, roles.

efforts should be of the latter sort. This distinction is exceptionally elementary, but because this understanding is at the very heart of effective postventive work, these rudimentary ideas need to be made explicit. The differences between the two can be charted in the form of some contrasts between ordinary talk (e.g., ''I'm so sorry to hear about the death.'' ''Please accept my most sincere condolescences.'' ''Time will heal the wounds.'') and a professional exchange.

Conversation	*Professional Exchange*
1. Content	
Substantive content, i.e., the talk is primarily about things, events, dates—the surface of the world.	Affective (emotional) content, i.e., the exchange focuses (not constantly but occasionally) on the feelings and the emotional tone of the patient, sometimes minimizing the ''facts.''
2. Level	
Manifest level, i.e., conversation focuses on what is said, the actual words that are uttered, the facts that are stated.	Latent level, i.e., the professional person listens for what is ''between the lines,'' below the surface, what is implied, not expressed or only unconsciously present.
3. Meanings	
Conscious meanings, i.e., in ordinary speech we deal with the other person as though what was said was meant and as though the person were ''a rational man'' and that he ''knows his own mind.''	Unconscious meanings, i.e., there is a whole flow of the mind that is not immediately available at any given moment to the person and that there are unconscious meanings and latent intentions in human exchanges. We listen for double entendre, puns, hidden meanings, latent implications, and so on.
4. Abstraction	
Phenotypic abstraction, i.e., there is concern with the ordinary interesting details of life, where no set of details necessarily bears any relationship to any other set.	Genotypic abstraction, i.e., the therapist is always looking for congruencies, similarities, commonalities, *generalizations* about the patient's psychological life. These constitute the understanding

of the therapist (and are the resevoir of his possible interpretations to the patient).

5. Role

Social role, i.e., in a conversation or ordinary discourse people are co-equals(like neighbors or friends) or depend on the prestige of age, rank, status, and so on, but essentially the relationship is between two people who have equal right to display themselves.

Transference, i.e., a professional exhange is not talk between two co-equals. Rather it is a very special kind of exchange between one person who wishes help (and tacitly agrees to play the patient's role) and another person who agrees to proffer help (and thus is cast in the role of physician, priest, father, magician, witch doctor, helper). Much of what is effective in the exchange is the patient's "transference" onto the therapist. Some of the effectiveness of the therapeutic exchange lies in the power of the "self-fulfilling prophecy."

Another retrospective example may be useful. Late one afternoon a beautiful 19-year-old girl was stabbed to death by an apparent would-be rapist in a government building. Within an hour her parents were shattered by the news given to them by two rather young, well-meaning but inexperienced policemen. The victim was the couple's only child. Their immediate reactions were shock, disbelief, overwhelming grief, and mounting rage, most of it directed at the agency where the murder had occured.

A few days later, right after the funeral, they were in the office of a high official who was attempting to tender his condolences when the mother said in an anguished tone: "There is nothing you can do!" To which, with good presence of mind, he answered that while it was true that the girl could not be brought back to life, there was something that could be done. Whether he knew the term or not, it was postvention that he had in mind. He brought them, personally, to my office.

I began seeing the parents, usually together, sometimes separately. The principal psychological feature was the mother's anger. I permitted her to voice her grief and to vent her rage (sometimes at me), while I retained the role of the voice of reason: empathizing with the parents' state, recognizing the legitimacy of their feelings when I could but not agreeing when in good conscience I could not agree. I felt that I was truly their friend, and I believed that they felt so too. I had insisted that each of them see a physician for a physical examination. A few months after the brutal murder, the mother developed serious symptoms that required major surgery, from which she made a good recovery. The situation raises the intriguing (and unanswerable) question in my mind whether or not that organic flurry would have occurred if she had not suffered the shock of her daughter's death.[26] In the year following her daughter's death the mother had two extended hospitalizations. Several months after the tragedy the parents seemed to be in rather good shape, physically and emotionally, everything considered. They still had low-level grief and no doubt always will. Here is an edited verbatim portion of a session exactly one year after the death.

DR. S: Is today a year?

MRS. A: Exactly one year. And just about this time when she was killed . . .

DR. S: Where are you both today? Can you sketch the course of your grief?

MRS. A: Well, at first it was extremely intense. It was actually a physical pain. For a couple of months I went around and it hurt—it actually hurt in here. And I felt like I was carrying the world on my shoulders and inside of me.

MR. A: I don't think the pain was physical, it was . . .

MRS. A: No, it wasn't. I mean I felt it physically, but it was a mental pain too.

MR. A: There are times when the pain is still there. It's hard to describe it, it's just there, feeling of pain. I guess it's part of sorrow. We had a very bad day yesterday, much more so than today.

MRS. A: You can't just cut off 19 years in one day. It was like losing an arm or a leg or a head or something. Or a head, because you can do without an arm, and you learn to do in a way, without a daughter. It sounds trite when you say it that way.

MR. A: I think one of the things that has happened in the past year is that, as far as I'm concerned, I don't think I've discussed it too much, but I'm more capable of facing the situation, of thinking about it. I used to try to put it out of my mind. For a while there, the hardest thing I had to do was look at her picture.

DR. S: Do you still have that in your house, do you have it displayed?

MRS. A: Yeah.

MR. A: We have one in our bedroom on the bureau. It stays there all the time, but, uh, I don't get a shock anymore when I look at her picture.

MRS. A: I still turn around to look when I blonde hair bobbing up and down and I still turn to look, and then I realize how stupid it is. She couldn't look like that anymore. A little girl lives down the street, that I sometimes see, and she walks like she walked. And it still plays tricks, I still look to see if it's her. And sometimes the other children say or do something and it's always in the back of our minds, always in the back of my mind anyway. I think these meetings with you have been very good for us, because there was someone we could talk to. And someone that could show—in a way—take a different viewpoint. How can we see beyond our noses when we're so grief stricken and, oh, I don't know.

MR. A: That's what I was trying to bring out a while ago, that is that you've helped us, me in facing the truth.

DR. S: How was that done?

MR. A: I don't know; just the fact that I was discussing rather freely and maybe . . .

MRS. A: And we thought we could tell you anything and you wouldn't be angry or, I don't know exactly how to say it, but I always felt we could talk to you and we could tell you exactly what we thought and not face any recriminations or anything like that.

DR. S: Speaking of anger and recriminations, there was a time—isn't this so—that you were just terribly angry?

MRS. A: Yes.

DR. S: What has happened to that anger?

MRS. A: It's dissipated. At first, in the beginning, I was ready to kill everybody and anybody.

DR. S: Including me.

MRS. A: Including you because you represented the government to us.

MR. A: No, really?

MRS. A: Yes, in a way he did because I blamed the government for her death. I still feel that somebody here helped. Somebody here helped, and he must know. Whoever it is; who helped, did his part in getting her killed. By not patroling the building, by not doing—a sin of omission is just as big as a big sin of comission. I mean they knew darn well that the building was not safe.

DR. S: So there are still certainly reservoirs of anger and blame.

MRS. A: At the time I wanted the murderer caught and killed. Now I would just like him stopped, but I don't want him killed. Will that bring her back? But people were afraid of us. They were afraid to talk to us.

MR. A: Some still are.

MRS. A: Some of them still are because they didn't know what to say. It was a difficult thing; it's a difficult thing for most people to find words of sympathy. What do you tell parents whose daughter is killed like that? Another thing that in a way you taught me is to take one day at a time.

DR. S: How did I teach you that?

MRS. A: I don't know how, but that's what I've been doing, taking one day at a time. You were able really to show us in a proper perspective. That's one of the things you did; you were always the one to look at things in a straight manner. How could we when we were so prejudiced about anything—I mean about what happened to her. We are so close to the forest, we can't see the trees.

MR. A: I think you've also managed to curtail her anger in general to a certain extent. Because she was mad at the whole world at the time—any reason. She'd get mad, get ready to prosecute her soup.

DR. S: Have there been some changes in your general character?

MRS. A: I think so, I've probably been a little bit more tolerant.

DR. S: What do you think will happen now in the next year or two?

MRS. A: We get more used to it. I suppose. He will become more resigned to it; that she isn't here, she won't come back, and that going to the cemetery won't hurt so much. But I try not to make this a special day because what's to celebrate? But it is in a way a special day.

DR. S: It is an occasion to memoralize.

MRS. A: It was sad to come home last night and find my husband was crying.

MR. A: It was just a defense mechanism. I was crying to keep you from crying, so you would feel sorry for me for a change.

MRS. A: I suppose in a way it made me less intolerant of other people. But what a price to have to pay. What a pity. All those years. There is something so final now. I used to feel that there was continuity, that she would have children and in a way live on. My husband is the last of his line. The last male of his line. The last one of his family.

MR. A: It's the end of the name anyway.

DR. S: There is a sense of being cut off from the future, isn't there?

MR. A: I imagine there is going to be a lot of hurt when we have to attend weddings or births.

MRS. A: Somehow it is very hard to think that when you die, that's the end. But it's not as bad as I used to be afraid of death. I am no longer afraid of death personally. It's no longer such a terrible thing. It was terrible, I suppose, because it was unknown. Another time I would have been afraid when I went into the hospital. I was so unafraid that I believed the doctor when he told me before the operation that it wasn't going to hurt. How naive can you be? I wanted to believe it. I don't think, I mean, I'm sure, I could have gone through this past year without my husband.

DR. S: I think you have helped each other in a marvelous way.

MRS. A: I'm really sure that I could never have come through it.

MR. A: Except for one time when she almost walked out on me.

MRS. A: That's different. That didn't count. To get through the impossible days and even longer nights. We weren't perfect, and she was not perfect. Of course, no one will ever bring up any of her faults now.

DR. S: That's so. One doesn't speak ill of the dead.

MRS. A: No. Everybody, when they do talk about her, glosses over any of her faults. No one wants to talk about them. I don't know of anyone who has voluntarily brought up her name but you. Why is there such a taboo? It's been a whole year.

DR. S: Do you feel more than a year older?

MR. A: Very much. We were discussing this not too long ago, and we both felt we had missed out on middle age, that we went from youth to old people.

DR. S: Really. You feel that way?

MRS. A: Most of the time I feel so old and I caught myself talking to my brother and I said when we were young, and he said, "Hey, you are talking about a couple of years ago."

DR. S: Well, what we need to work on is to bring back the sense of youthful middle age.

MRS. A: I don't thing that will ever come back. I always felt inside that I was about 19 or 20 and now I feel 60 years old. I said we could talk to you and tell you anything. You have taught us a great deal, and not to worry about recriminations.

MR. A: There were times when I felt that you were trying to make her mad at you.

DR. S: I never did that. I have always liked you.

MRS. A: I always felt that you liked me. It was that feeling. I remember the look on your face when I showed you her picture. I will never forget it.

DR. S: I can't describe what went through me.

MRS. A: You showed it. It was like hitting you, and you absolutely recoiled as though I had hit you. I miss you when I don't see you.

DR. S: How often do you think we ought to meet now? Should we make the next meeting in a month?

MR. A: They've been almost about a month apart.

MRS. A: I would hate to think about our meetings finishing, ending.

Principles of Postvention

What can be noted in this exchange are some general principles of postventive work:

1. In working with survivor victims of abrasive death, it is best to begin as soon as possible after the tragedy, within the first 72 hours if that can be managed.
2. Remarkably little resistance is met from the survivors; most are either willing or eager to have the opportunity to talk to a professionally oriented person.
3. Negative emotions about the decedent or about the death itself—irritation, anger, envy, shame, guilt, and so on—need to be explored, but not at the very beginning.
4. The postvener should play the important role of reality tester. He is not so much the echo of conscience as the quiet voice of reason.
5. Medical evaluation of the survivors is crucial. One should be constantly alert for possible decline in physical health and in overall mental well-being.
6. Needless to say, pollyannish optimism or banal platitudes should be avoided—this statement being a good example.
7. Grief work takes a while—from several months (about a year) to the end of the life, but certainly more than three months or six sessions.
8. A comprehensive program of health care on the part of a benign and enlightened community (or a first-rate hospital) should include preventive, interventive, and *postventive* elements.

REFERENCES

1. Kraus A, Lilienfeld A: Some epidemiologic aspects of the high mortality rate in the young widowed group. J Chronic Dis, 10:207–217, 1959
2. Young M, Benjamin B, Wallis C: The mortality of widowers, Lancet, 2:454–456, 1963
3. Parkes C: Bereavement and mental illness. Br J Med Psychology, 38:1–26, 1964
4. Rees W, Lutkins S: Mortality of bereavement. Br Med J, 4:13–16, 1967
5. Parkes C, Fitzgerald R: Broken heart: A statistical study of increased mortality among widowers. Br Med J, 1:740–743, 1969
6. Stein Z, Susser M: Widowhood and mental illness. Br J Prev Soc Med, 23:106–110, 1969
7. Parkes C: The first year of bereavement. Psychiatry, 33:442–467, 1970
8. Parkes C: Psychosocial transitions: A field for study. Social Sci Med, 5:101–115, 1971
9. Parkes C: Bereavement. New York, International Universities Press, 1972
10. Freud S: Mourning and melancholia, in the Standard Edition of the Complete

Psychological Works of Sigmund Freud, vol. 14. London, Hogarth, 1957

11. Lindemann E: Symptomatology and management of acute grief. Am J Psychiatry, 101:141–148, 1944
12. Bowlby J: Processes of mourning. Int J Psychoanal, 42:317–340, 1961
13. Caplan G: Principles of Preventive Psychiatry. New York, Basic Books, 1964
14. Lifton R: Death in Life: Survivors of Hiroshima. New York, Vintage, 1969
15. Silverman P: Intervention with the widow of a suicide, in Cain A (ed): Survivors of Suicide. Springfield, Ill., Thomas, 1972
16. Weisman AD: On Dying and Denying. New York, Behavioral Publications, 1972
17. Shneidman ES: Deaths of Man. New York, Penguin, 1974
18. Shneidman ES: Suicide, sleep and death, J Consult Psychol, 28:95–106, 1964
19. Shneidman ES: Recent developments in suicide prevention, in Shneidman ES (ed): The Psychology of Suicide. New York, Science House, 1970
20. Lindemann E, Greer I: A study of grief: Emotional responses to suicide, in Cain A (ed): Survivors of Suicide. Springfield, Ill., Thomas, 1972
21. Lindemann E, Vaughn WT, McGinnis M: Preventive intervention in a four-year-old child whose father committed suicide, in Cain A (ed): Survivors of Suicide. Springfield, Ill., Thomas, 1972
22. Varah C: The Samaritans. New York, Macmillan, 1966
23. Wolfenstein M: Disaster: A Psychological Essay. New York, Macmillan, 1957
24. Friedman P, Lum L: Some psychiatric notes on the *Andrea Doria* disaster. Am J Psychiatry, 114:426–432, 1957
25. Wallace A: Tornado in Worcester: An Exploratory Study of Individual and Community Behavior in an Extreme Situation. Washington, DC, National Research Council, 1956
26. Rahe RH: Subjects' recent life changes and their near-future illness reports. Ann Clin Res, 4:250–265, 1972

PART IV

Liaison Psychiatry and Medical Education

Louis Jolyon West

Introduction

Psychiatrists are physicians, responsible for preservation and restoration of health and dedicated to professional excellence and professional values. These values require deep commitment to the needs and lives of people. In this commitment psychiatrists give of themselves no less than do other physicians; in some ways they may give even more.

However, while the medical profession generally enjoys society's respect, and most Americans still consider doctors the most reliable people in an unreliable world, psychiatry is in trouble. Despite its remarkable progress, this relatively young specialty faces a profound crisis of confidence.

Literary arts often reflect main currents of contemporary public thought. Not long ago psychiatrists were given a rather positive image in autobiographies, novels, theatricals, and films such as *Fight Against Fears, Captain Newman, M.D., The Search, Spellbound,* and *Lady in the Dark*. More recently, however, in *A Clockwork Orange,* the psychiatrist is a sadistic manipulator; in *One Flew Over the Cuckoo's Nest,* a brutal bungler; in *Candy,* a crazy pervert; in *Terminal Man,* an insensitive technocrat; in *The Exorcist,* merely useless.

Meanwhile, in real life, the coverage of psychiatric disorders under various national health insurance proposals requires a major struggle. The various reorganizations of our national institutes have progressively separated psychiatry from alcoholism, drug abuse, mental retardation, and child development. Many new general hospitals lack psychiatric beds. Many community mental health centers, which once generally enjoyed psychiatric leadership, are now dominated by professionals from other disciplines and by laymen, while medical participation shrinks to a minimum.

Funds for psychiatric education and research dwindle. Internships disappear. Time for psychiatry and the behavioral sciences decreases in many

259

medical school curricula. Nonprofessional mental healers attract followers by the tens and hundreds of thousands. Other physicians widely express dissatisfaction with psychiatry, making fewer referrals and requesting fewer consultations. Widely read books declare mental illness a myth or tout weird treatments or proclaim the death of psychiatry.

Much of this trouble stems from the disillusioned backlash of an oversold public, the displaced hostilities of a turbulent, frustrated society, and psychiatry's own failures of vision, of effort, of nerve, and of organization. It is ironic that these troubles come at the very time when our field is making the most rapid progress in its history and has far more to offer than ever before. It now seems to me that the greatest and most basic problem of psychiatry—a nutritional deficiency state that complicates and exacerbates all our other ailments—has been psychiatry's drift away from the mainstream of medicine.

During this period of drift, our limited work with patients being primarily cared for by physicians who are not psychiatrists has represented a valuable link with the mainstream. Such work may incorporate much that was good from the early tradition of psychosomatic medicine and of psychiatric consultation services in general hospitals. Today, however, the broader implications of psychiatry's interface with the rest of medicine are becoming more clear in the context of what is now called liaison psychiatry.

SCIENTIFIC CONTEXT OF LIAISON PSYCHIATRY

Progress in psychiatry can be expected to derive naturally from new knowledge produced by basic and applied research in the biomedical and behavioral sciences and from ongoing clinical investigation in various disciplines. As this progress continues, all physicians must become increasingly well equipped to utilize a knowledge of psychiatry in the practice of medicine, whether or not they become psychiatrists. In this utilization the liaison psychiatrist will play an important part.

The biomedical information explosion is reaching incredible proportions. Biochemistry, biophysics, genetics, membrane physiology, immunology, molecular biology, and developmental biology are progressing so fast that it is difficult to grasp the significance of their advances. Nevertheless, psychiatry's responsibility, at least in a general way, must be to comprehend scientific progress in the biological sciences, to integrate it meaningfully with the behavioral sciences (where there is also an information explosion gonig on), and creatively to seek applications of the resulting compound that will be relevant to mental health and the practice of medicine.

Therefore the modern psychiatrist should strive to become a creative *integrator* of knowledge and technique in applied psychobiology. He must undertake to master the tools of synthesis. He will need an exceptionally broad scientific and biomedical vocabulary. He will need to develop familiarity with communication theory, information theory, general systems theory, and the like. He will need a working knowledge of the most useful conceptual models about human nature. Furthermore he must be prepared to apply these integrative talents, not only to the treatment of mental illness, but to general medicine and in all clinical specialties. This means working in liaison with other specialties to a far greater degree than is presently the case. It also means offering more than psychodynamic formulations and psychotherapeutic recommendations. These, while always a valuable part of the liaison psychiatrist's contribution, will be supplemented in the future by many other theoretical and practical elements in his role.

The liaison psychiatrist is increasingly concerned with the immediate state of the patient, the patient's most probable state at a specified future time, and the psychobiological requirements for maintaining or improving the patient's current level of adaptation. Assessments must be made through increasingly accurate biochemical, psychophysiological, and behavioral monitoring. I expect that clinical psychophysiological assessment will increasingly employ on-line auto-correlation techniques (e.g., spectral analysis) for predicting future states from ongoing data flow.

Rapid progress in psychiatric practice and theory can be expected to accompany sounder (albeit more complex) basic assumptions about man as a biosocial entity. Therefore, the present heavy emphasis on technical methodology in psychophysiological recording must give way to more integrative types of analysis of patients in terms of multiple adaptive processes and their interactions. In this context the liaison psychiatrist should become increasingly interested in autonomic and endocrine profiles, these to be understood as interactions between the state of autonomic and endocrine balance, acquired behavior, and adaptive requirements. Such an approach can be quite valuable in the solution of clinical problems. It will permit, for example, the most rational and effective employment of neuroleptic drugs as these increase in number and specificity. And let there be no doubt about one thing: the liaison psychiatrist of the future must be an expert clinical psychopharmacologist.

Great progress is being made in the analysis of psychobiological periodicity. More and more psychiatric interest focuses upon the mechanisms of variability in circadian rhythms and biological clocks. These and related observations are contributing to advances in diagnosis, prognosis, and treatment of illness. For example, studies of diurnal periodicity have led to a growing appreciation of how sleep and its associated bioelectrical and metabolic rhythms—both fast and slow—provide a unique window through which to assess the state of the patient. The implications of such research for psychiatry in its liaison relationship to the rest of medicine are numerous and profound. Sleep analysis soon may be a fundamental technique in clinical psychopathology, in psychosomatic diagnosis, and in following a patient's clinical course from the interdisciplinary or liaison point of view.

Psychiatry's preoccupation with patients' pathological reactions to noxious stimulation and stress has been modified increasingly by consideration of other implications such as the adaptation to stress through time and the mechanisms enhancing or diminishing such adaptation. Our fascination with the psychodynamics of neurosis and psychosis is yielding to a greater emphasis on understanding the total biosocial dynamics of developing and maintaining good health. Psychiatrists are now beginning to scrutinize the longitudinal development of health-significant conditional responses during human life, with special emphasis on early experience and on transactions between the maturing brain and the changing environment that take place during critical periods of growth and development. The applications of new knowledge along these lines have obvious significance for psychiatry's liaison relationship with pediatrics.

Recently there has been a resurgent interest of psychiatrists in problems of consciousness including areas long neglected, such as epilepsy. It may be that soon every young psychiatrist will understand how to employ computerized EEG analyzers as well as the correspondingly automated successors to electromyography, electro-oculography, and the cortical evoked potentials displayed by computers of average transients (CATs). These devices will be widely utilized in the study of problems of consciousness and other clinical problems, ranging from measurement of changing psychopathology to prediction of behavioral response patterns. The meaning of any given set of recordings one day may be obtained by processing it in relation to centralized banks of analyzed and coded bioelectric recordings. Applications of these techniques can be seen to psychiatric liaison work, not only with neurology, but to a number of other clinical areas (such as endocrinology) as well.

PROFESSIONAL CONTEXT OF LIAISON PSYCHIATRY

In recent years I have often expressed my opinion that while psychiatrists must and shall become more and more firmly identified with the profession of medicine, we should remember that the rest of medicine is also undergoing many significant changes. To relate meaningfully to these changes through liaison relationships, the psychiatrist of tomorrow must be much more of a neuroscientist than he is today; he must also be more of a social and behavioral scientist as well.

Moreover, as the increasingly scientific roots of psychiatry steadily replace empiricism, they will necessitate substantial changes in education, not only for the psychiatrist but for all physicians. After all, psychiatry is a fundamental part of all medical practice. And I must reiterate that the practice of medicine is in a state of flux.

For example, relationships are changing, not only between medical specialists but also between physicians and non-physicians in most health-related fields. Much of what is done by physicians today may be done by others tomorrow. This trend can be seen throughout the medical profession; many specialties are involved.

Psychiatry is already well along in this process of change. We should expect that in the relatively near future, most of the straightforward psychotherapy—of both individuals and groups—will probably be done by clinical (or medical) psychologists. Social workers and psychologists with special training in human sexuality and group dynamics will be doing more of the marriage and family counseling. Community consultation services on many health-related matters will increasingly be provided by experts from fields other than medicine. Epidemiologists, applied sociologists, criminologists, specialists in community medicine, and others are already becoming more and more involved.

It is likely that the future will find more and more hospitals, mental health centers, and mental health-related community programs directed by specially trained non-physicians such as executives with advanced university degrees in health administration. Educators, educational psychologists, school counselors, nurses, and even new paraprofessionals (e.g., mental health engineers) will soon be doing a considerable amount of preventive psychiatry. Ministers will be increasingly involved in group encounter work.

Meanwhile, a great deal of general office psychiatry, including the prescription of medication, will be carried out by physicians practicing specialties other than psychiatry. Family medicine, emergency medicine, internal medicine, pediatrics, and obstetrics comprise only a partial list.

I do not see these changes as a threat to psychiatry as a specialty. On the contrary, psychiatrists will be in greater demand than ever. They will be consulting and working in liaison relationships with colleagues in all of the foregoing activities. They must therefore be prepared to provide the increment of additional expertise and depth that true specialists can offer to colleagues who have received less, or different, training than their own. As this happens, the liaison psychiatric relationship will become fundamental to excellence both in the field of mental health and generally in the practice of medicine.

Meanwhile the psychiatrist as an individual will be occupied to a growing degree with the complicated cases, the serious psychopathologies, the major mental illnesses. He will care for such patients in intensive psychiatric treatment units of general hospitals, in community mental health centers, and in relatively small psychiatric hospitals, both public and private. He will be using his own office for examination, diagnosis, consultations by referral, prescription of a wide variety of therapies (not only drugs) according to clinical indications and contraindications, follow-up work, and increasingly in supervisory sessions with colleagues regarding psychiatric aspects of their work— that is to say, in liaison activities. In other words, liaison psychiatry not only takes us to the other fellow's shop; it may also bring him to ours.

Of course the psychiatrist will still engage in office psychotherapy, but with more highly selected cases. These will be patients having unusually complicated or severe problems—patients that family physicians or other non-psychiatrists cannot manage. The psychiatrist will more and more often be called upon in liaison to help with the patient whose physical disease has psychiatric complications, the dying patient and his survivors, the self-defeating or uncooperative patient, the mysterious or baffling case.

EDUCATIONAL CONTEXT OF LIAISON PSYCHIATRY

There are major implications of this changing prospect for the medical curriculum, the medical student, and the residency programs of tomorrow. Much new material must be included at all levels, from premedical courses to the increasingly important postresidency programs of continuing education in all specialties. The liaison relationship is a two-way street, and our colleagues themselves must be better educated and able to take full advantage of it.

With this in mind I predict the early development of a more broadly comprehensive general curriculum for undergraduate medical students. There will be a movement away from currently fashionable early specialized tracks. We know that virtually all medical students henceforth will go on to become specialists of some type, even in primary care which has itself become a specialty. Therefore the medical school years should provide the opposite of narrow specialization. Instead, medical education should insure the development of persons who are well rounded both as clinical scientists and as humane physicians. Our students (specialists-to-be) should learn as much as possible about man, his nature, and his culture in health and disease.

Medical schools should provide the broadest, soundest general groundwork to insure that every graduate will be reasonably prepared to utilize liaison relationships with specialties other than his own. Solid grounding in the behavioral sciences can help to make physicians more than simply high-level health-and-disease technologists. They will have the rest of their long lives for refinement of specialization. Today only about 5 percent of the average medical school curriculum comprises the behavioral sciences as such. Clearly more is needed.

These goals are incompatible with recent trends toward abbreviated pre-medical and medical education. Therefore I foresee a return to a full four-year college degree as a requirement for admission to medical school. Following this, four calendar years of diligent study should be expected in order to earn a medical degree, with educational *enrichment* rather than acceleration for the more gifted student. Recently a number of new medical schools have been created, and more are being built. It should not be necessary to cheapen medical education by overcrowding the existing schools, abbreviating the curriculum, educationally shortchanging the students, and debasing the intellectual currency of medical practice.

The disappearance of the internship is a matter of grave concern to many psychiatric educators. Psychiatrists lacking internships (or equivalent experiences in caring for physically ill patients) will unquestionably be handicapped in undertaking liaison work. Many other specialties (neurology, ophthalmology, radiology, etc.) share this concern. Perhaps we should be devising a universal or rotating first-year residency that would provide every new physician a general clinical background of experience, most of which would by design be outside the field of his planned specialization. If every physician possesses a modicum of experience in clincial medicine outside of his own specialty, he will be a better colleague, a more useful consultant, and certainly a more effective liaison participant.

At most medical schools today, psychiatrists mainly teach psychopathology, diagnosis, and clinical therapeutics of the mentally and emotionally ill. This teaching usually takes place on psychiatry services of various kinds. However, I think there will soon be a greatly increased emphasis upon liaison teaching by psychiatrists on other clinical services. Eventually psychiatry will be taught both on psychiatry services and on pediatric, medical, surgical, and obstetrical services, to the extent that was envisioned years ago by John Romano. For many years liaison teaching has been carried out at Rochester under the distinguished direction of George Engel. But in general the development during the 1950s and 1960s of special psychiatric consultation services and circumscribed psychosomatic units may actually (now seen in retrospect) have stultified rather than fulfilled the goals of Romano, Engel, Harold Wolff, Roy Grinker, Stewart Wolf, Franz Alexander, Arthur Mirsky, Spurgeon English, and other pioneers.

The fact is that even a large psychosomatic service cannot meet the needs of a modern teaching hospital for psychiatric liaison activities if the potentialities of the liaison approach are to be fully realized. Therefore, in tomorrow's university hospital, most if not all of the full-time psychiatric faculty should be actively involved in liaison teaching. Nearly every member of the department of psychiatry should be attached, for several scheduled hours weekly, to one of the various other hospital service units. He should become, in effect, the permanent liaison psychiatrist to that unit. He should make rounds regularly with its house staff and clinical clerks. Psychiatric residents, when learning liaison psychiatry (including consultation service and psychosomatic medicine), should be assigned to work with such faculty members in the context of an ongoing liaison relationship with that unit. The relationship naturally includes consultations regarding emotionally disturbed patients or those with psychosomatic problems. But it also involves considerations of the dynamics of the unit (or service); work with the staff in terms of their reactions to the patients and—on occasion—to each other; and teaching at all levels: nurses and other health professionals, medical students, residents, and even fully trained colleagues as well. For the liaison psychiatrist should be providing a useful continuing education exercise for his faculty counterpart in the other specialty, just as the specialist will certainly be providing one for him. All this will come just as fast as we are able to provide the psychiatric manpower; in my experience the liaison psychiatric program is welcomed by other specialties with enthusiasm.

I also expect that in every medical school the division or department of behavioral science will, in addition to providing a substantial didactic curriculum for medical students, create liaison arrangements with the other basic biomedical sciences. Such arrangements will further insure that the behavioral implications of basic medical sciences become part of the education of every physician and that students during their subsequent clinical clerkships on *all* services will have the necessary background—both biological and behavioral—to take full advantage of the psychiatric liaison teaching that they receive.

CONCLUSION

The necessity now facing the field of psychiatry is nothing less than to generate a new basic confidence in our specialty. To endure, this confidence must be fully justified. To achieve it, psychiatrists, their organizations, and their educational programs must undergo some changes.

We psychiatrists must satisfy the community's desire for more relevant and helpful contact with us and our work. We must develop more interesting and effective psychiatric continuing education, emphasizing clinical applications of progress in biomedical and behavioral sciences, social issues, and self-evaluation. We must exert vigorous leadership in all social and political arenas where decisions concerning psychiatry are made. We must improve communications (including positive interpretations of our values and practices) with the public, other disciplines, government, and among ourselves.

Most important of all, we must resubstantiate our medical professional identity.

Through all this we must wisely preserve the best in our professional tradition, cheerfully undertake appropriate change, and boldly work toward a challenging future. In no contemporary sphere of our specialty is this challenge greater than in liaison psychiatry.

Chase Patterson Kimball

20
The Challenge of Liaison Medicine

CONCEPTUAL APPROACH OF LIAISON MEDICINE

The challenge of liaison medicine is to effect within the body medicine an integration and synthesis of those sciences and arts that relate to the study and treatment of human discomfort. As such, its role is a presumptive one. Nevertheless, its heritage, in terms of its pioneers and present-day exponents, has been to seek and understand relationships between the different conceptual approaches utilized in the care of the ill. Whereas originally these relationships were seen as simple one-to-one correlations between ''factual'' phenomenon conceptualized in different language systems, for example, between psychology and physiology, in time they came to be viewed as sequential in terms of cause and effect. By and large, this has been only relatively useful in furthering our therapeutic approaches to illness, partly because there is intrinsic difficulty in relating observations made in two different language systems that may in essence be describing the same phenomenon. Furthermore, the selection process relating single variables is arbitrary and overly simplistic. Linear causality relating two events is a nineteenth-century phenonemon that is less and less useful in twentieth-century medicine. For the most part, we have outgrown two-dimensional linear models in favor of three-dimensional cyclical ones. We no longer view disease as determined by single factors but rather by multiple ones, occurring in a time and space relationship to one another in terms of an individual's life. It is the elaboration and further definition of this embryonic philosophical position within the framework of medicine that liaison medicine has come to espouse. As such, the name is less than adequate. The terms comprehensive, holistic, psychosomatic, psychosocial medicine have been little better in their time. Each has been compartmentalized off from the central body of medicine. It remains that this approach to illness is vested in a relatively small number of individuals in a few teaching hospitals. These individuals, in a

269

clinical setting, reside most frequently in departments of psychiatry or at best at the interface of psychiatry and medicine.

The immediate historical predecessor of liaison medicine was psychosomatic medicine, perhaps best espoused by Franz Alexander and his designation of the "holy seven" as the psychosomatic diseases. The emphasis on a selected number of illnesses served to exclude consideration of the psychosocial aspects of other illness states, a situation that has gradually been reconsidered over the past several decades.[1] At present the emphasis is that all illness states may be conceptualized from a psychosocial perspective. There is less concern with causality, which, as far as medicine is concerned, seems to have been a phenomenon adopted from its religious and philosophical derivation. Rather, the concern is with the relationship of those aspects of an individual's illness state that lend themselves to biological, psychological, and sociological conceptualizations that lead to a remediation of the disequilibrium imposed upon that individual's usual state of health. We may view the individual as we would a multifaceted diamond, utilizing a number of language systems to describe his state of health.

At this point in history our best developed language systems in describing individual human behavior (of which illness is one part) are biology, psychology, and sociology and their respective subgroups. No health state for an individual is adequately described until it has been subjected to the observational methods appropriate for the formulation of that state according to each of these approaches. The liaison physician's role is to assist other physicians and health professionals in utilizing a multidimensional approach in conceptualizing an individual's problems, defined as illness, and then selecting the applicable approach most likely to lead to the amelioration of that problem. To this extent, the liaison physician serves as a general systems analyst in the analysis of an illness state and the determination of the appropriate models for therapeutic intervention after all the component factors have been assessed.[2,3] This model restores to all facets of medicine an emphasis that has diminished over the past century, namely the emphasis on comprehensive diagnosis prior to the institution of therapy. With the increasing specialization that has characterized medical practice, presumably growing out of a single cause–single effect model of disease, diagnosis has largely become compartmentalized and biased by the specific persuasion or specialty practice of the therapist; thus, all patients are seen as diabetic by the endocrinologist until proven otherwise. The liaison physician would tend to engage in a more global assessment of a patient's problem prior to the selection of one or more therapeutic approaches.

THE ROLE OF THE LIAISON PHYSICIAN

Since the philosophical bases of liaison medicine has been suggested, it is pertinent to consider the training and specific activities of the liaison physician.

Ultimately, I suppose, this relates to a predisposition or particular orientation of the mind dependent on early child development and patterns of observations and their subsequent relatedness. Subsequently, learning processes that augment and partially shape these tendencies play a major role in determining those individuals who will be attracted to this orientation. It behooves medical educators to assess those personality patterns and educational processes that underlie and contribute to a student's acceptance of a multidimensional approach to a patient's problem.[4] It is possible that the relativity concepts that characterize modern physics, but as yet have hardly penetrated medical thinking, may serve as a more appropriate educational background for students of medicine than the rigid deterministic sciences of the nineteenth century. The medical curriculum, both in terms of organization and content, especially in its early and later phases, is antithetical to such an approach.[5] Basic science courses are most frequently taught in terms of specific cause and effect with little emphasis on conceptual models for thinking about illness phenomenon. In the initial clinical work emphasis may be on the whole patient. However, by the time of electives and residency specialization the emphasis has become one oriented toward specific causation. Those students who escape adherence to a specificity model are mostly lost from clinical medicine to essentially nonclinical activities in social and community medicine, public health, psychiatry, or novel writing.

In an attempt to espouse the philosophical basis of a multidimensional approach for the study and practice of medicine, liaison physicians have gradually placed emphasis upon working with students beginning in the first year in medical school.[6] The sine qua non of this approach has been the development of seminars in interviewing and approaches to the patient in the first quarter of the first year.[7, 8, 9] In these the student in a clinical setting with peers interviews a patient about the latter's illness problem. Subsequently, the interview is discussed from the standpoint of interviewing process, the patient as person, his problem, and his reaction to illness. Conceptualization of the patient and his problem are formulated in terms of biological, psychological and social perspectives. At this phase of development students voice concern about ethical issues relating to their relationship to patients as well as to the treatment of the patient's problem.

It is not by accident that liaison physicians have become concerned with the teaching of medical ethics in an extension of these seminars throughout the first year. Reinforcement of these basic approaches are present in the liaison physician's participation in introductory courses in human behavior, in which the latter is examined in terms of its biological, social, psychological bases, and in second-year interviewing courses in association with courses in physical diagnosis. In the third year clerkships in psychiatry frequently return the student to the medical and surgical units to study patients from a psychosocial perspective in addition to the biological one.[10] Emphasis is placed on the psychosocial aspects of illness. Liaison physicians may also hold conferences with students during their medical clerkship in which a patient's problem will be scrutinized from a psychosocial perspective.

In psychiatric residencies increasing attention and time is given to the training of the psychiatrist for his role as a consultant to other physicians and health professionals. Rather than applying psychiatric disease labels to medical patients, the emphasis is on the patient's reaction to illness in terms of the other things going on in his life, the illness setting, the treatment environment, and his underlying personality characteristics as well as staff relationships. In order to do this effectively, the liaison psychiatrist needs to obtain a thorough grounding in the patient's total problem, familiarizing himself with the progression of symptoms and signs, their meaning in terms of biological as well as a psychological formulation.

Among the challenges for the liaison physician is the inspection of the medical school curriculum for openings in which he may gain a toe hold, capitalizing on affect-laden situations in which the student's awareness of his own reactions can be a legitimate area for discussion and subsequently utilized to make him more empathic with patients.[11] We need to assess whether there is merit in beginning discussions about dying and death in the anatomy laboratory, about human experimentation in the physiology labs, and about patient rights and informed consent in our initial interviewing sessions, among others. Would our presence at a clinical correlation presentation serve to allow the student to discuss his frequent reaction to the clinician's lack of concern in relating with the presented patient in any way other than around the disease he wishes to discuss? What can the liaison physician learn about the development of student attitudes and values as they are affected by their experiences in medical education?[12] Can an identification of these lead to exercises and programs that would keep the student from foreclosing too abruptly his reaction to and comprehensive orientation to patients and their problems? Finally, does the liaison physician present an identifiable model for a small nucleus of students who may choose to emulate this approach?

CONTENT OF LIAISON MEDICINE

The subject matter that engages the clinical attention and academic interest of the liaison physician is ubiquitous, which is the most exciting challenge of this field. This general systems analyst–liaison physician might be viewed as an anthropologist let loose among a strange people in a strange environment utilizing a somewhat removed and different from usual focus in looking at ill patients. His attention is drawn to other than the usual relationships. He becomes absorbed in the relationships between individuals: doctors and patients, patients and families, families and nurses, nurses and doctors, doctors and doctors. He notes the effect of different environments on patients' reactions, for example, the intensive care unit.[13] He studies the relationship of individual's reactive states to illness and procedures in terms of premorbid personality characteristics.[14] He identifies covert and overt emotional states as they affect and are affected by relationships, environments, and illness. He becomes absorbed with the still too little studied altered states of consciousness, that characterize so many patients observed on medical and surgical units.[15] He is repeatedly challenged by that elusive and ubiquitous phenomenon, the conversion process.[16] He becomes intrigued with the relationship of loss, patterns of grieving and the onset of illness;[17, 18, 19] with the development of similar illnesses in patients of similar personality characteristics and behavioral patterns.[20] He is the great initial observer and subsequent explorer of the "new diseases of medical progress—for example, the intensive care unit syndrome,[21] hemodialysis,[22] open-heart surgery,[23] ileal bypass procedures,[24] contraception, abortion, and sterilization,[25] and the effects of new patterns of medical care on patients and physician. Still requiring further study are pehnomena such as hope and denial and their relationship to adaptation or maladaptation to illness.

At the same time it behooves the liaison physician not to become bogged down in the phenomenon as an entity in and of itself, as though it were another disease, but to stay patient-, student-, and peer-oriented, or more simply human-oriented. The liaison physician's challenge is that of becoming a seminal force in the teaching hospital and medical school at every level, emphasizing human concerns and elaborating how these can be objectively identified and utilized in understanding and treating the ill patient. His role, while based essentially in teaching, will also be through committee activity, especially the curriculum, admissions and health services training committees in which he may communicate his approach to other physicians.

RESEARCH IN LIAISON MEDICINE

Structure, discipline, and integration are brought to this field through the liaison physician's engagement in ongoing clinical research. His research begins at the patient's bedside, in the student seminar room, at the curriculum meeting, in the anatomy lab. It depends on his acumen in attending to phenomenon observed, perceiving it in a different way, asking the naive question, refining this into a simple hypothesis, adopting a suitable methodology for structured observations, and isolating variables in order to arrive at supporting conclusions or new hypotheses. These resulting conclusions or hypotheses should allow his colleagues in related fields to subject his observations to different levels of analysis in the laboratory utilizing specific biological, social and psychological techniques.

CHALLENGES OUTSIDE THE UNIVERSITY

As though the limits of the liaison physician's concerns were narrow, he may be criticized with having become overly absorbed with the hospitalized patient and not concerned enough with the patient and the physician working in the emergency unit, the outpatient clinics, and the community. With the increasing emphasis on prepaid health and primary care programs and facilities, there is developing a whole new clinical laboratory for the liaison physician's teaching and research interests. In these settings the liaison physician may turn his observations to the well individual and to individuals at a different phase in the well-sick spectrum. He may participate in longitudinal observations relating these with greater clarity to social and family situations. In longitudinal studies he may identify prospectively new relationships between behavioral patterns, early psychophysiological markers, and subsequent pathophysiological processes as well as the effect of different environmental constellations upon the development of these.

As the liaison physician moves out of the university hospital into community settings and new patterns of health care, he will need to develop new approaches to his educational methods, which will include (1) an assessment of needs of primary care and family physicians, (2) an identification of objectives, (3) a selection of appropriate educational methods, and (4) a procedure for the evaluation of the effect of his teaching. The challenges of continuing education and postgraduate programs for the general physician are the latest of challenges for the liaison physician.

REFERENCES

1. Kimball CP: Conceptual developments in psychosomatic medicine, 1939–1969. Ann Intern Med 73:307–316, 1970
2. von Bertalanfly L: General systems theory and psychiatry, in Arieti S (ed): American Handbook of Psychiatry, vol III. New York, Basic Books, 1966
3. Grinker RR, Robbins FP: The field concept of psychosomatic medicine, in Psychosomatic Case Book. New York, Blakiston, 1954
4. Kimball CP: On admission policies and medical education. J Med Educ 47:365–367, 1972
5. Kimball CP: The challenge of medicine in the 70's: Health care through education. JAMA 216:2124–2127, 1971
6. Kimball CP: Liaison psychiatry in the university medical center. Compr Psychiatry 14:241–249, 1973
7. Kimball CP: Techniques of interviewing. I. Ann Intern Med 71:147–153, 1969
8. Kimball CP: Techniques of interviewing. II. Setting up an interviewing course. Psychiatry Med 1:167–170, 1970

9. Kimball CP: Techniques of interviewing. III. The patient's personality and the interview process. Medical Insight 4:26–40, 1970

10. Kimball CP: A liaison department of psychiatry. Psychother Psychosom 22:219–225, 1973

11. Kimball CP: Medical education as a humanizing experience. J Med Educ 48:71–77, 1973

12. Kimball CP: The growth and development of the medical student. Selected Papers, Council on Medical Education AMA 70th Annual Congress on Medical Education 1974, pp 79–83

13. McKegney FP: The intensive care unit syndrome: The definition, treatment and prevention of a new "disease of medical progress." Conn Med 30:633–636, 1966

14. Kahana R, Bibring G: Personality types in medical management, in Zinberg NE (ed): Psychiatry and Medical Practice in a General Hospital. New York, International Universities Press, 1964

15. Engel GL, Romano J: Delirium, a syndrome of cerebral insufficiency. J Chronic Dis 9:260–277, 1959

16. Engel GL: "Psychogenic pain" and the pain-prone patient. Am J Med 26:899–918, 1959

17. Lindemann E: Symptomatology and management of acute grief. Am J Psychiatry 101:141–148, 1944

18. Holmes TH, Rahe RH: The social readjustment scale. J Psychosom Res 11:213–218, 1967

19. Engel GL, Schmale AH: Psychoanalytic theory of somatic disorder: Conversion, specificity and the disease onset situation. J Am Psychoanal Assoc 15:344–365, 1967

20. Friedman M, Rosenman RH: Association of a specific overt behavior pattern with blood and cardiovascular findings. JAMA 169:1286–1296, 1959

21. Kornfeld DS, Zinberg S, Malm JR: Psychiatric complications of open-heart surgery. N Engl J Med 273:287–292, 1965

22. Kaplan-DeNour A, Shaltiel J, Czaczhes J: Emotional reactions of patients on chronic hemodialysis. Psychosom Med 30:521–533, 1968

23. Kimball CP: Psychological response to the experience of open heart surgery. I. Amer J Psychiatry 126:348–359, 1969

24. Solow C, Silverfarb PM, Swift K: Psychosocial effects of intestinal bypass surgery for severe obesity. N Engl J Med 290:300–304, 1974

25. Talan KH, Kimball CP: Characterization of 100 women psychiatrically evaluated for therapeutic abortion. Arch Gen Psychiatry 26:571–578, 1972

Daniel B. Auerbach

21
Liaison Psychiatry and the Education of the Psychiatric Resident

Psychiatric education is currently in a state of extreme flux. There is wide discussion and disagreement about the role that psychiatry should play in the future and, thus, about what should be taught and emphasized during the residency years and beyond. There is ample evidence that consultation-liaison psychiatry contains within it unique opportunities to learn what many feel the psychiatrist of the future must know as well as the opportunity to learn more comprehensively the traditional aspects of psychiatry.

However, the residents themselves often react negatively to a consultation-liaison rotation and turn away from this type of work when they complete their training. An analysis of the realities of a present-day consultation-liaison service in a general hospital reveals that the aspects that can be so valuable to some are the same cited by others to explain their negative reactions. This discussion will attempt to further elucidate these differing views and their meaning for psychiatric education.

DEFINITIONS AND REALITIES OF CONSULTATION-LIAISON PSYCHIATRY

In evaluating the role of consultation-liaison psychiatry in residency education, the first inquiry should be, What is it about the structure of a consultation-liaison service that makes it potentially a fertile field for teaching psychiatry?

In general, any clinical, teaching, or research activity by a mental health professional in a nonpsychiatric location where acute or chronic care is offered comes under the purview of consultation-liaison psychiatry.[1, 2, 3] With regard to current residency education, however, the designation refers almost exclusively to the role of the psychiatrist on the wards and in the clinics of a general hospital.

The designations "consultation" and "liaison" reflect the multiple role expected of psychiatry on a medical or surgical service.[1] Consultation, in the strict sense, refers to the request by the primary physician to the psychiatrist for his opinion on some aspect of the patient's behavior that the primary physician feels indicates disturbed mental function.[4] Liaison is defined as a linking up or connecting of the parts of a whole, intended to bring about proper coordination of activities, especially intercommunication.[5]

In reality, however, the questions and needs of the primary physician can rarely be answered without considering the operational group of which the patient is a part.[4] It is in this way that the psychiatrist functions as liaison between various components of the hospital unit. Therefore, the psychiatrist tries to discover the significant interactions occurring between the patient, doctor, nurses, and family.[4] The usual conclusion is that the problem rarely exists just with the patient. A sick person stimulates extreme tensions and feelings in the hospital environment, and the patient's disturbing behavior is often just the most obvious manifestation of problems emanating from others. [2, 3, 4, 6] The inseparability of consultation and liaison has definite implications for residency education.

Another reality relevant to residency education is that consultation-liaison work presents the psychiatrist with different kinds of clients. First, the patient usually does not initiate the consult and is resentful that others feel that it is necessary. Second, the physician or nurse may feel strongly that the patient has the problem, and their problem is the patient. They are not initially interested in, and often react defensively to, the suggestion that they play a role in the onset of the disturbed behavior or can act to allieviate it.

Since there is often such a discrepancy between the perceptions of the patient and other members of the ward milieu, the psychiatrist, in order to fulfill his function, must teach the other care providers to understand more of the aspects of their interactions with the patient.[1, 2] This need to teach is further indicated by the types of problems that the psychiatrist is most often asked to see. A significant number are behavior problems defined as disturbing by the primary physician.[2, 3] It may be, however, that the behavior that the patient's doctor views as mental disturbance, the psychiatrist may view as being a temporary upset.[4] This difference of opinion, unless resolved, can have a profound influence upon the support that the patient is given. Current realities in medicine make it likely that it will be the psychiatrist, not the primary physician, who has the firmer grasp on the various psychosocial factors influencing the patient, and if he does not point them out (that is, teach) to the staff, usually they go unheeded.[1]

Thus, the medical and surgical house staff as well as nursing staff and other ward personnel become both a primary focus and a primary source of reinforcement for the work of the consultation-liaison psychiatrist.[7] If their consciousness is raised with regard to better patient care, then this can be the most potent justification for the work.

The need to work as a participant observer within an operational group as well as the need to teach in order to fulfill the primary goal of improved patient care can be seen as the unique educational opportunities of a consultation-liaison service. They are in addition to the knowledge gained from observing and responding to patient's with severe illness. There are those who feel that these opportunities are consistent with the new direction psychiatric education should take. These opportunities should be an inherent part of the program as well as experience in more traditional areas of psychiatry.

THE ROLE OF THE CONSULTATION-LIAISON SERVICE IN RESIDENCY EDUCATION

Recent commentaries on residency education call for a change in emphasis in psychiatry toward the rediscovery of its roots in medicine and the rejoining of medicine's pursuit of more effective methods of comprehensive health care delivery.[8, 9, 10] As well, the future may require the psychiatrist to be that medical specialist who can integrate what will become increasingly known about brain function with behavior to apply a true biosocial approach to medicine.[8]

At the very least, it is generally agreed that a psychiatrist should be able to provide competent consultation when called upon to do so by nonpsychiatric agencies in general and other physicians in particular.[6, 11] This skill may come to have increasingly practical significance. The current career goal for most psychiatric residents is still traditional private practice. However, it is likely that the current models of practice and delivery of mental health services may soon be obsolete. If the newly trained psychiatrist is not to become an isolated bystander in the evolution of mental health services, his repertoire of skills must be broadened for different styles of private practice.[12]

There is little doubt that there is no better place in current psychiatric education than a consultation-liaison service to emphasize psychiatry's role in medicine and to teach consultation skills. As already stated, a consultation-liaison service offers added opportunities to learn other areas of psychiatry. The most apparent is social and community psychiatry because liaison psychiatry is, in many respects, a part of social and community psychiatry. A medical or surgical service contains within it not only most of the elements and strata of any community, but also the added problems associated with a community that functions on the basis of providers and consumers. In addition, part of the sanction and legitimacy for the community psychiatrist comes from his identity as a physician and psychiatrist.[13] An initial experience on a consultation-liaison ward is an excellent way to prepare a resident for consultation with community agencies. It allows the resident to learn how to retain his identity in a nonpsychiatric milieu while functioning as a participant observer in that milieu. This learning process occurs in an environment most familiar to the resident and his primary identity as a physician.

Not so obvious as the close relationship between social and community psychiatry and consultation-liaison psychiatry is the role that the latter can play in the further learning of dynamic psychiatry. This role is best looked at from two perspectives. The first is the generally agreed opinion that in order to function effectively in a consultation role, one must first be a good psychiatrist. This means that one must have a firm grounding in dynamic psychiatry. This is not a universal opinion, however. Some feel that residents may turn to consultation psychiatry to escape the painful confrontations emanating from intensive psychotherapy.[12] It is difficult, however, to see how a resident on a consultation-liaison rotation could easily hide behind traditional roles and jargon, or could he exert as much authority as is possible on a psychiatric service.[7, 12] The demand on the resident is to sharpen his understanding of psychodynamics, his grasp of the various therapeutic techniques, and perhaps most importantly, an understanding of himself as a therapeutic instrument.[12]

The second perspective, related to the first, is that a consultation-liaison service can offer the resident many unique opportunities to further his understanding of dynamic psychiatry not found in quite the same way elsewhere.[11] One of these opportunities stems from conducting psychotherapy with acutely and chronically ill patients on an inpatient service. Illness, serious enough to require hospitalization, is a significant stress. It often activates unresolved conflicts and requires more primitive mechanisms of defense not as clearly seen (but just as significant) in a physically healthy outpatient.[11]

In the course of working with hospitalized patients, a resident is sometimes overwhelmed by a wealth of physiological and psychological findings. He feels compelled to devote his attention to one or the other. He may rationalize that because of the physical illness the case is too complex for dynamic interpretation.[14] He then devotes himself to the physiological aspects only. The capacity to overcome this "double vision" and comprehend the absolute interrelationship between psychological and physiological functions can lead to an expanded understanding of the manner in which patients perceive their bodies and use them to express psychological conflicts.[14]

A consultation-liaison rotation also offers the opportunity to experience countertransference in a different way and to learn the limitations of psychiatric intervention.[7, 15]

Consultation-liaison work is frustrating, and it can lead to affects of pessimism, hopelessness, and despair. Being exposed to the despair in patients with serious illness, as well as the wide ranging and frustrating way many patients have of dealing with illness, can make it difficult for a resident to define for himself a comfortable role in this milieu.[15] This reality is both a danger and an opportunity. It can lead to a permanent pessimism or can be worked through and seen as both a reflection of what the patient and the people caring for him must also feel.[15] This disjunctive affect is probably experienced more intensively in the complex environment of a hospital ward than almost anywhere else, but the same feelings will also be aroused less intensely in therapy with individual patients. If a resident can understand the meanings and uses of these disjunctive affects and other countertransference feelings on a consultation-liaison service, he will undoubtedly be better able to use them as a therapeutic instrument in psychotherapy.

Finally, in medicine generally, and certainly in psychiatry, possible goals often fall short of optimal ones, and psychiatric intervention has only limited efficacy.[7] In order to function effectively on a consultation-liaison service, a resident must be able to admit his limitations without feeling inadequate or subject to criticism. In so doing he can learn that a positive service is often performed just by doing what is possible under the circumstances.[7]

RESIDENT DISAFFECTION WITH CONSULTATION-LIAISON PSYCHIATRY

Thus, there seems to be ample evidence that consultation-liaison psychiatry has an entirely valid and important place in residency training. Yet, in actuality, all is not well. Even though the importance of consultation-liaison work is generally acknowledged, there is low motivation for psychiatrists to remain in the field and there is an obvious shortage of consulting psychiatrists in teaching centers and community hospitals.[7] In spite of its benefits, there is a good deal about liaison work that is frustrating and can cause even the most enthusiastic or experienced person some moments of despair.[1, 2, 7] It is obvious, therefore, that these frustrations would be more intense for a resident still in the process of achieving a professional identity.

In our experience, indeed, there is more disagreement as to the value of the consultation-liaison service than any other part of the training program for residents. It is clear that the very same realities of the service that can be so valuable are responded to by many residents as the most negative aspects.

Perhaps the major frustration is the attitude of the nonpsychiatric house staff and attendings. The feeling of our disaffected residents is probably most succinctly expressed by Kaufman's statement that with some exceptions the attitude of the medical and surgical staff runs the gamut "from frank and open hostility to complete lack of interest."[16] Our unhappy residents do not agree that working with hostile or indifferent colleagues is a legitimate part of psychiatric training. Psychiatry residents recognize the need for a team approach, but they do not feel it is their job to teach, convince, or deal with the anxiety of others when this is the job of the staff attendings or of medical school education.

This group of residents also point out that in a significant number of cases the patient does not really have a psychiatric problem at all. Rather the behavior and symptoms defined by the primary physician as disturbing are the end result of poor management by the very same doctor. Yet the request is to define the patient as psychopathologic, and "fix" him so he will stop bothering the doctor. Many do not feel that the resistance within the operational group is a legitimate clinical problem with which they should have to, or want to, deal.

Perhaps most significantly, many residents perceive their feelings of pessimism and despair not as a challenge but as a natural and unchangeable response to the reality of the hospital ward. They feel that the bitter helplessness and despair of critically ill and dying patients is understandable under the circumstances and conclude that they really cannot do anything to meaningfully change the situation. The demands of consultation-liaison work do, in fact, overwhelm some residents, and not finding a comfortable role or function there, they withdraw and look elsewhere.

The conclusion, however, is not that the rotation is totally without value. Our residents uniformly enjoy their interaction with the nursing staff and medical students and their one-to-one work with some of the patients. However, given all there is to learn in psychiatry, they steadfastly maintain that working in a liaison role takes unfair advantage of them, asks them to perform a function that more legitimately should be shouldered by others, and requires an inordinate expenditure of time that far outweighs any learning benefits.

The questions for psychiatric education are clear: All residents face the same problems, so why is it that some respond to these problems as a challenge and feel that working them through is one of the most enjoyable parts of the rotation and others respond so negatively? What can be done to assist residents in overcoming their anxiety about working in a liaison role?

RESIDENT FRUSTRATIONS AND THE IMPORTANCE OF ROLE MODELING

In order to answer these questions, the first step is to find out how consultation-liaison psychiatry as a division in a department of psychiatry is really viewed in practice. Mendel, in a 1966 study, noted that whereas most residency programs require some consultation experience, relatively few have a formal program.[17] McKegney has pointed out that everyone speaks well of consultation-liaison psychiatry, but he expresses the thesis that "consultation-liaison psychiatry is still a stepchild of psychiatry and medicine. It is provocative but difficult to manage, promising but largely unwanted and not a very healthy offspring."[7]

If this is the state of consultation-liaison psychiatry, then the negative feelings of disaffected residents can be viewed from an important perspective. Probably the most significant variable in the identity formation of the psychiatrist and thus in the way he practices is role modeling.[7, 18] A rotation on a consultation-liaison service is complex, frustrating and anxiety provoking, and a resident experiences it at a time when his professional identity is very fluid. He is told by his department that there are educational benefits to working with medical and surgical house staff who are indifferent or hostile. If modeling is so important for the psychiatry resident, then it is obviously just as important for trainees in other specialties. It is clear, therefore, that what psychiatry has to offer medicine and surgery must come first through the teaching of the medical and surgical attending staff. If this is not so, what the psychiatrist teaches and models can be quickly undone by the attitudes and behavior of other clinicians.[16]

Thus, liaison between the department of psychiatry faculty and the nonpsychiatric faculty would seem an essential prerequisite to asking a resident to form a liaison relationship with his counterparts on the house staff. If this is not so, then the resident is not only being asked to do something his mentors will not, but also without friendly working relationships between department faculty he is unlikely to counteract the prevailing attitudes on the service.

What is necessary, of course, is that the consultation-liaison division be a formally established and permanent administrative entity within the department, and that members of the faculty form permanent liaison relationships with the various nonpsychiatric services.[1] Then residents would work directly with the faculty member in charge. How this should be accomplished is open to disagreement. There are those who feel that all members of the full-time psychiatry faculty should have some liaison responsibility.[7, 8] There are others who feel it is counterproductive to attempt to decree competence or interest in consultation-liaison work; thus, it is better to depend upon a core group who choose the work freely.[1] There, however, are secondary considerations to the primary need to involve the department in some permanent, consistent, and significant way.

There are many possible answers and even more questions, but one aspect seems clear—that for those involved in psychiatric education it is time to avoid the attitude of "do what I say, not what I do." If liaison education is not given the emphasis many feel it deserves, then the most that can be expected is that those residents drawn to the field will be so drawn no matter what the department does, but perhaps an equal number whose professional identities are still in flux will never have the chance to find out.

REFERENCES

1. Lipowski ZJ: Consultation-liaison psychiatry: An overview. Am J Psychiatry 131:623–630, 1974
2. Lipowski ZJ: Review of consultation psychiatry and psychosomatic medicine. I. General principles. Psychosom Med 29:153–171, 1967
3. Lipowski ZJ: Preview of consultation psychiatry and psychosomatic medicine. II. Clinical aspects. Psychosom Med 29:201–224, 1967
4. Meyer E, Mendelson M: Psychiatric consultations with patients on medical and surgical wards: Patterns and processes. Psychiatry 24:197–220, 1961
5. Webster's New World Dictionary of the American Language (col ed). New York, World, 1960
6. Barnes RH, Busse EW, Bressler B: The training of psychiatric residents in consultative skills. J Med Educ 32:124–130, 1957
7. McKegney PF: Consultation-liaison teaching of psychosomatic medicine: Opportunities and obstacles. J Nerv Ment Dis 154:198–205, 1972
8. West LJ: The future of psychiatric education. Am J Psychiatry 130:521–528, 1973
9. Raskin DE: Psychiatric training in the 70's—toward a shift in emphasis. Am J Psychiatry 128:1129–30, 1972
10. Romano J: The teaching of psychiatry to medical students: Past, present, and future. Am J Psychiatry 126:1115–1126, 1970
11. Fox HM: Psychiatric residency on a medical service. Arch Gen Psychiatry 11:19–23, 1964
12. Pattison ME: Residency training issues in community psychiatry. Am J Psychiatry 128:1097–1102, 1972
13. Karno M: Liaison psychiatry—an experience in community consultation. Panel discussion: Liaison Psychiatry, A Resident Educative Process? 126th Annual Meeting American Psychiatric Association, Honolulu, May 9, 1973
14. Hoppe KD: Liaison psychiatry—a component experience in learning dynamic psychiatry. Panel discussion: Liaison Psychiatry, A Resident Educative Process? 126th Annual Meeting American Psychiatric Association, Honolulu, May 9, 1973
15. Mendelson M, Meyer E: Countertransference problems of the liaison psychiatrist. Psychosom Med 23:115–122, 1961
16. Kaufman MR: The teaching of psychiatry to the nonpsychiatrist physician. Am J Psychiatry 128:610–616, 1972
17. Mendel WM: Psychiatric consultation education—1966. Am J Psychiatry 123:150–155, 1966
18. Kardner SH, Fuller M, Mensh IN, Forgy EW: The trainees viewpoint of psychiatric residency. Am J Psychiatry 126:1132–1138, 1970

L. Robert Martin

22

Liaison Psychiatry and the Education of the Family Practitioner

There was little formal training in the basics of psychosocial medicine to the beleaguered family physician until the advent of the specialty of family practice with its three-year postdoctoral residency training program. Much of his advice was intuitive, and little is known regarding its effect on the patient's morbidity or satisfaction. Liaison psychiatry should assume the leadership role in the delineation of objectives and provide the faculty to implement these objectives in family practice residency training programs.

NEED FOR PSYCHIATRIC TRAINING
FOR THE FAMILY PHYSICIAN

In its "Essentials" for residency training in family practice, the AMA states that "this discipline [psychiatry] is one of the necessary bases for a family practice program" and continues "in the family practice unit, most of the pertinent knowledge and skill can best be acquired through a program in which psychiatry is integrated with medicine, pediatrics, and other disciplines."

The incidence of mental and psychological disease in family practice has been reported to vary from 3.9 to 17.2 percent.[2, 3, 4, 5] Deckert in an unpublished paper states that, of every 100 patients seen by the average family physician, "50 will present with symptoms that relate directly to emotional, psychological, or sociological problems; 25 will suffer from a variety of illnesses where psychological factors are significant either as etiological variables or management problems; 25 will suffer from a variety of illnesses where psychological factors are *not* particularly significant."[6] Intuitively judged, Deckert's figures probably more closely approximate the actual daily office experience.

INTEGRATION OF PSYCHOSOCIAL MEDICINE
AND FAMILY PRACTICE

The problems of implementing behavioral science or psychosocial medicine into the postgraduate training curriculum for family practice residents are multiple and include difficulties in taxonomy, developing appropriate objectives, methods of teaching and systems of evaluation. In 1966 the Willard Commission noted that it was not clear how best to incorporate the behavioral sciences into education for family practice.[7] It still is not clear how to incorporate such a program into such an educational format. Two suggestions have been made.

Bock and Egger have developed a conceptual behavioral science model that is conceived as a hierarchy of thought, beginning at the top level of the model with an overall view of health and proceeding down through succeeding levels to the operational level, ultimately to the presentation of content to the family practice residents.[8] McWhinney, in developing an experimental model, states that the "failure to integrate behavioral science with clinical medicine is due to a lack of a schema for classifying patient behavior."[9] He classifies such behavior at the point of physician contact into five categories: attendance with (1) symptoms or problems that have reached the limit of tolerance, (2) symptoms that provoke action not because of their distress but because of their implications, (3) problems of living presenting as symptoms, (4) administrative problems, and (5) reasons other than illness. He also suggests a taxonomy of social factors in illness that defines the patient's behavioral interreaction with his environment: "loss, conflict, change, maladjustment, stress, isolation, and failure."

One of the major responsibilities of the psychiatric liaison service, then, is to assist in the development of appropriate conceptual and experiential objectives for those trainees in the family practice residency training program. These objectives should relate to the need of the trainee not only to acquire a core of basic academic knowledge oriented to psychosocial medicine, but also to provide him with an experiential education that simulates the problems with which the practicing family physician is confronted daily.

Psychosocial medicine is the study and treatment of those diseases related to the psyche, which includes psychosis, psychoneurosis, neurosis and their etiological forces — physical illnesses and sociological problems. Behavioral science is the study of human behavior or an integrated study of the biological, psychological, and social-cultural facets of human behavior. Bishop states that "there is a trend to reassemble data about human beings from all disciplines (the social-cultural, psychological, biological, and physical environment) into a holistic framework and label it *Human Ecology*. This holistic approach seems most appropriate to family medicine.[10]

Ambulatory psychosocial medicine may occur in the context of continuing or crisis care. The intermingling of the two concepts of "continuity of care" and "psychosocial medicine" should occur within the ambulatory-care family practice center.

An identifiable provider of health care is responsible for the care of the patient's illnesses and psychosocial problems. This longitudinal training format, assuming responsibility over a period of time, provides the resident with constant feedback regarding the effectiveness of his counseling and patient satisfaction as well as a perspective of both physical and psychosocial health care, each having an impact on the other and each requiring simultaneous therapeutic efforts, thereby causing the physician to deal with them in concert rather than as separate entities.

Crisis-oriented community psychosocial medicine is best observed and appreciated while functioning on "hot lines," in "crash pads," in drug abuse clinics, in suicide centers, in centers for alcoholics, in VD clinics, in free clinics, and in many others.

In both continuity of care and crisis intervention formats of delivery the family physician of the future will be called upon not to "fly by the seat of his pants" in a very complex "traffic pattern," but to respond to and synthesize his knowledge of communication skills, counseling techniques, sources and availability of community resources, appropriate consultation and referral patterns, and basic psychosocial medicine.

The family practice resident should appreciate the definition of a family and its variants.[11] He should be appreciative of the intra-family dynamics and their relationship to states of "disease" within members of the family.[12] Furthermore, he should be skilled in family interviewing and therapy.[13]

Resident training programs should be so constructed as to provide the trainee with a maximum amount of time in supervised counseling, utilizing a format that includes a pre-encounter discussion to establish counseling objectives and goals, direct observation, and an immediate postencounter evaluation period.

Referral patterns to psychiatric specialists are clearly defined when one is confronted with a major psychiatric problem. In those psychosocial situations that are classified as intermediate or minor the family physician might consider referral to other allied health professionals with psychiatric training or experience.

Since counseling is the major psychosocial therapeutic modality that will be used by the family physician, during his period of resident training he should develop effective skills in these basic counseling situations: premarital, marital, sexual, teenage, drugs and alcohol, anxiety tension states, depression, pathological personalities, hysteria, and situational problems.

TRAINING IN MANAGING PSYCHOSOCIAL PROBLEMS OF BOTH PATIENT AND FAMILY

The family practice resident should experience a sufficient inpatient exposure to provide him with the knowledge and skills to identify and treat psychiatric emergencies as the physician of first contact. There is no need to require prolonged inpatient psychiatry rotation for him because psychiatric problems that confront the family physician are for the most part ambulatory.

During his training period the resident in family practice should be provided with the opportunity of managing under supervision acute, chronic, and situational psychosocial problems that occur within the patient or the family during hospitalization.

The family physician is responsible for the integration of the patient's feelings with the physical, sociocultural, psychological, biological, and environmental problems that confront the patient during hospitalization; that is, he maintains the patient's human ecological balance. Responsible continuity of care requires that the family physician function as the integrator of all ecological factors in order to assess the impact of the diagnosis or procedure on his patient's and his family's mental health.[14] To prepare the family practice resident for this responsibility, it is required that the resident meet and consult with the family of each of his hospitalized patients, providing them with explanation, advice, and emotional support. During these discussion periods the resident observes the family's reaction for denial, confusion, anxiety and resentment. He learns to be particularly sensitive to observing anger or resentment directed toward the patient and allows the family to feel comfortable in expressing their frustrations. He involves the family in the discharge process. Additionally, residents rotate on the Psychiatric Liaison Service, the objectives of which are similar to those of the psychiatric residency. These objectives follow:

1. To be aware of the goals of any given consultation request.
2. To be able to conduct a comprehensive interview, utilizing specific techniques of interviewing physically ill patients.
3. To possess a theoretical knowledge that permits the resident/consultant

    a. To develop hypotheses about the complex mind-body relationships.
    b. To understand the dynamic meaning and function of a given illness in terms of the patient's personality structure.
    c. To understand the significance of a given illness in the historical as well as present-day experience of the patient.
    d. To evaluate the capacity for and appropriateness of various treatment modalities.

4. To undertake the supervised psychotherapeutic treatment for an extended period of
    a. At least one patient with psychosomatic illness.
    b. One terminally ill patient.

It is anticipated that the future role of the family physician in the hospital setting will include not only the responsibility for functioning as the primary physician, but also that of being requested as a consultant in psychosocial medicine, for it is family practice that can best integrate the problems of the physical, emotional, and sociological states of "dis-ease."

OPPORTUNITY FOR PSYCHOSOCIAL INTROSPECTION FOR THE PRACTICING PHYSICIAN

The family practice resident should during his period of postgraduate training be provided with the opportunity of identifying the frames of reference and life-styles that compose his personality and the effect each of these has on his professional career life-style, his counseling situations, and his personal life-style.

A physician's vulnerabilities extend beyond the demands of his profession. He is at high risk only when he demands of himself more than he has been given, such as the physician from a barren childhood who becomes overly burdened by the demands of his dependent patients.[15]

To the practicing physician, psychosocial introspection is threatening to his ego as well as to his perception of his interrelationship with his peers; therefore, he usually requests counseling only in times of stress and crisis. The opportunity for the resident to identify and verbalize his anxieties, depressions, and frustrations should tend to destroy this negative attitude toward psychiatric counseling. As a result, he will become more effective in handling his patients with serious illnesses[16] and presumably more effective in coping with his personal problems.

COMMUNICATION SKILLS ARE ESSENTIAL
FOR THE FAMILY PHYSICIAN

"What the scalpel is to the surgeon, words are to the clinician."[17] The family practice trainee must acquire and develop identifiable communication skills using verbal and nonverbal (body language) techniques and physiological responses to emotion to evaluate properly the patient's state of "dis-ease." He should be competent in communicating with patients, families, peers, society and himself.

People approach a physician with a multiplicity of concerns regarding the process as well as the outcome of the encounter. Individuals have a set of anticipations when they seek out a physician, be it relief of symptoms, advice, empathy, or cure. They come not only with their expressed concerns, but also with a myriad of unexpressed concerns (anxiety, fear, tension, depression, guilt) and unexpressed social identification (cultural, religious, economic, nutritional, educational). It is in this milieu that meaningful dialogue and communication must occur. Is it any wonder that communication is probably the most important skill that a training program must impart to the family practice trainee?

Appropriate communication provides the physician with an accurate data base from which he can extrapolate certain probables relating to the patient's condition. This process of extracting information never ceases in the family physician's clinical practice. The physician imparts information either to reinforce the patient's behavioral attitudes or to change such attitudes. His major role is to assist the patient to understand and to gain the patient's acceptance of either behavioral change or reinforcement. Compliance with such counsel requires explanation, patient understanding, and motivation. Patient motivation relates directly to the physician's communicative skills, commitment, and the level of congruity in the encounter. Korsch and Negreti found that there was indeed a problem in patient-physician communication and that "the need for understanding the problem of communication and coping with it is increasing as the delivery of medical care is taken over more and more by the specialized professionals and technicians, so that the patient must relate to a galaxy of different health workers."[18]

In addition to the problems with the verbal skills, the physician may well have similar problems in providing appropriate diagnosis and therapy because of difficulty, not with his medical technique, but with his inability to translate what the patient's behavior is telling him.[19]

The successful family physician is an observer and a listener. Communication has often been described as a two-way street. Verbalization is one side, and observation and listening are the other. One will never hear the still of the night (or depression) unless one listens attentively.

OBSERVATION-DISCUSSION TEACHING MODELS

The UCLA psychiatric consultation-liaison training program for family practice residents is patterned according to the student-conceived precepts that the best teaching and assessment devices are those that provide direct experience for the student and observation followed by discussion.[20]

In accordance with these concerns, the floor plan of the Family Practice Center at University of California at Los Angeles was designed with an observation/discussion teaching module. The observation rooms are equipped with tapedecks, earphone listening devices, and one-way visual screens, despite some observers' concerns.[21] The center also has available for teaching purposes hand-carry television cameras with 20-minute to 60-minute reel-to-reel capability. Residents receive two months of formal training in ambulatory psychosocial medicine during their 36-month training program. The curriculum content is determined by representatives from the Psychiatric Consultation-Liaison Service and the Division of Family Practice. The format consists of both assigned reading and review of literature and direct observation of the trainee in an interviewing and/or counseling situation, with a specific point guide to assist the observer in evaluation.[22] Each interview is followed by an evaluation session between the observer and the interviewer.

The interview is time structured in a manner similar to other authors' suggestions[23, 24] and follows the following format:[25]

10 minutes	Review of chart prior to patient encounter
	Formulation of interview goals with preceptor
20 minutes	Approach to patient
	Greeting of patient with warmth, concern
	Ascertaining of patient's immediate concerns and expectations
	Interview
	Formulation of presenting problem with patient
	Assessment of immediate situation
	Examination
	Development of treatment plan
	Ascertaining of patient's feelings toward care and treatment plan
	Termination of encounter
20 minutes	Composition of brief note in problem-oriented fashion
20 minutes	Evaluation: preceptor and interviewer

This interview format is oriented to the multiple patient/physician encounters in which time is a major constraint. During such encounters the family physician must extract from the patient the salient features of the presenting complaint, delve into this complaint to an appropriate depth, assess the situation, develop and implement a plan, and evaluate the patient's comprehension. This vignette is played repeatedly in every family physician's office in the world. It requires the highest level of communicative skill, clinical comprehension, and knowledge of the patient's psychosocial substratum in order to perform at an acceptable level.

Repeated experience in such encounter situations, which are monitered directly and immediately assessed, are invaluable to the quality, efficiency, and confidence of the family physician's delivery of health care.

Psychosocial counseling is taught using a similar format:

10 minutes	Review of chart prior to patient encounter
	Formulation of counseling goals with preceptor
40 minutes	Patient/physician encounter
10 minutes	Composition of chart note
	Formulation of presentation to preceptor
30 minutes	Assessment and evaluation with preceptor

Direct observation is reinforced or replaced by television replay. The encounter may be replayed to the benefit of both the trainee and the observer or the film may be used in group teaching conferences. The effectiveness of this mode of education is well documented.[26-31] Other formats which have been used or considered are teaching with simulated patients and use of a computer to simulate patients.[32]

CONCLUSION

The role of the family physician in the practice of psychosocial medicine is of considerable magnitude. Such patients as frightened primips, hyperactive children, concerned parents, "lost" young adults, lonely senior citizens, dying patients as well as those with intrafamily discords and other identifiable emotional problems constitute a considerable portion of the family physician's daily practice. The training program for physicians who anticipate coping with such multivariable concerns must be structured with ongoing responsibility for both clinical and psychosocial decision making oriented to the resident physician, relevance to the physician's daily ambulatory care routine, and evaluation techniques that are immediate and substantive. Educators in the specialty of family practice, as well as those in psychosocial medicine, should assume the responsibility of providing the family practice trainee with the self-assurance, insight, and technical skills necessary to deliver quality comprehensive health care to his patients and their families.

REFERENCES

1. Department of Graduate Medical Education; Essentials. Chicago, The American Medical Association
2. Cooper B, Fry J, Kalton G: A longitudinal study of psychiatric morbidity in a general practice population. Br J Prev Soc Med 23:210–217, 1969
3. Wentz HS, Tindall HL, Zervanos NJ: Primary care research in a model family practice unit. J Fam Pract 1:52–59, 1974
4. Metcalfe DHH, Sischy D: Patterns of referral from family practice. J Fam Pract 1:34–38, 1974
5. Geyman JP: The Modern Family Doctor and Changing Medical Practice. New York, Appleton-Century-Crofts, 1971
6. Deckert GH: Man as he behaves. University of Oklahoma (unpublished manuscript)
7. Meeting the challenge of family practice: Report of the Ad Hoc Committee on Education for Family Practice of the Council on Medical Education. Chicago, AMA, 1966
8. Bock WB, Egger R: The development of a behavioral science model for a family practice program. J Med Educ 46:831–836, 1971
9. McWhinney IR: Beyond diagnosis: An approach to the integration of behavioral science and clinical medicine. N Eng J Med 287:384–387, 1972
10. Bishop FM: Behavioral science in family medicine. Presented at the American Academy of General Practice Workshop for Consultants in Family Practice, Kansas City, October 1969
11. Eiduson BT, Cohen J, Alexander J: Alternatives in child rearing in the 1970's. Am J Orthopsychiatry 43:720–731, 1973
12. Bauman MH, Grace NT: Family process and family practice. J Fam Pract 1:24–26, 1974
13. Satir V: Conjoint Family Therapy (rev ed). Palo Alto, Calif., Science & Behavior Books, 1967
14. Martin LR: Is family practice becoming an ambulatory care specialty? Symposium on Undergraduate Training in Family Practice, American Academy of Family Physicians, Kansas City, August 1974
15. Vaillant GE, Sobowale NC, McArthur C: Some psychologic vulnerabilities of physicians. N Engl J Med 287:372–375, 1972
16. Artiss KL, Levine AS: Doctor-patient relation in severe illness. New Engl J Med 288:1210–1214, 1973
17. Tumulty PA: What is a clinician and what does he do? New Engl J Med 283:20–24, 1970
18. Korsch BM, Negreti VF: Doctor-patient communication. Sci Am 227:66–74, 1972
19. Roose LJ: What are you and your patient really saying to each other? Medical Insight 24–35, 1971
20. Miller AA, Burnstein AG, Leider RJ: Teaching and evaluation of diagnostic skills. Arch Gen Psychiatry 24:255–259, 1971

21. Smith SR: In opposition to the use of the one-way mirror. J Med Educ 44:1161–1164, 1969
22. Miller AA, Burnstein AG, Leider RJ: Teaching and evaluation of diagnostic skills. Arch Gen Psychiatry 24:255–259, 1971
23. Froelich RE: A course in medical interviewing. J Med Educ 44:1165–1169, 1969 self-instructional programmed videotapes. J Med Educ 48:676–683, 1973
30. Patterson WB, Hitchens PJ, Cloud LP, et al: A portable TV studio for medical education. J Med Educ 48:691–692, 1973
31. Jason H, Kagan N, Werner A, et al: New approaches to teaching basic interview skills to medical students. Amer J Psychiatry 127:1404–1407, 1971
32. Friedman RB: A computer program for simulating the patient-physician encounter. J Med Educ 48:92–97, 197efjoxff

Donald H. Naftulin

23

Liaison Psychiatry:
A Refuge for the Medical Model
in Continuing Education in Psychiatry

In a southwestern United States survey of psychiatrists' continuing-education interests psychosomatic medicine ranked fifth behind an intensive review for American Board of Psychiatry and Neurology examinations, adolescent psychiatry, psychiatry and the law, and community psychiatry.[1] In the four years after the survey's completion annual courses were offered in these interest areas. In two of those four years only two psychiatrists enrolled in courses in psychosomatic medicine for all physicians. Among twenty-six courses offered, only one, and that classifiable within psychosomatic medicine, was canceled for lack of sufficient registrants. When psychiatrists who received the course announcements were randomly surveyed to determine reasons for not register-ing, most admitted that the course was of general importance but little relevance to their psychiatric practice needs. Given the low attendance of psychiatrists in courses related to psychosomatic medicine generally, one is forced to ask of what relevance this interest area is to the practice needs of most psychiatrists.

If findings from the exhaustive study of psychotherapists' characteristics by Henry, Sims, and Spray[2] are sufficiently generalizable, one can infer that the psychiatrists who felt the canceled psychosomatic medicine course was not relevant to their practice needs actually practiced more in terms of psychosocial intervention than the medical model of health care. Henry and his associates state that the distinction between types of patients treated by their four groups of psychotherapists (psychiatrists, psychoanalysts, psychologists, and social workers) is not based on medical or nonmedical training of the psychotherapists per se. Rather the distinction is influenced by the finding that a number of general psychiatrists are viewed by the overall psychotherapist sample as relying on their medical background as a basis for treating mental illness. Others are not. Thus, their reliance on medical training not only sets some psychiatrists apart from nonmedical therapists but also from those psychiatrists who eschew the medical model.

Further implications of this study suggest that it is psychiatry's predominant use of psychosocial intervention that does not allow one to distinguish operationally what psychiatrists do with patients that is different from what various other mental health professionals do. If American psychiatrists really practice more in the psychosocial than medical model, the arguments against training separately disciplined mental health professionals are persuasive and call into question the necessity that the optimal mental health professional be trained as a physician. Such views are hardly heretical in mental health literature.[3]

CHALLENGING THE MEDICAL MODEL

With the start of the 1970s some investigators seriously questioned the primacy of the psychiatrist in areas traditionally dominated by physicians. Dorken, in a high response survey of public mental health program administrators, convincingly documented the extent to which psychologists direct mental health care programs in many states. Looking to the future, he writes, "While the existence of a visible cadre of a profession in an area helps to develop a sense of public acceptance, it is also true that when critical posts that are traditionally filled by psychiatrists are vacant, public agencies will in time make alternate arrangements." [4] Dorken states this at a time when the national stream of psychiatry training is trickling but baccalaureate degrees in psychology are pouring forth from the college arts and sciences campuses. Lest the dispassionate reader feel such writing applies only to the undergraduate psychologist and the public sector of mental health care, in 1970 the number of first-year psychology graduate students reached 12,000. This number approximated that of all first-year medical students in the same year. If the trend continues, roughly 5000 psychology Ph.D.s will graduate annually beginning in 1977.[5] Academic posts and public human services can hardly absorb them all.

The precedent of licensing nonphysician professionals for limited drug-prescribing privileges is established among dentists, podiatrists, and some physician extenders in various states. It may still be considered heresy to suggest that nonmedical psychotherapists will eventually be accorded similar limited prescribing privileges. Heretical or not, Abroms and Greenfield feel, "Considering the quantities of tranquilizers now being indiscriminately prescribed by physicians, we wonder how a new professional could possibly do worse." [6] At the time of this writing at least two state legislative committees are wondering similarly, and they are studying the feasibility of such a suggestion.

These studies and their legislative implications strike at the very heart of the issue raised in the introduction as well as Parts III and IV of this book— whether we as psychiatrists have anything so more unique and so more effective to offer patients than do differently trained professionals.

The vast but not too generalizable literature in psychotherapy does little to establish psychiatry's therapeutic uniqueness. Mental health program administration is no more the realm of the qualified psychiatrist than it is of other equally qualified mental health professionals or professional administrators. And it is probable that the biological breakthroughs in the major mental illnesses will be largely attributable to the efforts of basic scientists in combination with clinicians investigating such efforts through applied behavioral studies. Person power for such efforts cuts across professional training tracks. One is forced to ask whether any function of a psychiatrist's training qualifies him more uniquely than other health or mental health professionals in the performance of any of his current roles. One answers rather tentatively that a task for which the psychiatrist is uniquely suited by training and function is that of consultation-liaison psychiatry.

EVOLUTION OF A CONCEPT

Mental health professionals, including psychiatrists, tend to confuse psychosomatic medicine and consultation-liaison psychiatry. One can argue that psychosomatic medicine is sufficiently different from consultation-liaison psychiatry so as not to be considered the same subspecialty. A strong historical case can be made for consultation-liaison psychiatry as a practical outgrowth and sensible application of the various theories, tested and untested, formerly sheltered under the umbrella of psychosomatic medicine. Since the popularization of the term by Alexander,[7] psychosomatic medicine has had brief comfort, partial acceptance, and final field study rejection as the embodiment of specificity theory. With Malmo[8] and the Laceys[9] psychosomatic medicine evolved into a discipline that was less theory bound and more subject to bench and clinical research requirements of validity and reliability testing. Because of multiple, frequently unidentifiable and uncontrollable, variables entailed in researching the better questions raised in the field, such testing has proved less than gratifying. Inconsistent findings that were rarely generalizable frustrated the researcher in the same manner that specificity theory of psychosomatic medicine frustrated the practical clinician.

However, psychosomatic medicine's future as a body of inquiry rests more with its application of scientific method than its earlier promise as a practical art. It appears that psychosomatic medicine as conceptualized in the 1950s has evolved into two separate but occasionally related disciplines, psychophysiologic medicine and consultation-liaison psychiatry. It is the latter with which the rest of this chapter is concerned.

CONSULTATION-LIAISON PSYCHIATRY

Consultation-liaison psychiatry can be viewed as the application of psychiatric principles to the care and environment of the medically ill, often hospitalized, patient. Its respectability as an emerging subspecialty area of psychiatry has in large measure been attributable to the scholarly clinical definition and theory building of Lipowski.[10] Its proponents and practitioners are primarily those psychiatrists who are comfortable with the medical model. But as we have discussed, it is this very comfort that sets them apart from their psychiatric colleagues who do not share it. It is quite probable that early socialization patterns and personality characteristics as well as values and attitudes that distinguish these two groups of psychiatrists may some day explain their relative adherence or avoidance of the medical model in mental health care. However, these are points of departure for future research. They are included only to emphasize what most of us already know, that the consultation-liaison psychiatrist is a different breed of mental health cat.

IDENTIFYING CONSULTATION-LIAISON SKILLS

The identification of skills for the consultation-liaison function requires a description of what the consultation-liaison psychiatrist actually does. The consultation-liaison psychiatrist must combine a problem-solving practical approach to psychosocial patient care with a substantive basis for understanding the patient's organic illness. One can oversimplify the former part of this combination as the liaison function of the psychiatrist and the latter as the consultation role he performs.

Consultation Role

The psychiatrist consultant is usually called when the physically ill patient presents problems of a behavioral nature not understandable or manageable by the consultee or ward staff. Once having identified whether the nature of the consultation request is primarily of the patient's cerebral/affective dysfunction associated with a brain syndrome, a superimposed psychiatric problem associated with physical disorder, or the consultee/staff response to the patient's behavior, or a combination of the three, the consultant has various options available to him.

If his discussion with the consultee and key ward staff, chart and medication review, physical and mental status examination suggest symptoms of brain syndrome, the psychiatrist consultant addresses himself to the various associated factors giving rise to it. A slick acronym for not inadvertently missing any of these factors is DAVID MIT (degenerative, avitaminotic, vascular, intoxicating, demyelinating, mytotic, infectious, traumatic). The initials subsume all of the probable etiologies involved in the brain syndromes and will facilitate the consultant's ability to recommend practical solutions. Since in many cases the consultee will probably have already identified the factors associated with the disorder, the consultant's primary role will be in recommending solutions, be they withdrawing nonlife support medications, initiating psychotropics, increasing sensory stimuli, or educating ward staff. It is the latter role that defines the psychiatrist's liaison function.

Liaison Function

The challenge of identifying the multiple associated factors of a brain syndrome or functional psychiatric disorder and recommending the manner in which they may be palliated is difficult enough. But the task of dealing with the staff ultimately responsible for the care of a patient with such disorder is usually greater. The staff conflict may be the covert reason behind the request for consultation and thus requires the psychiatrist's shift from the substantive understanding of functional and organic illness to the problem-solving role of addressing sensitive process-oriented issues among staff who are working to get patients well. A prerequisite of addressing such an issue is that the psychiatrist must have established a liaison with the staff in an effort to win their trust and alliance in solving a problem that has now become identified around a particular patient. In this effort the psychiatrist utilizes the traditional interpersonal skills fundamental to the doctor-patient relationship—judicious authoritative listening and intervention combined with empathy, professional warmth, and genuine concern. These imply effective use of interpersonal skills more covertly emphasized in traditional psychiatry residency programs. The liaison function is to impart them to the staff through appropriate modeling, curbstone exploration of staff feelings and motives, and follow-up staff meetings and patient visits. Some may view this liaison function as therapeutic, others as educational, for the consultee and staff. Whatever one's view, the psychiatrist working in this capacity must early identify the problem, define it in behavioral nonpunitive terms, address it utilizing the principles basic to interpersonal skills, and maintain the optimal liaison necessary for his future usefulness as the staff meet other vexing situations in patient management.

CONTINUING EDUCATION IN
CONSULTATION-LIAISON FOR
PSYCHIATRISTS

The effort of continuing education in consultation-liaison psychiatry for psychiatrists, based on what such a psychiatrist actually does, is then essentially twofold: (1) keeping abreast of the substantive issues in medicine that help explain organic and emotional components of the patient's disorder and (2) enhancing interpersonal skills and expanding them to hospital groups (staff/ patient) and systems (staff/patient/administration) in an effort to expedite the patient's therapy. Since a cornerstone of consultation-liaison psychiatry is the recognition and distinction of the interplay between functional and organic psychopathology, an organized rather extensive review of neurophysiology and general clinical neurology as it relates to psychiatric disorders is advisable. Among 60 psychiatrists enrolled in such a course in 1971, 90 percent felt that the course would help their practice and professional competence, but as many as 38 percent felt none of their patients would benefit from their having had this course. How many of these psychiatrists were actually functioning as consultation-liaison psychiatrists or identified more in the medical or psych-osocial model was not determined. However, the data suggest that although important to the consultation-liaison function, a review of neurology is profes-sionally enhancing but considered by almost half of the psychiatrist-participants as not useful for most patients seen by them.

In addition to a neurology update, it is to the consultation-liaison psychia-trist's advantage to be abreast of general pharmacology and psychopharmacol-ogy, especially drug side effects and synergy of new medications as the latter relate to the central nervous system. An annual refresher course in fluid and electrolyte balance is also beneficial for the psychiatrist who consults on any unit with acute postsurgical, intensive care, chronic dialysis, or burn patients. An ongoing review of psychological studies involving sensory deprivation and perception can provide the consultation-liaison psychiatrist with a greater inferential base on which to understand the physically ill patient and suggest remedies for him. With the exception of the psychological studies review, these educational means are currently available through the teaching conferences of existing hospitals and are systematically conducted for the nonpsychiatry resident staff of most teaching hospitals. The motivated consultation-liaison psychiatrist is often invited and certainly welcomed as a participant and dis-cussant. Participatory and reciprocal learning among medical colleagues from other specialties may be the most effective ongoing education for the consultation function. It is especially so if most of the psychiatrist's consultation requests are generated from one or a few specialty areas.

Continuing education for the liaison function may also be better effected through ward and outpatient experience in general medical or specialty settings. The liaison psychiatrist not skilled in group process may do well to refresh himself in this area. Courses in medical administration and organizational structure may facilitate the psychiatrist's ability to deal with staff problems eventually attributable to conflict in these areas. Adequate knowledge and increased information about such seemingly remote issues as current hospital plans for union representation, community advisory boards, the employment of new professionals, and impending budget priorities may provide valuable clues and resources to the multiple covert consultation requests within the increasingly important function of liaison psychiatry.

The dual function of the consultation-liaison psychiatrist has been all too briefly described. The most effective ongoing education for the enhancement of the consultation-liaison role is experiential on-the-job learning and the inherent or acquired motivation of the psychiatrist.

LOOKING AHEAD

If national health insurance in the United States follows even partially the model in the United Kingdom and Canada, it is quite probable that much of the practice of psychiatry will again become based in the medical center. This does not necessarily mean inpatient psychiatry but rather ambulatory care for the sick, nearly sick, and worried well as is customary in all areas of medicine.[11] The review mechanisms and professional standards established for such levels of care will, for psychiatry, be increasingly determined through existing medical societies or professional review boards. As the national priorities and their accompanying funding patterns emphasize greater training for primary care medicine, various medical specialties will make greater paper efforts, and perhaps even real efforts, to define themselves as primary care specialties. Traditional psychiatry will have a more difficult time defining itself accordingly. Consultation-liaison psychiatry, however, in the acute walk-in clinic, the emergency room, and the hospital ward, may not. The National Institute of Mental Health has conceded this and placed consultation-liaison training and services among its top funding priorities. Since this occurs at a time when funds for psychiatry residency training are curtailed, it is predictable that program directors will be more attracted to resident applicants that show an inclination toward consultation-liaison work.

Earlier studies demonstrate that effective psychiatric consultation-liaison correlates with decreased hospital stay, increased ambulation, lesser ward personnel turnover, and greater staff and patient satisfaction.[12, 13] If these studies are sufficiently replicated, prepaid health plans should utilize psychiatry staff in consultation-liaison roles more extensively than direct one-to-one relationships with patients. The issue of whether another mental health professional can perform these functions as well or better will not be solved. But psychiatry's clinical base in medicine provides it with the unique opportunity of being in the right place at the right time despite its increasing abandonment of the medical model. Private psychiatric practice in a society as affluent as our own will always provide enough challenge and work for a sizable number of psychiatrists, but it is probable that the majority will spend most of their future professional time in some aspect of public sector health care. The extent to which their role in that sector differs from other mental health professionals and nonprofessionals will determine the extent to which psychiatry remains a medical specialty. For psychiatrists in both the private and public sector a redefinition of multiple roles and the identification of more specific professionally unique skills is in order. This will not be easy. If such roles are more narrowly defined and unique professional skills identified in areas such as consultation-liaison psychiatry, continuing education for the psychiatrist will mean for many remedial education in medicine.

In a wry indictment of psychiatric education for the family physician, Greengold referred to the "well worn homily" of the need for increased communication between psychiatrists and family physicians.[14] He noted, not quite tongue-in-cheek, that family physicians are solicited quarterly to attend courses on "psychiatry and general practice." He wrote that "although family physicians do not receive psychiatrists' registration (in medical courses), we are sure that psychiatrists are equally proselytized for courses on 'general practice in psychiatry'." Unfortunately, Greengold was mistaken. We in psychiatry rarely are proselytized to attend medical courses outside our specialty. His message, read more sympathetically, is that those psychiatrists calling for psychiatric principles in clinical care must reciprocally apply medical principles to psychiatric care in order to maintain professional credibility and therapeutic effectiveness. To work meaningfully with medical colleagues and their patients, psychiatrists have an obligation to continue their knowledge and skills in general medicine.

Serving as a critic from within, Robinson highlights this obligation with an uncomfortable metaphor: "There is the problem of whether to straddle the fence of the medical and other models, or to jump to one side or the other. In the forseeable future we cannot avoid straddling that fence. But it seems probable that psychiatry's crotch will endure many sharp pains as it veers first to this side, then to the other, in an effort to keep its balance. Perhaps the best solution lies in lowering the fence."[15]

In what was then a controversial editorial, Funkenstein predicted the siphoning of residents from the psychiatry applicant pool into those of primary care specialties as the latter gained status and an increasing concern "with the patient as a person."[16] The national growth of family practice and emergency medicine residency programs with simultaneous cutbacks in psychiatry resident positions has borne out his prediction. An increasing emphasis of the consultation-liaison role for psychiatry may serve to soften this trend. Psychiatry, in turn, may attract more residents whose interest is in maintaining their medical identity and utilizing their medical skills.

Psychiatry as a medical specialty may be at the threshold of its fourth revolution, that of ultimately delegating its numerous theories, practical process skills, and few substantive contributions to other disciplines for the expansion of its mission. As such, it is very likely that in the future more of the fewer psychiatrists in its ranks will contend with those issues of the emotionally and mentally disordered where such patients interface with medicine, in the service of consultation-liaison psychiatry.

REFERENCES

1. Naftulin DH, Ware J, Myers V: Psychiatrist interest in continuing education: Results of a southwestern survey. Arch Gen Psychiatry 24:260–264, 1971
2. Henry W, Sims J, Spray L: Public and Private Lives of Psychotherapists. San Francisco, Josey Bass, 1973
3. Kubie L: Need for a new subdiscipline in the medical profession. Arch Neurol Psychiatry 78:283–293, 1957
4. Dorken H: Utilization of psychologists in positions of responsibility in public mental health programs: A national survey. Am Psychol 25:953–958, 1970
5. Dorken H, Whiting F: Psychologists and health service providers. Prof Psychol 5:309–319, 1974
6. Abroms G, Greenfield N: A new mental health profession. Psychiatry 35:10–22, 1973
7. Alexander F: Psychosomatic Medicine. New York, Norton, 1950
8. Malmo R: Activation, in Bachrach A (ed): Experimental Foundations of Clinical Psychology. New York, Basic Books, 1962
9. Lacey J, Lacey B: The law of initial value in the longitudinal study of autonomic constitution: Reproducibility of autonomic responses and response patterns over a four year interval. Ann NY Acad Sci 98:1257, 1962
10. Lipowski ZD: Review of consultation psychiatry and psychosomatic medicine. I, II, III. Psychosom Med 29:153–171, 1967; 29:201–224, 1967; 30:395–422, 1968
11. Garfield S: The delivery of medical care. Sci Am 222:15–23, 1970
12. Follette W, Cummings N: Psychiatric services and medical utilization in a pre-paid health plan. Med Care 5:25–35, 1967

13. Cummings N, Follette W: Psychiatric services and medical utilization in a prepaid health plan. II. Med Care 6:31–41, 1968
14. Greengold M: To whom it may concern. Arch Gen Psychiatry 23:245–246, 1960
15. Robinson R: Criticism of psychiatry, in Usdin G (ed): Psychiatry: Education and Image. New York, Brunner/Mazel, 1973
16. Funkenstein D: A new breed of psychiatrist? Am J Psychiatry 124:226–228, 1967

Index

Abortions, counseling, 137, 141–142, 144
Abram, H., 151, 153
Abrams, H., 140
Abroms, G., 296
Acetylcholine, 75
ACTH (adrenocorticotrophic hormone), 79–81
Acupuncture, 215
Adaptation syndrome, 78
Adler, C. S., 95
Affective disorders, 75, 76, 162
Affects, cognitive elements and, 62–63
Aging people, brain changes, 221
Aggressive behavior, 184–185
  neurotransmitters and stress, 76
Akinetic mutism, 163
Albany (New York Hospital), 8
Alcohol intoxication, 181–184, 222
  delirium, 226
  diagnosis and treatment, 181, 185
Alcoholics Anonymous, 178, 188
Aldosterone, 79–81
Alexander, Franz, 13, 39, 40–41, 73, 266, 270, 297
Alpha conditioning, 89, 215
American Hospital Association, 9–10
American Journal of Psychiatry, 1n

American Psychiatric Association,
  Diagnostic and Statistical Manual of Mental Disorders, 33–34
Amine neurotransmitters, 76
Amnesia, hysterical, 163
Amnestic syndrome, 163
Amphetamines, 76, 181–182
Anorexia, 77
Anorexia nervosa, 77
Anticholinergic drugs, 181, 183, 225
Antidepressant medication, 180
  tricyclic, 76–77
Antidiuretic hormone (ADH), 79–81
Anxiety
  conflict situation and arousal of, 40, 43
  hysterical, 17
  "key" signs in interviews, 200–201
  physiological signs of, 63, 200
  psychotherapeutic approach, 180
  symptoms, 180
Archives of General Psychiatry, 47n
Aristotle, 37
Arrhythmias, cardiac, biofeedback techniques, 94
Arteriosclerosis, 221
Arteriosclerotic dementia, 163
Arthritis, 43, 65
Arthur, R. J., 24

305

a
b
5 c
6 d
7 e
8 f
9 g
0 h
1 i
8 2 j